Gapenski's

FUNDAMENTALS OF HEALTHCARE FINANCE

Gapenski's FUNDAMENTALS OF HEALTHCARE FINANCE

THIRD EDITION

KRISTIN L. REITER | PAULA H. SONG

GATEWAY TO HEALTHCARE MANAGEMENT

HAP

AUPHA

Health Administration Press, Chicago, Illinois
Association of University Programs in Health Administration, Washington, DC

Your board, staff, or clients may also benefit from this book's insight. For information on quantity discounts, contact the Health Administration Press Marketing Manager at (312) 424-9450.

22 21 20 19 18 5 4 3 2 1

Library of Congress Cataloging-in-Publication Data

Names: Reiter, Kristin L. (Kristin Leanne) author. | Song, Paula H., author.
Title: Gapenski's fundamentals of healthcare finance / Kristin L. Reiter, Paula H. Song.
Other titles: Fundamentals of healthcare finance
Description: Third edition. | Chicago, Illinois : Health Administration Press; Washington, DC : Association of University Programs in Health Administration, 2018. | Revision of: Fundamentals of healthcare finance / Louis C. Gapenski. c2013. 2nd ed.
Identifiers: LCCN 2018000639| ISBN 9781567939750 (alk. paper) | ISBN 9781567939774 (xml) | ISBN 9781567939781 (epub) | ISBN 9781567939798 (mobi)
Subjects: LCSH: Medical economics.
Classification: LCC RA410 .G37 2018 | DDC 338.4/73621—dc23 LC record available at https://lccn.loc.gov/2018000639

The paper used in this publication meets the minimum requirements of American National Standard for Information Sciences—Permanence of Paper for Printed Library Materials, ANSI Z39.48-1984.(∞)™

Acquisitions editor: Janet Davis; Project manager: Theresa L. Rothschadl; Cover designer: James Slate; Layout: Cepheus Edmondson

Found an error or a typo? We want to know! Please e-mail it to hapbooks@ache.org, mentioning the book's title and putting "Book Error" in the subject line.

For photocopying and copyright information, please contact Copyright Clearance Center at www.copyright.com or at (978) 750-8400.

Health Administration Press
A division of the Foundation of the American College of Healthcare Executives
300 South Riverside Plaza, Suite 1900
Chicago, IL 60606-6698
(312) 424-2800

Association of University Programs in Health Administration
1730 M Street, NW
Suite 407
Washington, DC 20036
(202) 763-7283

We dedicate this book to the memory of our dear friend and colleague, Louis C. Gapenski, whose textbooks have touched countless students of healthcare finance.

BRIEF CONTENTS

Part III: Financing and Capital Investment Decisions

Part IV: Reporting Results

DETAILED CONTENTS

PREFACE

Almost 30 years ago, Louis C. Gapenski published his first healthcare finance textbook, *Understanding Healthcare Financial Management*. Over time, his experiences prompted him to write others, including this book, *Fundamentals of Healthcare Finance*. When he passed away on April 20, 2016, the field of healthcare finance lost a gifted scholar, writer, teacher, mentor, and friend.

By traditional academic metrics, Lou was a successful scholar: many peer-reviewed articles, other publications and book reviews, and presentations at academic and professional conferences. However, Lou was best known for his compendium of best-selling textbooks on corporate finance and healthcare financial management. His collaboration with Eugene Brigham served as a textbook factory: Lou was a coauthor of five editions of *Financial Management: Theory and Practice* (translated into Bulgarian, Chinese, French, Indonesian, Italian, Portuguese, and Spanish), six editions of *Intermediate Financial Management*, and five editions of *Cases in Financial Management* (all three from Dryden Press). In the early 1990s, Lou turned his attention to the nascent discipline of healthcare financial management and was among the first to argue that the theory and application of corporate finance was both relevant and necessary to the training of healthcare managers. Over the next 25 years, Lou authored seven editions of *Understanding Healthcare Financial Management*, five editions of *Cases in Healthcare Finance*, six editions of *Healthcare Finance: An Introduction to Accounting and Financial Management*, and two editions of *Fundamentals of Healthcare Finance* (all four from Health Administration Press). By any standard, this was an extraordinary level of textbook productivity and was a constant source of amazement and curiosity among his colleagues.

Lou's textbooks and casebook in healthcare finance were novel and innovative in that they offered the rigorous finance training commonly found in business schools but using language and context that would speak to those whose passion was healthcare. In all of Lou's work, his commitment to teaching and learning was evident. While planning for new textbooks or new editions of existing books, Lou would reach out to colleagues, students, and individuals working in the field, seeking input on how to improve his books and the associated ancillary learning materials. He was eager to receive feedback, and he worked tirelessly to implement the recommendations of those around him. His creativity was apparent in the new features offered in each edition and in the stories and examples he included to engage students and draw them into the subject matter. When Lou originally approached us about becoming coauthors, we had no idea how much we would learn from him about writing textbooks—assessment of learning needs, clear exposition of complex concepts and calculations, development of ancillary learning materials, and the business of publishing itself. Better than anyone we know, Lou understood how to write a good textbook.

In this edition, we have worked very hard to build on Lou's original vision for the book: to provide a learning resource for students interested in how healthcare finance is used by clinical and operational managers as opposed to financial managers. We have provided updates and edits throughout to ensure that it remains a relevant and valuable learning tool for students and instructors. We hope that the book will continue to provide financial acumen to those who strive daily to improve healthcare delivery.

Note: Adapted from K. L. Reiter and G. H. Pink, 2016, "Remembering Louis C. Gapenski," *Journal of Health Care Finance* 43 (2): 1–4.

CONCEPT OF THE BOOK

Our goal in the third edition of *Fundamentals* was to create a text that introduces readers to those basic principles and applications of healthcare finance that are most important to entry-level clinical and operational managers. Thus, principles that are used primarily by financial staff personnel are covered either lightly or not at all. For example, background information about financial markets and securities is not included in this book.

The end result is a book that contains three introductory chapters, six accounting chapters, and four financial management (corporate finance) chapters. The idea here is that entry-level managers, who typically will be working at the department level or perhaps in a medical practice setting, need to understand those finance principles that they will encounter and work with on a daily basis, while other concepts can be learned later as needed. Although this book does cover some "organizational" finance issues, its focus is on topics that are most relevant to managers of clinical operations.

Another consideration in writing this book is that most readers will be seeing the material for the first time. Thus, the concepts here are explained as clearly and succinctly as possible. We have tried hard to create a book that readers will find user-friendly, enjoyable, and self-instructive. If students don't find a book interesting, understandable, and useful, they won't read it.

INTENDED MARKET AND USE

The book is not designed for any specific type of educational program. Rather, it can be used in a wide variety of settings: undergraduate and graduate, traditional and executive, on-campus and distance learning, and even independently for professional development. However, the book is ideal for undergraduate health administration programs, undergraduate and graduate public health and health science programs, and nursing administration programs and courses.

The key to the book's usefulness is not the educational program but the focus of the course. If the course covers the fundamentals of healthcare finance, with a concentration on operational management, this book will be a good fit.

Practicing healthcare professionals who need to gain a better understanding of healthcare finance may greatly benefit from this book as well. Such professionals include clinicians who have management responsibilities and clinical managers who require additional finance skills.

CHANGES IN THE THIRD EDITION

Since the publication of the previous edition of this book, we have received comments from students and users at other universities. The reaction of students, other professors, and the marketplace in general has been overwhelmingly positive—every comment received indicates that the basic concept of the book is sound. Even so, nothing is perfect, and the healthcare environment is evolving at a dizzying pace. Thus, we have made many changes to the book, the most important of which are listed here:

- The book was updated and clarified throughout. Particular care was taken to include the most recent information on the Affordable Care Act and to update the real-world examples. In addition, there is no doubt that text material improves as it is repeatedly edited. Like all books, the first two editions had some rough spots, and considerable effort was expended to improve these discussions and to clarify end-of-chapter problems.
- The section on service line costing in chapter 4 was expanded to include discussions of two additional methods used to cost individual services: the cost-to-charge ratio and relative value units.
- Financial accounting coverage was updated to conform to the latest American Institute of Certified Public Accountants formats. For example, in chapter 12, we added a discussion of upcoming changes to the presentation of net assets by not-for-profit entities.

- We added more examples to the financial accounting chapters so readers can compare and contrast the financial statements of different types of healthcare organizations, including not-for-profit hospitals and home health care providers.
- Chapter 14 was added to several already-available online chapters to provide further discussion of time value of money concepts.
- The lecture presentation material was updated and improved based on continual use and suggestions from adopters and students alike.

All in all, these changes improve the quality and value of the book without affecting its basic concept and approach to learning.

INSTRUCTOR RESOURCES

This book's instructor resources, which are fully described below, include PowerPoint slides, a test bank, cases, and solutions to the end-of-chapter questions and problems and the five online cases.

For the most up-to-date information about this book and its instructor resources, go to ache.org/HAP and browse for the book by its title or author names.

This book's instructor resources are available to instructors who adopt this book for use in their course. For access information, please e-mail hapbooks@ache.org.

ANCILLARY MATERIALS FOR INSTRUCTORS

- *PowerPoint slides.* The essential material in each chapter—concepts, graphs, tables, lists, and calculations—is presented in roughly 25 to 35 slides. Hard-copy versions (or the files themselves) can be provided to students as lecture notes. Instructors may use these slides as is or customize them to meet their own unique needs.
- *Test bank.* An online test bank is available to adopters. It consists of roughly 15–20 multiple-choice questions per chapter.
- *Selected cases.* Five cases are available to instructors who want to incorporate cases into their courses. These cases are not as complex as those in *Cases in Healthcare Finance*, and they come with questions intended to both guide students and keep them on track. (See the next section for details.)

- *Solutions*. Instructors also have access to solutions to the end-of-chapter questions and problems, and solutions to the five online cases.
- *Additional online chapters*. Instructors who want to go over concepts beyond the fundamentals covered in the text may access four chapters that are posted online. (See the next section for details.)
- *Sample course syllabus*.

ANCILLARY MATERIALS FOR STUDENTS

Students (and instructors) can find the following learning tools on the Health Administration Press website at ache.org/books/FinanceFundamentals3.

- *Additional online chapters*. These four chapters aim to expand the scope of study.
  - Chapter 14—Time Value Analysis
  - Chapter 15—Lease Financing and Business Valuation
  - Chapter 16—Distributions to Owners: Bonuses, Dividends, and Repurchases
  - Chapter 17—Capitation, Rate Setting, and Risk Sharing
- *Online appendixes*. These two appendixes (operational analysis ratios and financial analysis ratios) provide a more extensive list of ratios and their definitions than what is provided in this book.
- *Selected cases*. These cases are not overly complex, and they give students the opportunity to apply many of the concepts discussed in the book and in class. The cases contain a set of questions that guide students along a solution path as they work each case.
  - Case 1—The Dialysis Center: Cost Allocation Concepts
  - Case 2—University Hospital: Marginal Cost Pricing
  - Case 3—Panhandle Medical Practice: Activity-Based Costing
  - Case 4—Better Care Clinic: Breakeven Analysis
  - Case 5—Twin Falls Community Hospital: Capital Investment Analysis

ACKNOWLEDGMENTS

Special thanks are due to Jane Chaffee Makhoul, who helped revise the third edition. Colleagues, students, and staff at the University of North Carolina at Chapel Hill and the University of Florida provided valuable feedback and inspirational support during the development, class testing, and revision of this book. In addition, the Health Administration Press staff was instrumental in ensuring the quality and usefulness of the book.

ERRORS IN THE BOOK

In spite of the significant effort that has been expended by many individuals on this book, it is safe to say that some errors exist. In an attempt to create the most error-free and useful book possible, we strongly encourage both instructors and students to e-mail us with comments and suggestions for improving the book. We certainly welcome your input.

CONCLUSION

In the environment faced by healthcare providers today, good finance is more important than ever to the economic well-being of the enterprise. As such, clinical managers must be thoroughly grounded in finance principles and applications. However, this is more easily said than done.

We hope that *Fundamentals of Healthcare Finance* will help you understand the finance issues currently faced by healthcare providers and, more important, that it will provide guidance on how best to deal with them.

Kristin L. Reiter, PhD
1104-H McGavran-Greenberg Hall
Department of Health Policy and Management
University of North Carolina at Chapel Hill
Chapel Hill, NC 27599-7411
reiter@ad.unc.edu

Paula H. Song, PhD
1105-A McGavran-Greenberg Hall
Department of Health Policy and Management
University of North Carolina at Chapel Hill
Chapel Hill, NC 27599-7411
psong@unc.edu

PURPOSE OF THE BOOK

This book is designed to introduce the fundamentals of healthcare finance as practiced in health services organizations. This purpose has several important implications.

First, because the book assumes the reader has no prior knowledge of the subject matter, it is totally self-contained, with each topic explained in basic terms. Furthermore, because clarity is so important when first explaining concepts, the chapters have been written in an easy-to-read fashion. None of the topics is inherently difficult, but new concepts often take some effort to understand. This process is made easier by the writing style used and the learning aids contained in the text.

Second, because this book focuses on fundamentals, it presents a broad overview of healthcare finance rather than an in-depth treatment that might be found in accounting or financial management books.

Third, and most important, the book discusses tasks that are essential to the operational management of clinical services, as opposed to tasks that are exclusively financial in nature and hence the sole province of the financial staff. The balance of the content is overweighted on accounting material, especially those aspects that are most relevant to entry-level managers. Of course, even managers whose primary responsibility is nonfinancial, such as those in operations, marketing, or human resources, need to know something about the finance department. Thus, the book is sprinkled with information related to topics that typically fall under the purview of the financial staff, but only in light doses.

When you finish the book, you will not be expected to fully understand every nuance of every finance principle or practice that pertains to every type of healthcare organization. Nevertheless, you will have sufficient knowledge of healthcare finance to function better as an operational manager and to judge the quality of financial analyses performed by others.

PART I

FOUNDATION CONCEPTS

Three factors make the provision of healthcare services different from any other services. First, many healthcare organizations, especially hospitals, are organized as not-for-profit corporations as opposed to for-profit, investor-owned businesses. For example, in Gainesville, Florida, Shands Healthcare at the University of Florida is a not-for-profit hospital, while North Florida Regional Medical Center is a for-profit hospital owned by investors. Second, payment for services rendered by healthcare providers typically is made by third-party payers, such as Medicare and Blue Cross and Blue Shield, rather than by the patients who receive the services. Finally, because the health status of the nation's population is a national concern, there is significant government involvement in the provision of health services. By focusing on these differences, part I presents the unique framework for the practice of healthcare finance.

Chapter 1 discusses the institutional setting for the delivery of healthcare services, including the organization and role of the finance staff and the types of healthcare organizations.

Chapter 2 focuses on alternative forms of business organization and ownership and how taxes influence finance decisions. Here, the specific differences between not-for-profit and investor-owned businesses are explored. In addition, the chapter briefly describes the nature of a business and the types of finance decisions that it must make.

Chapter 3 covers the third-party payer system and alternative reimbursement methods. Healthcare managers at all levels must know who the payers are and what payment methods are used. These external factors have a profound influence on the operations of all healthcare organizations. In addition, chapter 3 discusses the impact of healthcare reform on health services organizations.

Some of you may already be familiar with much of the information presented in part I, either because you have taken other courses that introduced this material or you have worked in the field. If this is your situation, a quick review cannot hurt; after all, repetition is the key to learning. For the rest of you, part I plays an important role in your understanding of the healthcare finance concepts presented in the remainder of the book.

CHAPTER 1

INTRODUCTION TO HEALTHCARE FINANCE

THEME SET-UP: CAREERS IN HEALTHCARE MANAGEMENT

If you are using this book, you either are working in healthcare or are interested in a career in healthcare. Of course, numerous career opportunities are available in clinical fields, including medicine, dentistry, nursing, and occupational and physical therapy, which some of you are already practicing or will enter on graduation. However, most of you are considering careers in healthcare management. In addition, many clinicians find themselves balancing both clinical and administrative roles, and so healthcare management knowledge is important.

According to the Association of University Programs in Health Administration, an education in healthcare management will prepare you to enter the exciting and challenging healthcare field, the largest in the United States, representing more than 11 million jobs. Healthcare executives have the opportunity to make a significant contribution to improving the health of the population and to work in one of tens of thousands of healthcare organizations throughout the United States and the world.

An education in healthcare management can take you in many different directions. Career options for healthcare managers have never been more diverse or exciting. The kinds of entry-level jobs offered to a college graduate vary in terms of the individual's interests, skills, and experience. Today, an estimated 300,000 people serve in healthcare management positions (from entry level to middle management to leadership) and in organizations of all sizes (from a practice with several people to a major corporation that employs thousands). After gaining the requisite experience, many healthcare management graduates are in a position to shape the future of healthcare in the United States and across the globe.

All that probably sounds good, but what types of organizations might be interested in hiring a healthcare management graduate? By the end of the chapter, you will have an idea of the settings available. See if any of them appeal to you.

Learning Objectives

After studying this chapter, you will be able to do the following:

- Define the term *healthcare finance* as it is used in this book.
- Discuss the structure of the finance department, the role of finance in healthcare organizations, and how this role has changed over time.
- Describe the major players in the healthcare sector.
- List the key issues currently facing healthcare managers.

1.1 INTRODUCTION

In today's healthcare environment, where financial realities play an important role in many, if not most, decisions, healthcare managers at all levels must understand the fundamentals of finance and how that knowledge is used to enhance the financial well-being of the institution. In this chapter, we introduce you to the rationale that underlies this book. Furthermore, we present background information about healthcare finance and the different types of healthcare organizations. We sincerely hope that this book provides significant help in your quest to increase your professional competency in the critical area of healthcare finance.

Healthcare financing
The system that a society uses to pay for healthcare services.

Health services organizations
Organizations that provide patient care services. Examples include hospitals, medical practices, clinics, and nursing homes. Also called *providers*.

Accounting
The measurement and recording of events that reflect the operations, assets, and financing of an organization.

1.2 DEFINING HEALTHCARE FINANCE

What is healthcare finance? It can be surprising to find that there is no single response because the definition of the term depends, for the most part, on the context in which it is used. Thus, your understanding should begin with learning the scope and meaning of the term *healthcare finance* as it is used in this book.

To start, recognize that healthcare finance is not about financing the healthcare system. **Healthcare financing** is a separate topic that involves how society pays for the healthcare services it consumes. This issue is complex and politically charged, and we do not tackle it directly in this book. Of course, the manner of financing healthcare affects how hospitals and physicians are reimbursed for services and hence has a significant influence on healthcare finance.

Most users of this book will become (or already are) managers at healthcare organizations, such as medical group practices, hospitals, home health agencies, or long-term care facilities. Thus, to create a book that provides the most value to its primary users, we focused on finance as it applies in **health services organizations**. Of course, the principles and practices of finance cannot be studied in a vacuum but must be based on the realities of the current healthcare environment, including how healthcare services are financed.

In health services organizations, *healthcare finance* consists of both the accounting and financial management functions (see "Critical Concept: Healthcare Finance"). **Accounting**, as its name implies, concerns the recording, in financial terms, of economic events that reflect the operations, assets, and financing of an organization.

CRITICAL CONCEPT
Healthcare Finance

Healthcare finance can have many different definitions, depending on the setting. For our purposes, healthcare finance encompasses the accounting and financial management functions of healthcare organizations. Accounting involves the measurement, in financial terms, of a business's operations and financial status, while financial management (corporate finance) involves the application of theory and concepts developed to help managers make better decisions. In practice, the two functions blend, with accounting generating the data needed to make sound decisions and financial management providing the framework for those decisions.

In general, the purpose of accounting is to create and provide to interested parties—both internal (managers) and external (investors)—useful information about an organization's financial status and operations.

Financial management
The use of theory, principles, and concepts developed to help managers make better financial decisions.

Whereas accounting provides a rational means by which to measure a business's financial performance and to assess operations, **financial management** (often called corporate finance) provides the theory, concepts, and tools necessary to help managers make better financial decisions. Of course, the boundary between accounting and financial management is blurred; certain aspects of accounting involve decision-making, and much of the application of financial management concepts requires accounting data.

Self-Test Questions

1. What does the term *healthcare finance* mean?
2. What is the difference between accounting and financial management?

1.3 THE ROLE OF FINANCE IN HEALTH SERVICES ORGANIZATIONS

Chief financial officer (CFO)
The senior manager (or top finance dog) in a large organization's finance department. Also called *vice president of finance*.

The primary role of finance in health services organizations, as in all businesses, is to plan for, acquire, and use resources to maximize the efficiency (and value) of the enterprise (see "Critical Concept: Role of Finance"). As discussed in section 1.4 of this chapter, the two broad areas of finance—accounting and financial management—are separate functions at larger organizations, although the accounting function usually is carried out under the direction of the organization's **chief financial officer (CFO)** and hence falls under the overall category of finance.

CRITICAL CONCEPT
Role of Finance

The primary role of finance in health services organizations is to plan for, acquire, and use resources to maximize the efficiency of the organization. This role is implemented through specific activities such as planning and budgeting.

Finance Activities

Chapters 1 through 3 of this book provide foundational information that is helpful for understanding finance activities. The specific finance activities explored in the remaining chapters of this book include the following:

- *Costs and profitability, planning, and budgeting.* First and foremost, healthcare finance involves evaluating the financial effectiveness of current operations and planning for the future. Chapters 4 through 6 cover these functions.

- *Financial operations.* Healthcare organizations spend a lot of time managing cash and supply inventories as well as collecting money owed for services rendered. Proper management of these functions is necessary to ensure operational effectiveness and to reduce costs. Typically, managers at all levels are involved, to a greater or lesser extent, in these processes, which are discussed in chapter 7.
- *Financing decisions.* All organizations must raise funds to buy the assets necessary to support operations. Such decisions involve many issues, such as the choice between long-term and short-term debt and the use of leases versus conventional financing. Senior managers and the financial staff typically make the financing decisions, but these decisions have ramifications for managers at all levels. Business financing is the subject of chapter 8.
- *Capital investment decisions.* One of the most critical decisions managers make is the selection of new facilities (including land, buildings, and equipment). Such decisions are the primary means by which businesses implement strategic plans; hence, they play a key role in a business's financial future. Chapters 9 and 10 describe these decisions, which affect everyone in the organization.
- *Financial reporting.* For a variety of reasons, businesses must record and report to outsiders the results of operations and current financial status. This task is typically accomplished with a set of financial statements, which are explained in chapters 11 and 12.
- *Financial and operational analysis.* To achieve and maintain a high level of organizational performance, businesses must constantly monitor both financial and operational conditions and take actions as needed to ensure that goals are met. Chapters 7 and 13 address these topics.

In addition to those finance activities that involve operational managers, the following activities are accomplished primarily by the finance staff:

- *Contract management.* In today's healthcare environment, health services organizations must negotiate, sign, and monitor contracts with managed care organizations and health insurers. The finance staff typically has primary responsibility for these tasks, though operational managers clearly are affected by external contracts and must be involved in their negotiation and management.

- *Financial risk management.* Many financial transactions that take place to support the operations of a business can, in themselves, increase a business's risk. Thus, an important finance staff activity is to manage financial risk.

The Four Cs

The finance activities at health services organizations may be summarized by the four Cs: costs, cash, capital, and control (see "Critical Concept: The Four Cs").

> **CRITICAL CONCEPT**
> The Four Cs
>
> The finance activities in healthcare organizations can be summarized by the four Cs: (1) *cost* measurement and minimization, (2) *cash* management, (3) *capital* acquisition, and (4) *control* of resources.

The measurement and minimization of costs are vital activities to the financial success of all healthcare organizations. Rampant costs, compared to revenues, usually spell doom for any business.

A business might be profitable but still face a crisis because of a shortage of cash. Cash is the lubricant that makes the wheels of a business run smoothly; without it, the business grinds to a halt. In essence, businesses must have sufficient cash on hand (or the ability to raise it quickly) to meet cash obligations as they occur. In healthcare, a critical part of managing cash is collecting money from insurers for patient services provided. (This element is so important that some healthcare finance professors include *collections* as the fifth C.)

Capital represents the funds (money) used to acquire land, buildings, and equipment. Without capital, healthcare businesses would not have the physical resources needed to provide patient services. Thus, capital allows healthcare organizations to meet the healthcare needs of their communities.

Finally, a business must control its financial and physical resources to ensure that they are being wisely employed and protected for future use. In addition to meeting current mission requirements, healthcare organizations must plan to meet society's future healthcare needs.

Importance of Finance over Time

In times of high profitability and abundant financial resources, the finance function tends to decline in significance. For example, when most health services organizations were reimbursed on the basis of the actual costs they incurred, the role of finance was minimal. At that time, the most critical finance function was cost accounting because it was more important to account for costs than it was to control them. In response to payer (primarily Medicare) requirements, health services organizations (primarily hospitals) churned out a multitude of reports to comply with regulations and to maximize revenues. The complexities of cost reimbursement meant that a large amount of time had to be spent on cumbersome accounting, billing, and collection procedures. Thus, instead of focusing on value-adding activities, most finance work focused on bureaucratic functions.

In recent years, however, providers have redesigned their finance functions to recognize the changes that have occurred in the health services field. Billing and collections remain important, but to be of maximum value to the enterprise, the finance function must support cost-containment efforts, managed care and other payer contract negotiations, joint venture decisions, and integrated delivery system participation. In essence, finance must help lead organizations into the future rather than merely record what has happened in the past.

Although in this book our emphasis is on finance, we must stress that all organizational functions are important. In addition to finance, managers must understand some elements of many different functions, such as marketing, facilities management, and human resource management. All business decisions have financial implications, however, so all managers (whether in operations, marketing, personnel, or facilities) must know enough about finance to incorporate financial considerations properly into the plans and decisions in their specialized areas (see "For Your Consideration: Do Nonfinancial Managers Need to Know Finance?").

Self-Test Questions

1. What is the role of finance in today's healthcare organizations?
2. What are the four Cs?
3. How has the role of finance changed over time?

For Your Consideration
Do Nonfinancial Managers Need to Know Finance?

A much-debated topic at the water cooler is whether nonfinancial managers, including clinical managers, need to know much about finance. As outlined in the American College of Healthcare Executives (ACHE) 2018 Competencies Assessment Tool, healthcare managers should over time attain competencies in 24 areas of financial management. Among the areas listed are basic accounting principles, reimbursement principles, budgeting, revenue generation, performance monitoring, and applying financial planning to organizational objectives. Of course, financial management competencies represent only a small proportion of the complete list of management competencies assessed by the tool. Still, by including financial management in the assessment tool, ACHE considers it a key skill set for healthcare managers regardless of work setting or years of experience.

What do you think? Do nonfinancial general managers need financial management skills? What about clinical managers? Justify your answers.

1.4 THE STRUCTURE OF THE FINANCE DEPARTMENT

Comptroller (controller) The finance department manager who handles accounting, budgeting, and reporting activities.

Treasurer The finance department manager who handles capital acquisition, investment management, and risk management activities.

Business (practice) manager The manager responsible for the finance function in a small healthcare organization, such as a medical practice with one or a few clinicians.

The structure of the finance department depends on the type (e.g., hospital, medical practice) and size of the healthcare organization. Large organizations generally structure their finance departments in the following way.

The head of the finance department holds the title of CFO. (The title of vice president—finance is also used.) This individual typically reports directly to the organization's chief executive officer (CEO) and is responsible for all finance activities in the organization. The CFO directs two senior managers who help manage finance activities: the comptroller and the treasurer.

The **comptroller** (pronounced, and sometimes spelled, "controller") is responsible for accounting and reporting activities, such as routine budgeting, preparation of financial statements, and patient accounts management. For the most part, the comptroller is involved in activities covered in chapters 4 through 7, 11, and 12 of this text. The **treasurer** is responsible for the acquisition and management of capital (funds). In other words, the treasurer must raise the funds needed by the organization and ensure that those funds are effectively used. Specific activities include the acquisition of capital, cash and debt management, lease financing, financial risk management, and endowment fund management (in not-for-profits). In general, the treasurer is involved in those activities discussed in chapters 8 through 10 and chapter 13 of this book.

In large organizations, the comptroller and treasurer have managers under them who are responsible for specific functions, such as the patient accounts manager, who reports to the comptroller, and the cash manager, who reports to the treasurer. In small businesses, many of the finance responsibilities are combined and assigned to one individual. For example, in a small group practice, the finance function is managed by one person, often called the **business (practice) manager**, who typically is supported by one or more clerks.

? SELF-TEST QUESTIONS

1. Briefly describe the typical structure of the finance department in a large healthcare organization.
2. How does the size of the organization affect the finance department structure?

1.5 HEALTHCARE SETTINGS

Healthcare services are provided in numerous settings, including hospitals, ambulatory care offices and clinics, long-term care facilities, and integrated delivery systems. Before the 1980s, most healthcare organizations were freestanding and not formally linked with other organizations. Those that were linked tended to be part of **horizontal systems**, which control a single type of healthcare facility, such as a group of hospitals or nursing homes. Recently, however, many healthcare organizations have created **vertical systems**, which control different types of providers such as medical practices, hospitals, and nursing homes.

Horizontal system
A single business entity that owns a group of similar providers, such as hospitals.

Vertical system
A single business entity that owns a group of related, but not identical, providers such as hospitals, medical practices, and nursing homes.

Hospitals

Hospitals provide diagnostic and therapeutic services to individuals who require more than several hours of care, although most hospitals are actively engaged in ambulatory (walk-in) services as well. To ensure a minimum standard of safety and quality, hospitals must be licensed by the state and undergo inspections for compliance with state regulations. In addition, most hospitals are accredited by **The Joint Commission** (previously called the Joint Commission on Accreditation of Healthcare Organizations). Joint Commission accreditation is a voluntary process intended to promote high standards of care. Although the cost to achieve and maintain compliance with standards can be substantial, accreditation provides eligibility for participation in the Medicare and Medicaid programs, and hence most hospitals seek accreditation (chapter 3 discusses Medicare and Medicaid).

The Joint Commission
The accreditation body for hospitals and other health services organizations.

Recent environmental and operational changes have created significant challenges for hospital managers. For example, many hospitals are experiencing decreasing admission rates and shorter lengths of stay, resulting in reduced revenues and excess capacity. On the other hand, hospitals in fast-growing areas are hard-pressed to keep ahead of patient demand. In addition, all hospitals are being pressured to reduce costs by reimbursement rates that fail to keep up with inflation and to assume greater risk in their contracts with payers.

Hospitals differ in function, length of patient stay, size, and ownership. These factors affect the type and quantity of assets, services offered, and management requirements and often determine the type and level of reimbursement. Hospitals are classified as either general acute care facilities or specialty facilities.

General acute care hospital
A hospital that treats all conditions that require a relatively short hospitalization (e.g., fewer than 30 days).

General acute care hospitals provide general medical and surgical services and selected acute specialty services. Such hospitals, which account for the majority of hospitals, have relatively short lengths of stay, typically a week or less. **Specialty hospitals**, such as psychiatric, children's, women's, rehabilitation, and cancer facilities, limit the admission of patients to specific ages, sexes, illnesses, or conditions. The number of specialty hospitals has grown significantly in the past few decades because of the belief that such hospitals can provide better patient services than can hospitals that treat all conditions. In addition, specialty hospitals often experience lower costs than general hospitals because they do not require the overhead associated with providing many different types of services.

Specialty hospital
A hospital that treats patients with a common characteristic or condition, such as a children's or a cancer hospital.

Hospitals vary in size from fewer than 25 beds to more than 1,000 beds; general acute care hospitals tend to be larger than specialty hospitals. Although economists do not all agree, the general belief is that the optimal hospital size is about 400–500 beds. Smaller hospitals do not benefit from economies of scale, while larger hospitals are too big to manage efficiently (have diseconomies of scale). Small hospitals, those with fewer than 100 beds, tend to be located in rural areas. Many rural hospitals have experienced financial difficulties in recent years because they have less flexibility than large hospitals, limiting their ability to lower costs in response to tightening reimbursement rates. Most of the largest hospitals are academic health centers or teaching hospitals. These hospitals offer a wide range of services, including tertiary care, which consists of specialized services for patients with unusually severe, complex, or uncommon problems.

Government hospital
A hospital owned by a government entity. Federal hospitals are owned by the federal government, while public hospitals are owned (or funded) by state or local governments.

Hospitals are classified by ownership as governmental, private not-for-profit, or investor owned. **Government hospitals**, which make up about 22 percent of all hospitals, are broken down into federal and public (nonfederal) entities. Federal hospitals, such as those operated by the uniformed services or the US Department of Veterans Affairs, serve special purposes. Public hospitals are funded wholly or in part by a city, county, tax district, or state. In general, federal and public hospitals provide substantial services to indigent patients. In recent years, many public hospitals have converted to other ownership categories (primarily, private not-for-profit) because local governments have found it increasingly difficult to fund healthcare services and at the same time provide other necessary public services.

Private not-for-profit hospital
A hospital that is not governmental but is operated for the exclusive benefit of the community.

Private not-for-profit hospitals are nongovernmental entities organized for the sole purpose of providing inpatient healthcare services. Because of the charitable origins of US hospitals and a tradition of community service, roughly 73 percent of all private hospitals (58 percent of all community hospitals) are not-for-profit entities. In return for serving a charitable purpose, these hospitals receive numerous benefits, including exemption from federal and state income taxes, exemption from property and sales taxes, eligibility to receive tax-deductible charitable contributions, favorable postal rates, favorable tax-exempt financing, and tax-favored annuities for employees.

Investor-owned hospital
A hospital that is owned by investors who benefit financially from its operation. Also called a *for-profit hospital.*

The remaining 27 percent of private hospitals (21 percent of all community hospitals) are **investor-owned hospitals**, whose owners (typically shareholders) benefit directly from the profits generated by the business. Historically, most investor-owned hospitals were owned by physicians, but now most are owned by large corporations, such as HCA (Hospital Corporation of America), which owns approximately 174 hospitals in the United States and England; CHS (Community Health Systems), which owns nearly 137 hospitals; and Tenet Healthcare, which owns 77 hospitals. Unlike not-for-profit hospitals, investor-owned hospitals pay taxes and forgo the other benefits of not-for-profit status.

Despite the expressed differences in mission between investor-owned and not-for-profit hospitals, not-for-profit hospitals are being forced to place greater emphasis on the financial implications of operating decisions than in the past. This trend has raised concerns in some quarters that many not-for-profit hospitals are failing to meet their charitable mission. As this perception grows, some people argue that these hospitals should lose some, if not all, of the benefits associated with their not-for-profit status. (Chapter 2 discusses the differences between investor-owned and not-for-profit hospitals in detail.)

Hospitals are labor intensive because they provide continual nursing supervision to patients, in addition to the services given by other clinical, professional, and semiprofessional staff members. Physicians petition for privileges to practice in hospitals. While they admit and provide care to hospitalized patients, most physicians are not hospital employees and hence are not directly accountable to hospital management. However, physicians retain a major responsibility for determining which hospital services are provided to patients and how long patients are hospitalized. Thus, physicians play a critical role in determining a hospital's costs and revenues and hence its financial condition.

Ambulatory (Outpatient) Care

Ambulatory (outpatient) care encompasses services provided to patients who are not admitted to a hospital or nursing home. Traditional outpatient settings include clinics, medical practices, hospital outpatient departments, and emergency departments. Nontraditional settings, such as home health care, ambulatory surgery centers, urgent care centers, diagnostic imaging centers, rehabilitation and sports medicine centers, and clinical laboratories, have emerged and are seeing substantial growth. The latest innovation in ambulatory care is the retail clinic, a small clinic operated in a retail store (such as Wal-Mart) and staffed by a physician assistant or nurse practitioner. Compared to hospital-based services, these innovative settings offer patients more amenities and convenience and, in many situations, lower prices. For example, urgent care and ambulatory surgery centers are typically less expensive than their hospital counterparts because hospitals have higher overhead costs. (The same lower-cost logic applies to urgent care centers and retail clinics compared to medical practices.)

Ambulatory (outpatient) care Care that is provided to patients who are not institutionalized. Typical settings include physicians' offices, outpatient surgery centers, and walk-in clinics.

Many factors have contributed to the expansion of ambulatory services, with technology leading the way. Often, patients who once required hospitalization because of the complexity, intensity, invasiveness, or risk associated with certain procedures can now be treated in outpatient settings. In addition, health insurers have encouraged providers to expand their outpatient services by requiring authorization for inpatient services and instituting payment mechanisms that provide incentives to perform services on an outpatient basis.

Finally, starting a business that provides outpatient care is easier than starting a new hospital. Ordinarily, ambulatory facilities are less costly to operate and less frequently subject to licensure and certificate-of-need (CON) regulations (exceptions are hospital outpatient units and ambulatory surgery centers) than are hospitals, and they generally are not accredited. (Section 1.6 of this chapter discusses licensure and CON regulation in detail.)

As outpatient care consumes an increasing portion of the healthcare dollar and as efforts to control outpatient spending are enhanced, the traditional role of the ambulatory care manager is changing. Historically, ambulatory care managers have handled routine management tasks such as billing, collections, staffing, scheduling, and patient relations, while the owners, often physicians, have tended to the important business decisions. However, a more complex healthcare environment, coupled with growing competition, is forcing managers of ambulatory care facilities to become more sophisticated in making business decisions, including finance decisions.

Long-Term Care

Long-term care
Care that is provided in either an institutional or outpatient setting that covers an extended period.

Long-term care consists of healthcare (and some personal care) services provided to individuals who lack all or some functional ability, specifically in the activities of daily living such as eating, bathing, and locomotion. This type of care usually covers an extended period and may be given as an inpatient or outpatient service. Although the most common users of long-term care are the elderly, the services are available to individuals of all ages.

Individuals become candidates for long-term care when they become too mentally or physically incapacitated to perform daily living tasks and when their family members are unable to provide the help needed. Long-term care is a hybrid of healthcare and social services. Nursing homes are a major provider of such care.

Nursing home care is offered at three levels: (1) skilled nursing, (2) nursing, and (3) residential care. Skilled nursing facilities (SNFs) provide the level of care closest to hospital care. Services must be provided under the supervision of a physician and must include 24-hour daily nursing care. Nursing facilities (NFs) are intended for individuals who do not require hospital or SNF care but whose mental or physical conditions require daily continuity of one or more medical services. Residential care facilities are sheltered environments that do not provide professional healthcare services. Thus, most health insurance programs do not provide coverage for residential care.

Long-term care facilities are more abundant than hospitals. However, SNFs and NFs are smaller than hospitals, with an average of about 100 beds, compared with about 160 beds for hospitals. Large for-profit, long-term care companies exist (such as Brookdale Senior Living, which operates 1,121 facilities across the United States), but many nursing homes are mom-and-pop operations. Nursing homes are licensed and inspected by states, which also license nursing home administrators. Although The Joint Commission accredits nursing homes, only a small percentage of these facilities obtain accreditation because it is not required for reimbursement and the standards to achieve accreditation are much higher than licensure requirements.

The long-term care field has experienced tremendous growth in recent decades. In 1960, long-term care accounted for only 1 percent of US healthcare expenditures, but by 2012 it accounted for more than 9 percent. Demand increases are anticipated, as the percentage of the US population aged 65 or older is expected to grow from 15 percent in 2016 to 24 percent in 2060. The elderly are disproportionately high users of healthcare services in general and are major users of long-term care in particular.

Although long-term care is often perceived as nursing home care, many new services are less institutional, such as adult day care, life care centers, and hospice programs. These services tend to offer a higher quality of life, although they are not necessarily less expensive than institutional care. Home health care, provided for an extended period, is an alternative to nursing home care but is not as readily available in many rural areas. Furthermore, third-party payers, especially Medicare, have sent mixed signals about adequately paying for home health care. In fact, many home health care businesses have been forced to close in recent years as a result of a new, less generous Medicare payment system.

Finally, many Americans suffer from a long-lasting or chronic illness (from the Greek word *chronos*, meaning time). Some chronic diseases, such as cancer, can be life-threatening. Other chronic illnesses, such as asthma and diabetes, while often incurable, can be managed by the patient for many years with proper care.

In the traditional system, the treatment of chronic illnesses was fragmented, with primary care physicians, specialists, hospitals, and other providers separately contributing their services without much planning or coordination with the other parties. Today, practitioners have finally recognized that the most effective way to provide chronic care is using a long-term integrated approach, wherein a single case manager is responsible for the patient's care, regardless of the setting.

Have found that it doesn't guarentee better care

Integrated Delivery Systems

Many healthcare experts have extolled the benefits of providing hospital care, ambulatory care, long-term care, and business support services through a single integrated delivery system (see "Critical Concept: Integrated Delivery System"). The potential benefits of such a system include the following:

- Patients are kept in the corporate network of services (**patient capture**).
- Providers have access to managerial and functional specialists, such as reimbursement and marketing professionals.
- Information systems that track all aspects of patient care, as well as insurance and other data, can be developed more easily than under a disjointed care model, and the costs to develop them can be shared.
- Larger, multipurpose organizations have better access to capital.
- The ability to recruit and retain management and professional staff is enhanced.
- Healthcare insurers can be offered a complete package of services (one-stop shopping).

Patient capture
The concept that once a patient enters the system (e.g., a doctor's office), all services needed by that patient should be provided in the system.

- A full range of healthcare services, including chronic disease management and health-status improvement programs, can be better planned and delivered to meet the needs of a defined population. Many of these population-based efforts typically are not offered by stand-alone providers.
- Incentives that encourage all providers in the system to work together for the common good of the system can be created, which has the potential to improve quality and control costs.

CRITICAL CONCEPT
Integrated Delivery System

An integrated delivery system consists of a number of different types of healthcare organizations, such as hospitals, clinics, and nursing homes, owned and operated as a single entity. Although integrated delivery systems offer the opportunity to coordinate all aspects of patient care under a single umbrella, their complexity makes the overall management process much more difficult than in smaller organizations that focus on one type of service.

Although integrated delivery systems can be structured in many ways, the defining characteristic of such systems is that the organization has the ability to assume full clinical responsibility for the healthcare needs of a defined population. Because state laws typically mandate that the insurance function can be assumed only by licensed insurers, integrated delivery systems typically contract with insurers rather than directly with employers. Sometimes, the insurer, often a managed care plan, is owned by the integrated delivery system itself, but generally it is separately owned. In contracts with some insurers, the integrated delivery system receives a fixed payment per plan-covered life and hence assumes both the financial and clinical risks associated with providing healthcare services.

To be an effective competitor, integrated delivery systems must minimize the provision of unnecessary services, because additional services create added costs but do not necessarily result in additional revenues. Thus, the objective of integrated delivery systems is to provide all needed services to its member population in the lowest-cost setting (see "Healthcare in Practice: What We Spend on Healthcare"). To achieve this goal, integrated delivery systems invest heavily in primary care services, especially prevention, early intervention, and wellness programs. Thus, clinical integration among the various providers and components of care is essential to achieving quality, cost efficiency, and patient satisfaction.

In spite of the benefits of integration, health system executives have found that managing large, diverse enterprises is difficult. In many cases, the financial and patient care gains predicted were not realized, and some integrated delivery systems formed in the 1990s have broken up. However, healthcare reform legislation has created additional incentives that have fostered the rise of the accountable care organization. We discuss this new provider form, along with other features of reform, in chapter 3.

HEALTHCARE IN PRACTICE
What We Spend on Healthcare

Most people think that healthcare spending in the United States is out of control. For example, in 2015, almost 18 percent of the nation's total value of goods and services (gross domestic product [GDP]) was spent on healthcare. The proportion of GDP devoted to healthcare is expected to rise to more than 20 percent by 2025, an amount greater than the anticipated expenditure for housing and food combined. In effect, rapidly rising healthcare costs are squeezing out the spending on other goods and services. By comparison, most other industrialized nations, such as Germany, England, and Canada, currently spend about 8 to 10 percent of their GDP on healthcare.

Where does all this money go? Data from 2015 indicate that Americans spend healthcare dollars this way:

Hospital care	32.3%
Physician and other clinical services	22.5%
Prescription drugs	10.1%
Public health, research, and facilities	7.3%
Administrative costs	7.9%
Long-term care	4.9%
Other health and personal care	5.1%
Dental care	3.7%
Durable and nondurable medical equipment	3.4%
Home health care	2.8%
Total	100.0%

As you can see, the largest area of healthcare expenditure is hospital care; the second largest, physician and other clinical services, includes diagnostic imaging, outpatient surgeries, physical therapy, and chiropractic care. Combined, hospitals and ambulatory care providers consume more than half of each healthcare dollar.

The next biggest healthcare expense, at 10.1 percent, is prescription drugs. The proportion spent on prescription drugs is expected to increase over time as more and more individuals gain access to insurance programs that cover prescription drugs. However, commentators expect the increase in spending on prescription drugs to be mitigated by the increasing use of lower-cost generics and the potential for large insurers to negotiate lower prices.

(continued)

HEALTHCARE IN PRACTICE
What We Spend on Healthcare *(continued)*

Almost 8 cents of each healthcare dollar is spent on administrative costs. In 2015, more than $3.2 trillion was spent on healthcare, and about $252 billion of that money paid for government and insurance company administrative costs. Administrative costs can be defined and measured in numerous ways, but regardless of how they are measured, these costs eat up a great deal of money. Estimates vary, with some reaching more than 30 percent when all administrative costs, including those at provider organizations, are considered. One persuasive argument for establishing a universal or national healthcare system is that it can dramatically reduce administrative costs and hence make more money available for patient services.

Will we ever get healthcare spending under control? While there are current efforts aimed at reducing costs, predicting the long-term outcome of this problem is impossible. What we do know is that it cannot continue to grow at the current rate without causing financial damage to other parts of the economy. Thus, sooner or later, additional action will have to be taken.

Source: This Healthcare in Practice is based on National Health Expenditure data from the Centers for Medicare & Medicaid Services. See www.cms.gov/Research-Statistics-Data-and-Systems/Statistics-Trends-and-Reports/NationalHealthExpendData/index.html.

1.6 REGULATORY AND LEGAL ISSUES

Healthcare services are subject to many regulations. For example, pharmacy services are regulated by state and federal laws, and radiology services are highly regulated because of the handling and disposal of radioactive materials. Entry into the healthcare sector is also heavily regulated. Examples of such regulation include licensure, CON, and rate-setting and review programs.

Licensure
The process of granting "permission" for healthcare (and other) professionals to practice. Most professional licenses are granted by states with the goal of protecting the public from incompetent practitioners.

States require **licensure** of certain healthcare providers in an effort to protect the health, safety, and welfare of the public. Licensure regulations establish minimum standards that must be met to provide a service. Many types of providers are licensed, including entire facilities (e.g., hospitals, nursing homes) and individuals (e.g., physicians, dentists, nurses, even some managers).

Licensed facilities must submit to periodic inspections and review activities. Such reviews focus more on physical features and safety than on patient care and outcomes, although progress is being made to change this practice. Thus, licensure has not necessarily ensured that the public will receive high-quality services (see "For Your Consideration: Medical Malpractice").

FOR YOUR CONSIDERATION
Medical Malpractice

Many people have criticized the medical malpractice system in the United States for being expensive, adversarial, unpredictable, and inefficient. Physician advocacy groups claim that 60 percent of malpractice claims are dropped, withdrawn, or dismissed without payment, and only a small percentage of malpractice suits result in monetary awards. Yet, the direct cost of these suits, along with the incentive for providers to practice *defensive* medicine, significantly increases the cost of patient care. In total, an estimated 2–10 percent of healthcare costs are a result of the current malpractice system. Proponents of the current system say that it encourages providers to be more aware of patients' medical needs, creates incentives for the development of improved equipment and procedures, and provides a means for patients who have been wronged to seek compensation for damages.

What do you think? Should the current system be changed? If so, what are some potential changes? (Some observers have put forth such ideas as limiting lawyers' fees, capping awards for noneconomic damages, and decreasing the statute of limitations.)

Critics of licensure contend that it is designed to protect providers, not consumers. For example, licensed paramedical professionals (e.g., physician assistants, dental hygienists) usually are required to work under the supervision of a physician or dentist, making it impossible for paramedical professionals to compete with physicians or dentists. Despite the limitations of licensure, it is undoubtedly here to stay.

Certificate-of-need regulation was enacted by Congress in 1974 in an effort to control growing healthcare costs (see "Critical Concept: Certificate of Need"). CON legislation required providers to obtain state approval on the basis of community need for construction and renovation projects that either relate to specific services or exceed a defined cost threshold. This attempt to control capital expenditures by controlling expansion and preventing duplication of services lasted less than a decade before the Reagan administration began to downplay CON regulation and promote cost controls through competition. However, CON regulation, in one form or another, still exists in roughly 35 states.

Critics of CON regulation argue that it does not provide as much control over capital

CRITICAL CONCEPT
Certificate of Need

A certificate of need (CON) is the approval required by many states before a new healthcare facility can be constructed. CON proponents claim the system helps control costs by preventing excess capacity. Critics, however, contend that CON regulation impedes competition and the spread of new technologies while protecting established providers, even those that do not operate efficiently.

expenditures as originally envisioned and that it increases costs by requiring additional administrative expenditures when new facilities are needed. Perhaps the biggest criticism of CON is that it creates a territorial franchise for the services it covers; that is, it creates barriers for new entities entering markets, even though the new businesses may be more cost efficient and offer better patient care than the existing ones.

Cost-containment programs
State programs that require providers (primarily hospitals) to submit budgets each year for approval.

In addition to CON, many states enacted **cost-containment programs** at the time when most healthcare reimbursement was based on costs. By the late 1970s, nine states had mandatory cost-containment programs, and many other states had voluntary programs (those that did not mandate compliance). The primary tool for cost-containment programs is the *rate-review system*.

Three types of rate-review systems have been used: (1) detailed budget reviews with approval or setting of rates; (2) formula methods, which use inflation formulas to set target rates; and (3) negotiated rates, which involve joint decision-making between the provider and the rate setter. Some states that use rate-review systems have reduced the rate of cost increase to below the national average, while others have failed to do so. However, rate review, as a sole means of cost containment, has been criticized because it does not address the issue of demand for healthcare services.

Professional liability
The responsibility of organizations and individuals who provide professional services, such as hospitals and physicians, for losses that result from malpractice.

The primary legal concern of healthcare providers is **professional liability**. Malpractice suits are the oldest form of quality assurance in the US healthcare system, and today such suits are used to an extreme extent. Many people believe that the United States is in the midst of a malpractice insurance crisis. Total malpractice premiums, which have remained stable or decreased over the past five years, have been passed on to healthcare purchasers. On average, physicians pay $24,500 on malpractice premiums, although some specialist physicians pay malpractice premiums of more than $100,000 per year. However, the total number of paid medical claims and the amount paid for malpractice claims has been steadily decreasing over the past decade.

Although providers in some states have achieved tort reforms, malpractice litigation continues to be perceived as inefficient because it diverts resources to lawyers and courts and creates disincentives for physicians to practice in high-risk specialties and for hospitals to offer high-risk services. In addition, such litigation encourages the practice of defensive medicine, whereby physicians overuse diagnostic services in an effort to protect themselves from liability.

Professional liability is the most visible legal concern in healthcare, but the sector is subject to many other legal issues, including the typical general liability and antitrust claims. In addition, healthcare providers are confronted with unique ethical issues, such as the right to die or to prolong life, that are often resolved through the legal system.

? Self-Test Questions

1. What are some forms of regulation in the healthcare sector?
2. What is the most pressing legal issue facing healthcare providers today?

1.7 CURRENT CHALLENGES

In recent years, the American College of Healthcare Executives (ACHE) has conducted an annual survey of CEOs regarding the most critical concerns of healthcare managers. Financial concerns have headed the list of challenges in every year since the survey began in 2002. When asked to rank their specific financial concerns in 2015, CEOs listed the transition from fee-for-service to a value-based payment system as their primary challenge, with adequate reimbursement from Medicaid and bad debt also near the top of the list. (Reimbursement is discussed in chapter 3.)

Just as ACHE surveyed its CEO members, the Healthcare Financial Management Association surveyed CFOs in 2017 regarding their concerns for the future. Their most pressing issue was the need for increased investments in technology to improve revenue cycle management. Aside from increased budgets, CFOs cited the need to leverage technology better to link clinical and financial opportunities in order to optimize performance. Another top concern among the CFOs was the increase in uncompensated care as patients assume more responsibility for payments through high-deductible health plans.

Taken together, these surveys confirm the fact that finance is of primary importance to today's healthcare managers. The remainder of this book is dedicated to helping you confront and solve these issues.

Self-Test Question

1. What are some important issues facing healthcare managers today?

Theme Wrap-Up: Careers in Healthcare Management

What are some settings that require healthcare management graduates? The largest employers of healthcare managers are hospitals. In the United States, about 5,000 community hospitals, as well as Veterans Affairs, military, and public health facilities, are in operation. In hospitals, healthcare managers are needed in a multitude of functional areas, such as operations, marketing, human resources (personnel), facilities, information technology, and finance. About 40 percent of all healthcare management graduates initially take positions at hospitals. Most start their careers in operations, while some find they are better suited for one of the other functional areas and move quickly into specialized staff positions.

Another career opportunity is in medical practice management. Almost 1 million physicians practice in the United States in settings that range from one-physician (solo) practices to large group practices (such as Mayo Clinic, which has more than 3,800 physicians). Physicians practice within specialties, the largest of which is internal medicine. Other specialties include cardiology (heart), dermatology (skin), pediatrics (children), and surgery.

Some group practices consist of only one specialty, while other practices include physicians from several specialties (multispecialty practices). Obviously, the larger the group practice, the greater the need for management expertise.

The structure of the management staff at large group practices is similar to that at hospitals, while small practices may have only a practice manager and a few clerks. In addition to physician practices, other healthcare professionals, such as physical therapists and psychologists, may own stand-alone medical practices that require managerial skills beyond those possessed by the clinicians. The bottom line is that healthcare organizations need managers, and the larger the organization, the greater the need.

As the population ages and life expectancy increases, the requirement for long-term care will continue to grow at a rapid rate. As of 2014, about 15,600 nursing homes operated in the United States. These facilities require significant managerial expertise to prosper in an era of financial constraints, as do other institutional providers.

A multitude of career opportunities is also available in insurance, health services research, consulting, public health, and even homeland security.

Regardless of your specific healthcare management goals, knowledge of the fundamentals of healthcare finance is a critical skill. This book will help you obtain this professional competency.

Key Concepts

This chapter provides an introduction to healthcare finance. Here are the key concepts:

- The term *healthcare finance*, as it is used in this book, refers to the accounting and financial management principles and practices used in healthcare organizations to ensure the financial well-being of the enterprise.
- The primary role of finance in healthcare organizations, as in all businesses, is to plan for, acquire, and use resources to maximize the efficiency and value of the enterprise.
- Finance activities generally include the following: (1) *estimating costs and profitability, planning, and budgeting*; (2) *financial operations management*; (3) *financing decisions*; (4) *capital investment decisions*; (5) *financial reporting*; (6) *financial and operational analysis*; (7) *contract management*; and (8) *financial risk management.*
- Finance activities can be summarized by the *four Cs*: costs, cash, capital, and control.
- The size and structure of the finance department in healthcare organizations depend on the type and size of the provider entity.
- The finance department in large provider organizations is generally led by the *chief financial officer (CFO)*, who typically reports directly to the chief executive officer

(CEO) and is responsible for all finance activities in the organization. Under the CFO are the *comptroller (controller)*, who is responsible for accounting and reporting activities, and the *treasurer*, who is responsible for the acquisition and management of capital (funds).

- In large organizations, the comptroller and treasurer direct managers with responsibility for specific functions, such as the *patient accounts manager*, who reports to the comptroller, and the *cash manager*, who reports to the treasurer.
- In small healthcare businesses, the finance responsibilities are combined and assigned to one individual, often called the *business (practice) manager*.
- All business decisions have financial implications, so all managers (whether clinical or in operations, marketing, personnel, or facilities) must know enough about finance to incorporate its implications into their specialized decision processes.
- Healthcare services are provided in numerous settings, including hospitals, ambulatory care facilities, long-term care facilities, and even the home.
- Hospitals differ in function (general acute care vs. specialty), length of stay, size, and ownership (government vs. private, for-profit vs. not-for-profit).
- Ambulatory care, also known as *outpatient care*, encompasses services provided to noninstitutionalized patients. Outpatient settings include medical practices, hospital outpatient departments, ambulatory surgery centers, urgent care centers, diagnostic imaging centers, rehabilitation and sports medicine centers, and clinical laboratories.
- *Long-term care* entails healthcare services provided for an extended period, including inpatient, outpatient, and home health care, often with a focus on mental health, rehabilitation, or nursing home care.
- *Home health care* brings many of the same services provided in ambulatory care settings into the patient's home.
- The defining characteristic of an *integrated delivery system* is that it has the capability of providing all healthcare services needed by a defined population.
- Entry into the healthcare sector is heavily regulated. Examples of regulations include licensure, certificate of need (CON), and rate setting and review programs.
- Legal issues, such as malpractice, are prominent in discussions about controlling healthcare costs.
- Two recent surveys of healthcare executives confirm that healthcare managers view financial concerns as their most important current issue.

In chapter 2, we continue our discussion of foundation concepts and move on to finance-related topics, such as business basics, forms of organization, and taxes.

End-of-Chapter Questions

1.1 a. What does the term *healthcare finance* mean, as it is used in this book?
b. What are the two broad areas of healthcare finance?
c. Why is it necessary to have a book on healthcare finance as opposed to a generic finance book?

1.2 a. Briefly discuss the role of finance in the healthcare field.
b. Has this role increased or decreased in importance in recent years?

1.3 a. Briefly describe the following healthcare settings:
- Hospitals
- Ambulatory care
- Home health care
- Long-term care
- Integrated delivery systems

b. What benefits are attributed to integrated delivery systems?

1.4 What role does regulation play in the healthcare sector?

1.5 What is the structure of the finance function in healthcare organizations?

1.6 What is the primary legal issue facing providers today?

CHAPTER 2

HEALTHCARE BUSINESS BASICS

Theme Set-Up: Business Goals

Healthcare finance cannot be practiced in isolation. Rather, it must be guided by the goals of the organization. That concept is exactly what Jane Matthews, a recent healthcare management graduate, had in mind as she thought about two job interviews scheduled to take place in the next several days. The openings were for an entry-level management position at Southwest Healthcare, a for-profit (investor-owned) multispecialty group practice, and the same position at St. Jerome's Hospital, a not-for-profit organization. To prepare for the interviews, Jane studied the organizations and their goals. She wondered if the different ownership status of the providers resulted in a significant difference in mission, goals, and financial behavior.

Thanks to her healthcare management classes, Jane had a rough idea of the characteristics of different ownership types. Still, she thought long and hard about whether St. Jerome's was even a business. After all, as a Catholic hospital, it had a long history of providing charity care to society's less fortunate. Also, it had no well-defined owner group, so it could be thought of as being owned by the community at large.

On the other hand, Southwest was owned by its physicians and did not have the same tradition of serving the poor. Had the obligation to make money for the physician-owners influenced Southwest's mission and goals, creating differences between it and St. Jerome's? If so, does this fact mean its approach to financial decision-making differs? Jane wanted to answer these questions before she began her interviews.

By the end of this chapter, you will know more about the various types of provider organizations, their goals, and how these goals influence the finance function. See if your take on the situation is the same as Jane's.

Learning Objectives

After studying this chapter, you will be able to do the following:

- Define the concept of a *business* in financial terms.
- Describe the alternative legal forms of business.
- Articulate the key differences between for-profit and not-for-profit businesses.
- Explain how business goals are influenced by the form of organization and ownership.
- Briefly discuss the implications of tax laws for individuals, for-profit businesses, and not-for-profit corporations.

2.1 INTRODUCTION

Most of the basic concepts of healthcare finance are the same regardless of the specific sector (e.g., hospital vs. long-term care vs. medical practice) and organizational setting. However, some aspects of healthcare finance are influenced by the unique nature of particular types of healthcare organizations. In this chapter, we present the context in which health services finance is practiced.

First, we consider the nature of businesses. Is the provision of health services a business, and, if so, how are such businesses formed, and what are the implications of being a business as opposed to a pure charity? Then, we explore the consequences of being a health services business that is organized as a not-for-profit corporation. Does not-for-profit status influence an organization's goals and objectives, and, if so, does it affect the practice of finance?

These, along with a brief look at the impact of taxes, are some of the issues we explore in this chapter.

2.2 CONCEPT OF A BUSINESS

What is a business? If you asked this question of a group of accountants, the answer probably would involve financial statements, such as the income statement and balance sheet (which we cover in chapters 11 and 12). If you asked a group of lawyers, the answer likely would include legal forms of business, which we describe in the next section.

From a financial (economic) perspective, a business can be thought of as an entity—its legal form does not matter—that (1) obtains financing, or capital, from the marketplace; (2) uses those funds to buy land, buildings, and equipment (that is, assets); (3) operates those assets to create goods or services; and (4) sells those goods or services to create revenue. To be financially viable, a business has to generate sufficient revenue to pay all of the costs associated with creating and selling its goods or services.

Although this description of a business is surprisingly simple, it tells a great deal about the basic decisions that business managers must make. One of the first decisions is what legal form the business will take. The next decision is how the business will raise the capital it needs to get started. Should it borrow the money (use debt financing), raise the money from owners (or from the community if not-for-profit), or use some combination of the two sources? Next, once the start-up capital is raised, what assets (facilities and equipment) should be acquired to create the services (in the case of healthcare providers) that will be offered to patients?

Note that businesses are profoundly different from pure charities (see "Critical Concept: Business Versus Pure Charity"). A business, such as a hospital or medical practice, sustains itself financially by selling goods or services. Thus, it is in competition with other businesses for the consumer dollar. A pure charity, such as the American Heart Association, on the other hand, does not sell goods or services. Rather, it obtains funds by soliciting contributions and then uses those funds to supply charitable (free) services. In essence, a pure charity is a budgetary organization in that the amount of contributions fixes its budget for the year. Similarly, a government agency has a budget that is fixed by appropriations.

Of course, pure charities and government agencies must operate in a businesslike manner, but they do not operate like businesses because they do not obtain their operating funds by selling goods or services (see "For Your Consideration: Businesses, Pure Charities, and Government Entities"). Some healthcare providers do solicit contributions, and many provide some charitable care, but health services organizations primarily sustain themselves by selling services.

CRITICAL CONCEPT
Business Versus Pure Charity

A business is an entity that raises capital in the marketplace; invests those funds in assets; and uses those assets to create goods or services, which it sells. Businesses differ from pure charities in the sense that businesses sustain themselves by revenue obtained from sales, while pure charities are sustained primarily by contributions. In a sense, pure charities, as well as government agencies, are budgetary organizations in that their funding is constrained by external forces (contributions or appropriations), and each year they must operate within the budget. Businesses, however, are not so constrained; they can influence their "funding" by selling more products or services.

FOR YOUR CONSIDERATION
Businesses, Pure Charities, and Government Entities

A healthcare business relies on revenues from sales to create financial sustainability. For example, if a hospital's revenues exceed its costs, cash is being generated that can be used to provide new and improved patient services, and the hospital can continue to meet community needs. On the other hand, pure charities, such as the American Red Cross, rely on contributions for revenues, so the amount of charitable services provided (which typically are free) is limited by the amount of contributions received. Finally, most governmental units are funded by tax receipts, so, as with charities, the amount of services provided is limited, in this case by the taxing authority's ability to raise revenues. Yet, in spite of differences, all three types of organization must operate in a financially prudent manner.

What do you think? From a finance perspective, how different are these types of organizations? How does the day-to-day functioning of their finance departments vary? Is finance more important in one type of organization than in another?

? Self-Test Questions

1. Briefly describe a business from a financial perspective.
2. What is the difference between a business and a pure charity?

2.3 LEGAL FORMS OF BUSINESSES

Because the focus of this book is on the practice of finance in healthcare businesses, a good starting point is to understand the different legal forms of businesses (see "Critical Concept: Legal Forms of Businesses"). Many health services managers work for corporations, including not-for-profit corporations, because these businesses often are large and require extensive management structures. However, some healthcare managers choose to work for medical practices that are organized as proprietorships or partnerships—and hybrid forms (which have features of both partnerships and corporations) are becoming common in medical practices as well. Health services managers need to be familiar with all legal forms of businesses, regardless of the form of their own organization. To illustrate this point, hospital managers, whether at for-profit or not-for-profit hospitals, work closely with the physician staff, so knowledge of how physicians organize their practices is useful.

! CRITICAL CONCEPT
Legal Forms of Businesses

Business entities can be one of three basic legal forms: (1) proprietorship or partnership, (2) corporation, or (3) hybrid (a combination of the first two types). Each legal form has its advantages and disadvantages, but most large businesses, including all not-for-profits, are organized as corporations. Proprietorships and partnerships are easy to form, but sale of an ownership interest is difficult and owners have unlimited liability. For-profit corporations are more complex to set up, but they offer easier ownership transfer and limited liability. However, for-profit corporations are often subject to double taxation—once at the corporate level and again at the shareholder (owner) level. Hybrid forms tend to offer some advantages of each ownership type without the disadvantages.

Proprietorships and Partnerships

A **proprietorship** (or sole proprietorship) is a business owned by one person. Going into business as a proprietor is easy—the owner merely begins business operations. However, most cities require even the smallest businesses to be licensed, and state licensure is required for most healthcare professionals.

Proprietorship
A simple form of business owned by one person. Also called *sole proprietorship*.

The proprietorship form of organization is easily and inexpensively formed, is subject to few government regulations, and pays no corporate (business) income taxes. All earnings of the business, whether reinvested in the business or withdrawn by the owner, are taxed as personal income to the proprietor. In general, a sole proprietorship will pay lower total taxes than a comparable taxable corporation because corporate profits are taxed twice—once at the corporate level and again by shareholders (owners) at the personal level when profits are distributed as dividends or when the stock is sold.

Partnership
An unincorporated business that is created and owned by two or more people.

A **partnership** is similar to a proprietorship, but it is owned by two or more individuals. Partnerships may operate under different degrees of formality, ranging from informal oral agreements between the partners to formal agreements filed with the state in which the partnership conducts business. Like a proprietorship, a partnership can be advantageous because of its low cost and ease of formation. In addition, the tax treatment of a partnership is similar to that of a proprietorship; the partnership's earnings are allocated to the partners and taxed as personal income, regardless of whether the earnings are actually paid out to the partners or retained in the business.

Proprietorships and partnerships have several disadvantages, including the following:

- Selling an ownership interest in the business is difficult. There is no well-established market for selling an ownership stake in a proprietorship or partnership.
- Proprietors and partners have unlimited personal liability for the debts of the business, which can result in losses greater than the amount invested in the business. In a proprietorship, unlimited liability means that the owner is personally responsible for the debts of the business. In a partnership, it means that if any partner is unable to meet his obligation in the event of bankruptcy, the remaining partners are responsible for the unsatisfied claims and must draw on their personal assets if necessary to fulfill that obligation.
- The life of the business is limited to the life of the owners.

For these reasons, proprietorships and most partnerships generally are restricted to relatively small businesses.

The three disadvantages of proprietorships and partnerships listed earlier lead to the fourth, and perhaps most important, disadvantage from a finance perspective: the difficulty that proprietorships and partnerships have in attracting large amounts of capital. This hurdle is not high for a small business or when the proprietor or partners are wealthy, but in most situations the difficulty of attracting capital becomes a disadvantage if the business needs to grow substantially to take advantage of market opportunities. Thus, many for-profit businesses start out as sole proprietorships or partnerships but then ultimately convert to corporations.

For-Profit Corporations

A for-profit (investor-owned) business may be organized as a corporation, but a not-for-profit business must be organized as a corporation. In this section, we focus on the advantages and disadvantages of for-profit corporations. Not-for-profit corporations, along with additional facets of for-profit corporations, are discussed in section 2.4 of this chapter.

A **for-profit corporation** is a legal entity that is separate and distinct from its owners and managers. The creation of a separate business entity provides these primary advantages:

For-profit corporation
A legal business entity that is separate and distinct from its owners and managers.

- A for-profit corporation has unlimited life and can continue in existence after its original owners and managers have died or left the company.
- Transferring ownership in a for-profit corporation is easy because ownership is divided into shares of stock that can be easily sold (assuming the business is large and its stock is frequently traded).
- Owners of a for-profit corporation have limited liability. To illustrate, suppose Kate Anderson made an investment of $10,000 in a partnership that subsequently went bankrupt, owing $100,000. Because the partners are liable for the debts of the partnership, Kate could be assessed for a share of the partnership's debt in addition to the loss of her initial $10,000 contribution. In fact, if the other partners were unable to pay their shares of the indebtedness, Kate could be held liable for the entire $100,000. However, if the $10,000 had been invested in a corporation that went bankrupt, Kate's potential loss would be limited to her initial $10,000 investment. (Note that in the case of small, financially weak corporations, the limited liability feature of ownership is often fictitious because bankers and other lenders require personal guarantees from the shareholders.)

With these three major advantages—unlimited life, ease of ownership transfer, and limited liability—for-profit corporations can more easily raise money in the financial markets than sole proprietorships or partnerships can.

For-profit corporations have two primary disadvantages. First, corporate earnings typically are subject to double taxation—once at the corporate level, and again at the personal level, when dividends are paid or the stock is sold. Second, setting up a corporation and fulfilling the subsequent requirement to file periodic state and federal reports are more costly and time-consuming activities than are required to establish a proprietorship or partnership.

While participants in a proprietorship or partnership can begin operations without much legal paperwork, the founders, or their attorney, of a corporation must prepare a charter and a set of bylaws before launching operations. Today, attorneys have standard electronic forms for charters and bylaws, so they can set up a no-frills corporation with modest effort. Indeed, a number of websites help founders perform most of the set-up work themselves. Still, starting a corporation remains relatively difficult compared to a proprietorship or partnership, and it is even more difficult if the corporation has nonstandard features.

Liquid investment
An investment that can be sold quickly at a fair price.

C corporation
A traditional for-profit corporation.

S corporation
A for-profit corporation with a limited number of shareholders that, after filing an application with the Internal Revenue Service, is taxed as a proprietorship or partnership.

Hybrid form
A legal business entity that has features associated with both partnerships and for-profit corporations.

Limited partnership
A partnership in which the general partners have most of the control and unlimited liability while the limited partners have little control and liability that is limited to their initial contribution.

The value of any for-profit business, other than a small one, generally is maximized if it is organized as a corporation for the following reasons:

- Limited liability reduces the risks borne by the owners (shareholders). With all else the same, the lower the risk, the higher the value of the ownership investment.
- A business's value is dependent on growth opportunities, which in turn are dependent on the business's ability to attract capital. Because corporations can obtain capital more easily than other forms of business can, they are better able to take advantage of growth opportunities.
- The value of any investment depends on its liquidity (a **liquid investment**), which means the ease with which it can be sold for a fair price. Because an ownership interest in a for-profit corporation is much more liquid than a similar interest in a proprietorship or partnership, the corporate form of organization creates more value for its owners.

For tax purposes, standard for-profit corporations are called **C corporations**. However, if they meet certain requirements, one or a few individuals can form a for-profit corporation and elect to pay taxes as if the business were a proprietorship or partnership, hence avoiding double taxation. Such corporations, which differ only in how the owners are taxed, are called **S corporations** (the name comes from subchapter S of the tax code). Although S corporations are similar to two of the hybrid forms (discussed next) in terms of taxes, the hybrid forms provide more flexibility and benefits to owners.

Hybrid Forms

In addition to the two basic forms of organization—proprietorship/partnership and corporation—several **hybrid forms** of business are used by healthcare businesses.

To begin, two specialized types of partnerships have different characteristics from those of a standard partnership. First, limiting some of the partners' liabilities is possible by establishing a **limited partnership**, wherein certain partners are designated general partners and others are limited partners. The limited partners, as with the owners of a corporation, are liable only for the amount of their initial investment in the partnership, while the general partners have unlimited liability. However, the limited partners typically have restricted or no control; control rests solely with the general partners. Limited partnerships are quite common in some industries (think real estate). They are not very prevalent in the health services sector because finding one partner who is willing to accept all of the business's risk and another partner who is willing to relinquish control is difficult.

A **limited liability partnership (LLP)** is available in many states. In such a partnership, the partners have joint liability for all of its actions, including personal injuries and indebtedness. However, all partners enjoy limited liability regarding professional malpractice because partners are only liable for their own individual malpractice actions, not those of the other partners.

A **limited liability company (LLC)** has some characteristics of both a partnership and a corporation. The owners of an LLC are called members, and they are taxed as if they are partners in a partnership. However, a member's liability is similar to that of a shareholder of a corporation because liability is limited to the member's initial contribution in the business. Personal assets are only at risk if the member assumes specific liability, such as signing a personal loan guarantee.

A **professional corporation (PC)**, called a professional association in some states, is a corporate form of organization common among physicians and other individual and group practice healthcare professionals. All 50 states have statutes that prescribe the requirements for such businesses, providing the usual benefits of incorporation but not relieving the participants of professional liability. Indeed, the primary motivation behind a PC, which is a relatively old business form compared to the LLP and LLC, was to provide a way for professionals to incorporate yet be held personally liable for professional malpractice.

Limited liability partnership (LLP)
A partnership that limits the professional (malpractice) liability of its members.

Limited liability company (LLC)
A corporation that combines some features of a partnership with others of a corporation.

Professional corporation (PC)
A type of corporate business organization in which the owner or managers retain professional (medical) liability. Called a professional association in some states.

? Self-Test Questions

1. What are the three basic forms of business organization, and how do they differ?
2. What are the different types of partnerships?
3. What is the difference between a C corporation and an S corporation?

2.4 ALTERNATIVE FORMS OF OWNERSHIP

Unlike other sectors, not-for-profit corporations play a major role in the healthcare field. As we note in chapter 1, about 58 percent of community hospitals in the United States are private not-for-profit hospitals. Only 21 percent of all hospitals are for-profit (investor owned); the remaining hospitals are government operated. Not-for-profit ownership is also present in nursing home and home health care businesses. In this section, we compare and contrast the features of for-profit and not-for-profit corporations. We begin by offering additional detail on for-profit corporations.

Additional Information on For-Profit Corporations

When you think of a corporation, you probably think in terms of an investor-owned (for-profit) corporation (see "Critical Concept: Investor-Owned [For-Profit] Corporations").

> **CRITICAL CONCEPT**
> Investor-Owned (For-Profit) Corporations
>
> Investor-owned corporations are for-profit businesses whose ownership (stock) is either publicly traded (owned by a large number of investors) or privately held (owned by a small number of investors). The shareholders of for-profit corporations exercise control of the business by voting for the board of directors. Shareholders have a claim on the residual earnings of the business, which is the amount of revenue that remains after all expenses have been paid. All or a portion of the residual earnings may be paid out to shareholders as dividends or may be used to repurchase shares currently owned by shareholders. For-profit corporations must pay taxes, including property and income taxes.

Large businesses, such as Microsoft, Google, and General Electric, are investor-owned corporations. In healthcare, HCA and Tenet Healthcare are for-profit corporations in the hospital sector. Other healthcare examples include Apria Healthcare, which offers home health services, and Brookdale Senior Living, which provides long-term care.

Investors become owners of for-profit corporations by buying shares of common stock in the company. When stock is sold by the company, the funds raised from the sale go to the corporation. However, stock owners (shareholders) can sell their shares to other individuals. These sales typically take place on exchanges, such as the New York Stock Exchange, or in the over-the-counter market, which is composed of a large number of stockbrokers connected by a sophisticated electronic trading system. When shares are bought and sold by individuals through exchanges, the corporations whose stocks are traded receive no funds from the trades. Corporations receive funds only when the shares are first sold to investors.

Publicly held company
A for-profit corporation whose shares are held by the general public (a large number of shareholders) and traded on an exchange, such as the New York Stock Exchange, or in the over-the-counter market.

Investor-owned corporations may be publicly held or privately held. The shares of **publicly held companies** are owned by a large number of investors and are widely traded. For example, Hospital Corporation of America (HCA), which operated 166 general acute care hospitals in 2016, had more than 370 million shares owned by individual and institutional shareholders as of December 31, 2016. Another example is Kindred Healthcare, which operates nursing homes, home health services, long-term acute care hospitals, and rehabilitation services and has about 85 million shares owned by some 2,773 shareholders. Drug companies, such as Merck and Pfizer, are also publicly held corporations.

Privately (closely) held company
A for-profit corporation whose stock is owned by a small number of individuals—usually the business's managers—and is not publicly traded.

Conversely, the shares of **privately (closely) held companies** are owned by just a handful of investors and are not publicly traded. In general, the managers of privately held companies are major shareholders. For example, HCA was a publicly held company until November 2006. At that time, the outstanding stock of the company was purchased by a small group of investors, taking the company private. In reality, privately held companies are more similar to partnerships than to publicly held companies. Often, the privately held corporation is a transitional form of organization that exists for a short time between a proprietorship or partnership and a publicly owned corporation. A closely held corporation may be motivated to go public either by the need for additional capital or by the desire of the owners to cash out. In the case of HCA, the new owners sold off poorly performing hospitals, improved the operations of the remaining hospitals, and in 2011 took the company public again. By doing so, the shareholders who took the company private both recovered their investment in the hospital chain and earned a tidy profit.

Stockholders (shareholders) are the owners of investor-owned corporations. As owners, they have these basic rights:

Stockholders (shareholders)
The owners of a for-profit corporation by virtue of holding one or more shares of the company's stock.

- *The right of control.* Common shareholders have the right to vote for the corporation's board of directors, which oversees the management of the company. Each year, a company's shareholders receive a ballot, called a proxy, which they use to vote for directors and to vote on other issues proposed by management or shareholders. In this way, shareholders exercise control. In the voting process, shareholders cast one vote for each common share held.
- *A claim on the residual earnings of the firm.* A for-profit corporation sells goods or services and realizes revenue from the sales. To produce this revenue, the corporation must incur expenses for materials, labor, insurance, debt capital, and so on. Any excess of revenue over expenses—the residual earnings—belongs to the shareholders of the business. Often, a portion of these earnings is paid out in the form of dividends, which are cash payments to shareholders, or stock repurchases, whereby the company buys back shares held by shareholders. However, management typically elects to reinvest some (or all) of the **residual earnings** in the business, which presumably will produce even higher earnings in the future. (If you are interested in more information about how corporate earnings are distributed to shareholders, see online chapter 14, which is available at ache.org/books/FinanceFundamentals3.)
- *A claim on liquidation proceeds.* In the event of bankruptcy and liquidation, shareholders are entitled to any proceeds that remain after all other obligations of the business have been satisfied. In most liquidations, however, little or nothing is left for shareholders.

Residual earnings
The earnings (profits) of a business after all expenses have been paid.

In summary, for-profit corporations have three key traits. First, the owners (the shareholders) of the business are well defined and exercise control of the firm by voting for directors. Second, the residual earnings of the business belong to the owners, so management is responsible only to the shareholders for the profitability of the firm. Third, investor-owned corporations are subject to taxation at the local, state, and federal levels.

Not-for-Profit Corporations

If an organization meets a set of stringent requirements, it can qualify for incorporation as a not-for-profit (tax-exempt) corporation (see "Critical Concept: Not-for-Profit [Tax-Exempt] Corporation"). Such corporations are sometimes called *nonprofit corporations.* Because

CRITICAL CONCEPT
Not-for-Profit (Tax-Exempt) Corporation

Not-for-profit healthcare businesses must be incorporated under the provisions of Section 501(c)(3) of the IRS Tax Code. Because such corporations have no owners, none of their profits can be paid out as dividends. In essence, not-for-profit businesses are "owned" by the community at large and are controlled by a board of trustees, which generally includes community representation. In general, not-for-profit corporations are exempt from local, state, and federal income and property taxes.

nonprofit businesses (as opposed to pure charities, such as the American Red Cross) need profits to sustain operations, and because it is hard to explain why nonprofit corporations should earn profits, the term *not-for-profit* is used here, as it is more descriptive of such health services corporations.

Tax-exempt status is granted to healthcare businesses that meet the tax definition of a charitable corporation as defined by Internal Revenue Service (IRS) Tax Code section 501(c)(3). Hence, such corporations are also known as 501(c)(3) corporations. This section of the code specifies that "the exempt purposes set forth in section 501(c)(3) are charitable, religious, educational, scientific, literary, testing for public safety, fostering national or international amateur sports competition, and preventing cruelty to children or animals." Because the promotion of health is commonly considered a charitable activity, a corporation that provides healthcare services can qualify for tax-exempt status, provided that it meets the other requirements.

In addition to the charitable purpose, a not-for-profit corporation must be organized and operated so that it operates exclusively for the public, rather than private, interest. Thus, no profits can be used for private gain and no direct political activity can be conducted. Also, if the corporation is liquidated or sold to an investor-owned business, the proceeds from the liquidation or sale must be used for a charitable purpose. Because individuals cannot benefit from the profits of not-for-profit corporations, such organizations cannot pay dividends. However, prohibition of private gain from profits does not prevent parties, such as managers or physicians, from benefiting through salaries, perquisites, contracts, and so on.

Not-for-profit corporations differ significantly from investor-owned corporations. Because not-for-profit corporations have no shareholders, no single body of individuals has ownership rights to the firm's residual earnings or exercises control of the firm. Rather, control is exercised by a board of trustees, which, for all practical purposes, is not constrained by external parties (such as shareholders). However, unlike for-profit corporations, the boards of not-for-profit corporations are typically dominated by community leaders, who presumably are motivated to ensure that the organization meets community needs.

Not-for-profit corporations are generally exempt from taxation, including both property and income taxes, and have the right to issue tax-exempt debt. (The ability to issue tax-exempt debt means that not-for-profit corporations pay relatively low interest rates on their debt financing.) Finally, individual contributions to not-for-profit organizations can be deducted from taxable income by the donor, so not-for-profit corporations have access to tax-subsidized contribution capital. (The tax benefits enjoyed by not-for-profit corporations, including the benefits associated with tax-exempt debt, are discussed in more detail in section 2.6, which focuses on tax laws.)

For-profit corporations must file annual income tax returns with the IRS. The equivalent filing for not-for-profit corporations is IRS **Form 990**, Return of Organization Exempt from Income Tax. Its purpose is to provide both the IRS and the public with financial information about not-for-profit organizations, and it is often the only source of such information. It is also used by government agencies to prevent organizations from abusing their tax-exempt status. Form 990 requires significant disclosures related to governance and boards of directors. In addition, not-for-profit hospitals are required to file **Schedule H** to Form 990, which includes financial information on the amount and type of community benefits (primarily charity care or financial assistance) provided, bad debt losses, and collection practices. IRS regulations require not-for-profit organizations to provide copies of their three most recent Form 990s to anyone who requests them, whether in person or by mail, fax, or e-mail. Form 990s are also available to the public through several online services.

Form 990
A form filed by not-for-profit organizations with the IRS that reports on an organization's governance and charitable activities.

Schedule H
An attachment to IRS Form 990 filed by not-for-profit hospitals that provides additional information on the hospital's community benefit activities.

The financial problems facing federal, state, and local governments have caused politicians to take a close look at the tax subsidies provided to not-for-profit hospitals. Several bills that require hospitals to meet minimum levels of care to the indigent to retain tax-exempt status have been introduced in the US Congress. Such efforts by Congress have prompted the American Hospital Association to issue guidelines on tax-exempt status, which include, among other things, (1) charity care, or providing financial assistance for uninsured patients of limited means (without such requirements, self-pay patients often pay much higher rates than those paid by insurers); (2) communicating charity care and financial assistance policies; (3) ensuring fair and transparent billing and collections practices; (4) promoting community health and reporting **community benefits**, which encompasses the full range of services provided to the population served, such as health education and community outreach; and (5) improving **transparency**, or the ability of outsiders to understand a business's governance structure and policies, including executive compensation.

Community benefits
Services and initiatives taken by providers, such as financial assistance for uninsured patients of limited means and education programs, that enhance the health and well-being of the community.

In addition to congressional action, legislators in more than 20 states have proposed bills that mandate the amount of charity care provided by not-for-profit hospitals and the billing and collections procedures applied to the uninsured. For example, Texas has established minimum requirements for charity care that, in effect, hold not-for-profit hospitals accountable to the public for the tax exemptions they receive. The Texas law specifies four tests, and each hospital must meet at least one of them. The test that most hospitals use to comply with the law requires that at least 4 percent of patient revenue be spent on charity care and government-sponsored indigent care. In Illinois, not-for-profit hospitals are required to provide charity care or other specified services at levels equivalent to what they receive in property tax exemptions in order to maintain their tax-exempt status.

Transparency
The ability of outsiders to know what is happening in a business.

At the federal level, the IRS now requires all not-for-profit hospitals to report community benefit through their annual tax filings. Community benefit includes financial assistance and other resources, such as community health improvement services, that are reported on Schedule H of the IRS Form 990. Schedule H is designated solely for tax-exempt hospitals. Although the IRS collects these data, the federal government does not mandate minimum levels of community benefit that not-for-profit hospitals must provide in order to maintain tax-exempt status.

Finally, municipalities in several states have attacked the property tax exemption of not-for-profit hospitals that have "neglected" their charitable missions (see "For Your Consideration: Making Not-for-Profit Hospitals Do Good"). For example, tax assessors in several states have forced selected hospitals to pay property taxes, arguing that the hospitals had strayed too far from their charitable purpose. Such "voluntary" payment of property taxes by a not-for-profit entity, which is becoming more common, is called *payment in lieu of taxes*.

According to a recent study, the total value of tax exemption for not-for-profit hospitals exceeded $24 billion in 2011. This estimate includes the forgone value of federal, state, and local revenues associated with corporate income taxes, tax-exempt bonds, charitable contributions, and sales and property tax associated with not-for-profit hospitals.

Self-Test Questions

1. What are the major differences between investor-owned and not-for-profit corporations?
2. What pressures recently have been placed on not-for-profit hospitals to ensure that they meet their charitable mission?

For Your Consideration
Making Not-for-Profit Hospitals Do Good

Many people have criticized not-for-profit hospitals for not earning their charitable exemptions. In 2010, the Illinois Supreme Court concluded that Provena Covenant hospital, located in Urbana, Illinois, was not a charitable institution for property tax purposes. The court's opinion reasoned that the primary use of the hospital property was to provide medical services for a fee, while *charity* means providing a gift to the community. The opinion further pointed out that (1) the charity care being provided was subsidized by payments from other patients; (2) many patients granted partial charity care still paid enough to cover costs; and (3) the hospital's community benefit activities, such as a residency program and an education program for emergency responders, also benefited the hospital and thus were not truly gifts to the community. Therefore, the hospital property was not in charitable use.

FOR YOUR CONSIDERATION
Making Not-for-Profit Hospitals Do Good *(continued)*

Most not-for-profit hospitals today are, of course, primarily supported by payments for services rather than by charitable contributions. Under the opinion's reasoning, the property tax exemption may be hard to maintain. However, a partial dissent by two justices suggests that this case is not the end of the issue. The dissent argues that the plurality opinion impinges on the legislative function of setting specific standards for tax exemption, and the issue should be settled by legislative action rather than by courts.

What do you think? Should not-for-profit hospitals lose their property tax or income tax exemptions if they do not provide sufficient charity care? Should legislatures set standards that hospitals must meet to maintain their tax-exempt status? If so, how might such standards be specified?

2.5 ORGANIZATIONAL GOALS

Healthcare finance is practiced with some objective in mind. Finance goals must be consistent with, and support, the overall goals of the organization. Thus, in the next section we discuss goals by which to establish a framework for financial decision-making in healthcare organizations.

Small For-Profit Businesses

In a proprietorship or partnership, a small privately owned corporation, or any other form of for-profit small business, the owners generally are also the managers. In theory, the business can be operated for the exclusive benefit of the owners. If the owners want to work hard every day to maximize income and wealth, they can. On the other hand, if they want to devote every Wednesday to playing golf, they can do that instead. (Of course, the business still has to satisfy the needs of its customers, or else it will not survive.)

Typically, in small businesses, goals of income (wealth) and other benefits (such as leisure time) are blended in such a way as to satisfy the owners' wishes. In large publicly held corporations, where owners and managers are separate parties, organizational goals become important guideposts for managers.

Large For-Profit Businesses

From a finance perspective, the primary goal of large publicly held corporations is generally assumed to be shareholder (owners') wealth maximization (see "Critical Concept:

CRITICAL CONCEPT
Shareholder (Owners') Wealth Maximization

The primary goal of large investor-owned businesses is shareholder wealth maximization, or maximization of owners' wealth. For corporations, this goal translates to stock price maximization. Of course, many other managerial goals exist, such as the fair treatment of all parties to the business. Still, when alternative courses of action are considered, the impact on shareholder wealth typically plays the dominant role in the decision-making process.

Shareholder [Owners'] Wealth Maximization"), which translates to stock price maximization. Investor-owned corporations do, of course, have other goals. Managers, who make the actual decisions, are interested in their personal welfare, in their employees' welfare, and in the good of the community and society at large. Still, the goal of stock price maximization is a reasonable operating objective on which to build financial decision rules.

The primary obstacle to shareholder wealth maximization in large investor-owned corporations is the **agency problem**. An agency problem exists when one or more individuals hire another individual or group of individuals (agents) to perform a service on their behalf, thereby delegating decision-making authority to those agents. Such a problem occurs between shareholders and managers of large investor-owned corporations because the managers typically hold only a small proportion of the firm's stock, and hence they benefit relatively little from stock price increases. On the other hand, managers benefit substantially from such actions as increasing the size of the firm to justify greater salaries, bonuses, and fringe benefits; awarding themselves generous retirement plans; and spending excessively on office space, personal staff, and travel—actions often detrimental to shareholders' wealth. Many situations arise in which managers are motivated to take actions that are in their, rather than the shareholders', best interests.

Agency problem
The problem that arises when the managers of a for-profit corporation are separate from the owners. In this situation, managers are motivated to act in their own interests as opposed to the interests of shareholders.

Shareholders recognize the agency problem and counter it by creating compensation incentives, such as stock options and performance-based bonus plans, that encourage managers to act in shareholders' interests. In addition, other factors, such as the threat of takeover or removal, keep managers focused on shareholder wealth maximization.

Of course, managers of investor-owned corporations can have motivations that are inconsistent with shareholder wealth maximization. Still, sufficient incentives and sanctions exist to motivate managers to view shareholder wealth maximization as an important goal. Thus, shareholder wealth maximization is a reasonable goal for financial decision-making in investor-owned corporations in spite of the agency problem.

Benefit corporation (B corporation)
A type of for-profit corporation that allows managers to consider social and environmental goals ahead of shareholder wealth maximization.

Readers may be interested to note that a newer form of for-profit corporation, available in 33 states including California and New York, allows managers to consider social and environmental goals ahead of stock price. Such a corporation, called a **benefit corporation (B corporation)**, is primarily intended to allow corporate boards and managers more flexibility in balancing shareholder value and the greater good. Benefit corporations must specify their social and environmental goals in the company's bylaws. Furthermore, such corporations must publish an annual benefit report, which measures how well these goals are being met. An example of a B corporation in the healthcare field is Transplant Connect, which provides medical records and clinical management systems software that support organ, tissue, and eye donation and transplantation.

Not-for-Profit Corporations

Although not-for-profit corporations have no shareholders, a number of parties, called **stakeholders**, have a financial interest in the organization. For example, a not-for-profit hospital's stakeholders include the board of trustees, managers, employees, physicians, creditors, suppliers, patients, and potential patients, who may include the entire community. (An investor-owned hospital has the same set of stakeholders, plus owners, who dictate the goal of ownership wealth maximization.) While managers of investor-owned businesses have to please primarily one class of stakeholders (the owners) to keep their jobs, managers of not-for-profit businesses must please all of the organization's stakeholders because no single, well-defined group exercises control.

Stakeholder
A party that has an interest—typically financial—in an organization. For example, owners (in for-profit businesses), managers, patients, and suppliers are some stakeholders of healthcare businesses.

Some people argue that managers of not-for-profit corporations do not have to please anyone at all because they tend to control the actions of the board of trustees, who are expected to exercise oversight. Others argue that managers of not-for-profit firms have to please all of the firm's stakeholders to a greater or lesser extent because all are necessary to the successful performance of the business. Of course, even managers of investor-owned firms should not attempt to enhance shareholder wealth by treating other stakeholders unfairly, as such actions ultimately are detrimental to shareholders.

Typically, the goal of not-for-profit corporations is stated in terms of a mission statement. For example, here is the current mission statement of Mercyhealth, an integrated regional health system: "Exceptional health care services with a passion for making lives better."

Although this mission statement provides Mercyhealth's managers and employees with a framework for developing specific goals and objectives, it does not provide much insight into the goals of the hospital's finance function. For the hospital to accomplish its mission, its managers have identified the following three financial goals:

- Emphasize cost containment through efficient operations.
- Promote accountable care strategies to meet the changing needs of patients and purchasers of healthcare services.
- Enhance access to capital and achieve long-term success.

In effect, Mercyhealth's managers are saying that to achieve the hospital's commitment to excellence as stated in its mission statement, the hospital must remain financially strong and profitable. Financially weak organizations cannot accomplish their stated missions over the long run. What is interesting is that Mercyhealth's three financial goals are probably not much different from the finance goals of for-profit health systems.

Clearly, for-profit health systems have to worry about providing returns to shareholders; however, to maximize shareholder wealth, these systems also must maintain financial viability and have the financial resources to offer new services and technologies. Furthermore, competition in local markets for hospital services will not permit for-profit health systems to charge appreciably more for services than their not-for-profit competitors charge.

? Self-Test Questions

1. What is the difference in organizational goals between investor-owned and not-for-profit businesses?
2. How does a benefit corporation (B corporation) differ from a traditional for-profit corporation?
3. What is the agency problem, and how does it apply to investor-owned firms?
4. What factors tend to reduce the agency problem?

2.6 TAX LAWS

Personal (individual) taxes
Taxes paid by individuals to federal and state (in most states) authorities on wages, interest, dividends, capital gains, and proprietorship and partnership income.

The value of any investment—whether a security, such as a stock in an individual's retirement account, or a business's investment in new diagnostic equipment—depends on the usable cash flows that the investment is expected to provide. Because taxes affect usable cash flows, both individuals and managers of for-profit healthcare businesses must be concerned about taxes.

US tax laws are complicated and are constantly changing. Indeed, some tax law provisions automatically expire over time if not renewed by congressional action. As a consequence, covering even the most basic features of tax laws in an introductory healthcare finance book is nearly impossible. Still, healthcare managers must understand those features of the tax system that directly affect financial decision-making.

Capital gains
The profit that is generated when securities (or other investments) are sold for more than their purchase price.

Personal (Individual) Taxes

Individuals must pay **personal (individual) taxes** to federal and state (in most states) authorities that can approach 40 percent of income. Income from proprietorships and partnerships, as well as interest, dividends, and **capital gains** on securities investments, are reduced when personal taxes are taken into account.

To illustrate the impact of personal taxes, assume that Dr. Cynthia Morgan's tax rate is 35 percent and she receives $200,000 in partnership income from her medical practice. Using the letter T to represent tax rate, she must pay $T \times \$200,000 = 0.35 \times \$200,000 = \$70,000$ in taxes on that income, which leaves her with only $\$200,000 - \$70,000 = \$130,000$ in usable (after-tax) income. This tax analysis leads to the following useful impact of taxes equation:

$$\begin{aligned} AT &= BT - (T \times BT) \\ &= BT \times (1 - T), \end{aligned}$$

where AT = after tax and BT = before tax. Thus, Dr. Morgan's after-tax income can be calculated as follows:

$$\begin{aligned} AT &= BT \times (1 - T) \\ &= \$200,000 \times (1 - 0.35) \\ &= \$200,000 \times 0.65 \\ &= \$130,000. \end{aligned}$$

Note that this equation can be applied to interest rates as well as dollar amounts. (See problem 2.3 at the end of the chapter as an example.) Clearly, taxes will influence personal investment decisions, so any tax implications of investment alternatives must be considered in the decision process. This deliberation is especially important when two investments under consideration have differential tax implications.

Corporate Taxes

Corporate tax laws affect both for profit and not-for-profit businesses, but in different ways.

For-Profit Corporations

In addition to personal taxes paid by individuals, investor-owned (for-profit) corporations must pay both federal and state **corporate taxes**, which can account for up to 21 percent of taxable income. For-profit corporations pay taxes on earnings before dividends are distributed, so corporate income is subject to double taxation. (Income is taxed once when corporations pay their income taxes and again when shareholders pay their income taxes on dividends and capital gains.) Small corporations can avoid double taxation by filing with the IRS as an S corporation, which, for tax purposes only, prorates the corporate income among the owners to be taxed as personal income. Also, hybrid forms of business avoid double taxation.

Corporate taxes
Income taxes paid by for-profit (taxable) corporations to federal and state authorities.

Not-for-Profit Corporations

Not-for-profit corporations, for the most part, are not subject to income, property, or sales taxes. The exemption from taxes is, by far, the biggest benefit granted to not-for-profit health services organizations. In addition, such organizations enjoy two other tax benefits.

First, not-for-profit organizations are able to borrow funds (use debt financing) on which the interest payments are exempt from the lender's personal taxes. Thus, if Jake Jaworski buys a $5,000 bond issued by Mercyhealth, a not-for-profit corporation, the interest paid by the hospital to Jake is not subject to personal taxes.

To illustrate the advantage of being able to issue tax-exempt debt, first assume that Jake owns some bonds issued by HCA, a for-profit hospital system. These bonds have an interest rate of 10 percent, so Jake receives 0.10 × $100 = $10 in annual interest for every $100 worth of bonds he owns. If Jake pays 40 percent in federal and state income taxes, each $10 of interest provides him with $AT = BT \times (1 - T)$ = $10 × (1 – 0.40) = $10 × 0.6 = $6 of usable (after-tax) interest.

However, if the bonds had been issued by Mercyhealth, Jake would not have to pay taxes on the interest and hence would keep the entire $10. If investors truly require a $6 after-tax (usable) return, Mercyhealth can issue debt with an interest rate of only 6 percent and, with all else the same, investors (such as Jake) in the 40 percent tax bracket would be as willing to buy these bonds as they are the HCA 10 percent bonds.

Thus, the interest rate that Mercyhealth must set on its debt issues to entice lenders is lower than the rate that HCA must set because of the tax exemption on debt issued by not-for-profit corporations. This exemption appears to give not-for-profit healthcare businesses a big advantage over for-profit businesses, but we have not told the full story. For-profit providers can deduct their interest payments on debt financing from taxable income and hence gain a tax benefit that, over time, reduces the effective interest rate on for-profit hospital debt to about the same amount as paid by similar not-for-profit (tax-exempt) providers.

The second tax benefit not-for-profit organizations enjoy is that the contributions made by individuals to not-for-profit corporations are tax deductible to the donor. If Miguel Corales, who is in the 40 percent personal income tax bracket (including federal and state taxes), were to donate $1,000 to Mercyhealth, his taxable income would be reduced by $1,000. A reduction in taxable income of this amount would save Miguel T × $1,000 = 0.40 × $1,000 = $400 in taxes. Thus, the effective dollar cost of his contribution would only be $600, because he saved $400 in taxes by making the contribution. In effect, the government will pay Miguel 40 cents for every dollar he contributes. In this way, not-for-profit providers have access to a source of financing (contributions) that, for all practical purposes, is not available to investor-owned providers.

Because of the impact that taxes have on usable earnings of investor-owned businesses and because not-for-profit ownership has important tax consequences, we highlight and explain, as needed, these tax implications throughout the book. For now, recognize that taxes play a critical role in many finance decisions.

Self-Test Questions

1. Why must a finance book consider taxes?
2. What is the primary tax advantage of not-for-profit corporations?
3. Why is the ability to issue tax-exempt debt an advantage for not-for-profit corporations?
4. What advantage accrues to businesses that qualify for tax-exempt contributions?

Theme Wrap-Up: Business Goals

After conducting more research on forms of business organization and goals, here's what Jane Matthews concluded. For starters, the not-for-profit St. Jerome's Hospital is indeed a business. It must accomplish all of the actions associated with businesses: (1) raise capital; (2) invest the funds raised in land, buildings, and equipment; (3) provide patient services; and (4) earn enough profit to sustain and grow the organization. Even though it offers a significant amount of charity care, which is mostly funded from profits earned on services provided to those who do pay, the hospital must operate as a business, not as a pure charity.

Now, what about the difference in goals between Southwest Healthcare and St. Jerome's? Southwest's mission is to "provide timely, high-quality, and efficient healthcare to its service area in a competent and compassionate manner by offering a wide variety of services from primary care to specialized procedures." St. Jerome's mission is to "extend the Catholic healthcare ministry by continually improving the health and quality of life of the people in the communities we serve."

These mission statements are laudable, but do they translate to different financial goals? Probably not. Southwest does not address the issue of owners' wealth in its mission statement, but the physician-owners are concerned with earning a return on the capital they invested in the business. To succeed, the practice must offer the services needed by the communities in which it operates at a price and quality that make its services competitive in the marketplace. St. Jerome's must achieve the same goal. To accomplish its mission, the hospital needs to offer state-of-the-art technology and services at competitive prices.

Thus, both organizations must maintain the financial wherewithal to expand the number and types of services they provide to meet the changing needs of the populations they serve. In addition, each organization must be able to invest in new technologies to provide the best patient care and to remain competitive. As one prominent Catholic healthcare administrator said, "No margin, no mission," which simply means you have to be profitable to accomplish your mission.

In the end, Jane determined that the finance function at for-profit and not-for-profit healthcare providers must be executed in just about the same way. All businesses must maintain financial viability to be competitive in the marketplace.

Did you arrive at the same conclusion?

Key Concepts

This chapter presents background material on business organizations and goals. Here are the key concepts:

- A *business* maintains its financial viability by selling goods or services, while a *pure charity* relies solely on contributions.
- The three legal forms of business are proprietorship or partnership, corporation, and hybrid. Although each form of organization has unique advantages and disadvantages, most large businesses, and all not-for-profit entities, are organized as corporations.
- *Investor-owned corporations* have *shareholders* (or stockholders), who are the owners of the corporation. Shareholders exercise control through the proxy process, whereby they elect the corporation's board of directors and vote on matters of major consequence to the firm. As owners, shareholders have a claim on the residual earnings of the corporation. Investor-owned corporations are fully taxable.
- Healthcare organizations that meet certain criteria can be organized as *not-for-profit corporations*, which are governed by a board of trustees. Rather than having a well-defined set of owners, such organizations have a large number of stakeholders, who have an interest in the organization. In effect, not-for-profit corporations are owned by the communities they serve, although technically they have no owners.
- From a financial management perspective, the primary goal of investor-owned corporations is shareholder wealth maximization, which translates to stock price maximization. For not-for-profit corporations, a reasonable goal for financial management is to ensure that the organization can fulfill its mission, which translates to maintaining financial viability. Both goals lead to roughly the same managerial behavior.
- An *agency problem* is the conflict of interest that arises between the owners and managers (agents) of large for-profit corporations. The problem is mitigated by incentives created to motivate managers to act in the best interest of owners.
- The value of any income stream depends on the amount of *usable*, or *after-tax, income*. Thus, tax laws play an important role in financial management decisions.
- Individuals pay personal (individual) taxes to federal and state (in most states) authorities on proprietorship, partnership, interest, dividend, and capital gains income.

- *For-profit corporations* pay corporate income taxes to federal and state authorities. Because corporations pay taxes, and then individuals pay taxes on dividend and capital gains income, corporate income typically is subject to double taxation.
- Before-tax (BT) income can be converted to after-tax (AT) income using this equation:

$$AT = BT \times (1 - T),$$

  where T is the tax rate.
- Small corporations can file with the Internal Revenue Service for *S corporation status*, under which they are taxed as proprietorships or partnerships and hence avoid double taxation.
- Not-for-profit corporations generally are exempt from all levels of property, income, and sales taxes. Furthermore, not-for-profits can use *tax-exempt debt financing*, which means that lenders do not have to pay taxes on the interest earned. Contributions to not-for-profit corporations can be deducted from the donor's taxable income, which encourages such contributions.

Because managers of healthcare organizations must make financial decisions within the constraints imposed by the economic environment, we draw on the concepts described here throughout the remainder of the book.

End-of-Chapter Questions

2.1 a. From a financial perspective, briefly describe the concept of a business.
b. What is the difference between a not-for-profit business and a pure charity?

2.2 What are the three legal forms of business organization? What are their advantages and disadvantages?

2.3 What are the primary differences between investor-owned and not-for-profit corporations?

2.4 What is the difference between a standard corporation (C corporation) and a benefit corporation (B corporation)?

2.5 a. What is the primary goal of investor-owned corporations?
b. What is the primary goal of most not-for-profit healthcare corporations?
c. Are substantial differences found between the finance goals of investor-owned and not-for-profit corporations? Explain your answer.
d. What is an agency problem?

2.6 a. Why are tax laws important to healthcare finance?
b. What three major advantages do tax laws give to not-for-profit corporations?

End-of-Chapter Problems

2.1 Assume that Provident Health System, a for-profit hospital, has $1 million in taxable income for 2016, and its tax rate is 30 percent.

a. Given this information, what is the firm's net income? (Net income is what remains after taxes have been paid.)

b. Suppose the hospital pays out $300,000 in dividends. A shareholder, Carl Wu, receives $10,000. If Carl's tax rate on dividends is 15 percent, what is his after-tax dividend?

2.2 A firm that owns the stock of another corporation does not have to pay taxes on the entire amount of dividends received. In general, only 30 percent of the dividends received by one corporation from another are taxable. The purpose of this tax law feature is to mitigate the effect of triple taxation, which occurs when earnings are first taxed at the first firm, its dividends paid to the second firm are taxed again, and the dividends paid to shareholders by the second firm are taxed yet again. Assume that a firm with a 21 percent tax rate receives $100,000 in dividends from another corporation. What taxes must be paid on this dividend, and what is the after-tax amount of the dividend?

2.3 Theresa Davis is in the 40 percent personal tax bracket. She is considering investing in HCA (taxable) bonds that carry a 12 percent interest rate.

a. What is her after-tax yield (interest rate) on the bonds?

b. Suppose Twin Cities Memorial Hospital has issued tax-exempt bonds that have an interest rate of 6 percent. With all else the same, should Theresa buy the HCA or the Twin Cities bonds?

c. With all else the same, what interest rate on the tax-exempt Twin Cities bonds would make these bonds and the HCA bonds equally advantageous?

2.4 Aditi Patel currently holds tax-exempt bonds of Good Samaritan Healthcare that pay 7 percent interest. She is in the 40 percent tax bracket. Her broker wants her to buy some Beverly Enterprises taxable bonds that will be issued next week. With all else the same, what rate must be set on the Beverly bonds to make Aditi interested in making a switch?

2.5 George and Margaret Wealthy are in the 48 percent tax bracket, considering both federal and state personal taxes. Norman Briggs, the CEO of Community General Hospital, has been aggressively pursuing a contribution from them of $500,000 to the hospital's soon-to-be-built Cancer Care Center. Without the contribution, the Wealthys' taxable income for 2016 would be $2 million. What impact would the contribution have on the Wealthys' 2016 tax bill?

CHAPTER 3

PAYING FOR HEALTH SERVICES

THEME SET-UP: BIG SKY'S REVENUE SOURCES

Big Sky Dermatology Specialists is a small group practice in Jackson, Wyoming. The city is located in the scenic Jackson Hole Valley and is a major gateway to the Grand Teton and Yellowstone National Parks. In addition, it is home to the world's largest ball of barbed wire. (It is amazing what you learn when studying healthcare finance!)

Jen Latimer, a recent graduate of Idaho State University's healthcare administration program, was just hired to be Big Sky's practice manager. One of her first tasks was to review the group's payer mix. (Payer mix is a listing of the individuals and organizations that pay for a provider's services, along with each payer's percentage of revenues.) After all, revenues are the first step (of many) needed to ensure the financial success of any business.

To understand Big Sky's revenues more thoroughly, Jen focused on two questions. First, who are the payers? In other words, where does Big Sky's revenue come from? Second, what methods do the payers use to determine the payment amount? By gaining an appreciation of the group's revenues, Jen believed she could accurately judge the financial riskiness of the practice. Furthermore, she would be able to identify possible steps toward increasing the practice's revenues and reduce the riskiness associated with those revenues.

By the end of the chapter, you will have a better understanding of healthcare-provider revenue sources and how the specific payment method influences provider behavior. Specifically, you, like Jen, will know more about how these issues affect Big Sky.

Learning Objectives

After studying this chapter, you will be able to do the following:

- List the key features of insurance.
- Describe the major types of third-party payers.
- Discuss, in general terms, the reimbursement methods used by third-party payers, and the associated incentives and risks for providers.
- Explain how clinical and procedural coding affects reimbursement.
- Define the specific reimbursement methods used by Medicare.
- Describe the key features of healthcare reform.

3.1 INTRODUCTION

In most industries, the consumer of the product or service (1) has a choice among many suppliers, (2) can distinguish the quality of competing goods or services, (3) makes a (presumably) rational decision regarding the purchase on the basis of quality and price, and (4) pays for the full cost of the purchase.

The provision of healthcare services does not follow this general model, as healthcare is delivered under unique circumstances. First, often only a few individuals or organizations provide a particular service. Second, judging the quality of competing providers is difficult, if not impossible. Third, the decision (or at least recommendation) on which provider to use for a particular service typically is not made by the consumer but rather by a physician or some other clinician. Fourth, the bulk of the payment to the provider is not normally made by the user (the patient) but by an insurer. Finally, for most individuals, the purchase of health insurance is paid for (or heavily subsidized) by employers or government agencies, so many patients are insulated from the true cost of healthcare services.

This highly unusual marketplace significantly influences the supply of and demand for healthcare services. To gain a better understanding of the unique payment mechanisms involved, we must examine the healthcare reimbursement system.

3.2 BASIC INSURANCE CONCEPTS

Because insurance is the cornerstone of healthcare reimbursement, an appreciation of basic insurance concepts will help you better understand the marketplace for healthcare services.

A Simple Illustration

Assume that no health insurance exists and that you face only two medical outcomes in the coming year:

Outcome	Probability	Cost
Stay healthy	0.99	$ 0
Get sick	0.01	50,000
	1.00	

What is your expected healthcare cost (in the statistical sense) for the coming year? To find the answer—$500—multiply the cost of each outcome by its probability of occurrence and then sum the products:

$$\begin{aligned}\text{Expected cost} &= (\text{Probability of outcome 1} \times \text{Cost of outcome 1}) \\ &\quad + (\text{Probability of outcome 2} \times \text{Cost of outcome 2}) \\ &= (0.99 \times \$0) + (0.01 \times \$50{,}000) \\ &= \$0 + \$500 = \$500.\end{aligned}$$

CRITICAL CONCEPT
Risk Aversion

Risk aversion is the tendency of individuals and businesses to dislike financial risk. Risk-averse individuals and businesses are motivated to use insurance and other techniques to protect against risk. For example, a favorite tool to control risk is diversification, which in the context of revenues means lowering risk by having different sources of income. By not depending on one source—say, Medicare patients—a provider can reduce the uncertainty (riskiness) of its revenue stream. Insurance is another way to limit risk. Individuals buy insurance on the houses they own to limit the consequences of calamitous events, such as fires or hurricanes.

Now, assume that everyone else faces the same medical outcomes and hence faces the same odds and costs associated with healthcare. Furthermore, assume that you, and everyone else, make $60,000 a year. With this salary, you can easily afford the $500 expected healthcare cost. The problem, however, is that no one's actual cost will be $500. If you stay healthy, your cost will be zero; if you get sick, your cost will be $50,000, and this amount could force you, and most people who get sick, into personal bankruptcy, which is a ruinous event. (Do not forget that you have to pay all of your living expenses out of your $60,000 annual income in addition to any healthcare costs.)

Now, suppose an insurance policy that pays all of your healthcare costs for the coming year is available for $600. Would you take the policy, even though it costs $100 more than your "expected" healthcare costs?

Most people would, and do. Because individuals are risk averse (see "Critical Concept: Risk Aversion"), they are willing to pay $100 more than their expected benefit to eliminate the risk of financial ruin. In effect, policyholders are passing the costs associated with the risk of getting sick to the insurer who, as you will see, is spreading those costs over a large number of subscribers.

Would an insurer be willing to offer the policy for $600? If the insurer could sell enough policies, it would know its revenues and costs with some precision. For example, if the insurer sold a million policies, it would collect 1,000,000 × $600 = $600 million in health insurance premiums; pay out roughly 1,000,000 × $500 = $500 million in claims; and have about $100 million to cover administrative costs. It could provide a reserve in case claims are greater than predicted and make a profit. By writing a large number of policies, the financial risk inherent in medical costs can be spread over a large number of people, reducing the risk for the insurance company (and for each individual).

Basic Characteristics of Insurance

The simple example discussed earlier illustrates why individuals seek health insurance and why insurance companies are formed to provide such insurance. Next, we will dig a little deeper into insurance basics.

Pooling
The spreading of losses over a large group of individuals (or organizations).

Insurance typically has four distinct characteristics:

1. *Pooling of losses.* The **pooling** (sharing) of losses is the heart of insurance. Pooling means that losses are spread over a large group of individuals so that

each individual realizes the average loss of the pool rather than the actual loss incurred. In addition, pooling involves the grouping of a large number of homogeneous exposure units (people or things having the same risk characteristics). Thus, pooling implies (a) the sharing of losses by the entire group and (b) the prediction of future losses with some accuracy based on the law of large numbers. (The law of large numbers implies that predicting outcomes is easier when many identical trials are involved. For example, if a coin is flipped only once, you do not know whether the results will be heads or tails. However, if the coin is flipped 1,000 times, the result will be very close to 500 heads and 500 tails. In other words, you cannot predict the results of a single toss with any confidence, but you can predict the aggregate results if you have a large pool of tosses.)

2. *Payment only for random losses.* A **random loss** is unforeseen and occurs as a result of chance. Insurance is based on the premise that payments are made only for losses that are random. We discuss the moral hazard problem, in which losses are not random, in a later section.

Random loss
An unpredictable loss, such as one that results from a fire or hurricane.

3. *Risk transfer.* An insurance plan almost always involves **risk transfer**. The sole exception to the element of risk transfer is self-insurance, whereby an individual or a business does not buy insurance. (Self-insurance is discussed in a later section.) Risk transfer means that the risk is shifted from the insured to the insurer, which typically is in a better financial position to pay the loss than is the insured because of the premiums collected. In addition, because of the law of large numbers, the insurance company is better able to predict its losses.

Risk transfer
The passing of risk from one individual or business to another (usually an insurer).

4. *Indemnification.* **Indemnification** is the reimbursement of the insured if a loss occurs. In the context of health insurance, indemnification occurs when the insurer pays, in whole or in part, the insured or the provider for the expenses related to an insured's illness or injury.

Indemnification
The agreement to pay for losses incurred by another party.

In summary, we applied these four characteristics to our insurance example: (1) The losses are pooled across a million individuals, (2) the losses on each individual are random (unpredictable), (3) the risk of loss is passed to the insurance company, and (4) the insurance company pays for any losses.

Real-World Problems

Insurance works fine when the four basic characteristics are present. However, if any of these characteristics is violated, problems arise. The two most common problems are adverse selection and moral hazard.

> **CRITICAL CONCEPT**
> Adverse Selection
>
> Adverse selection, in its simplest form, means that individuals most likely to need healthcare services are most likely to buy health insurance. This tendency creates a problem for insurers because it drives the costs of healthcare for a defined population to higher-than-anticipated levels.

Adverse Selection

Adverse selection occurs because those individuals and businesses likely to incur losses are more inclined to purchase insurance than are those less likely to incur losses (see "Critical Concept: Adverse Selection"). For example, an otherwise healthy individual without insurance who needs a costly surgical procedure is more apt to get health insurance if she can afford it, whereas an identical individual without the threat of surgery is less likely. Similarly, consider the health insurance purchase likelihood of a 20-year-old versus that of a 65-year-old. All else the same, the older individual, with much greater health risk because of age, will probably obtain insurance. (Individuals aged 65 or older consume, on average, more than three times the dollar amount of healthcare services that younger individuals do.)

If the tendency toward adverse selection goes unchecked, a disproportionate number of sick people, or those most likely to become sick, will seek health insurance, causing the insurer to experience higher-than-expected claims. This increase in claims will trigger a premium increase, which worsens the problem, because healthier members of the plan will either pursue cheaper rates from another company (if available) or forgo insurance.

> ***Underwriting***
> The selection and classification of candidates for insurance.

One way health insurers attempt to control adverse selection is by instituting **underwriting** provisions. Thus, smokers may be charged a higher premium than nonsmokers. Another way is by including preexisting condition clauses in contracts, although this strategy was disallowed by the passage of the Affordable Care Act in 2010. (A preexisting condition is a physical or mental condition of the insured individual that existed before the issuance of the policy.) A typical clause might state that preexisting conditions are not covered until the policy has been in force for some period—say, one or two years. Preexisting conditions present a true problem for the health insurance field because an important characteristic of insurance is randomness. If an individual has a preexisting condition, the insurer no longer bears random risk but rather assumes the role of payer for the treatment of a known condition.

Because insurers tend to avoid paying large predictable claims, the US Congress passed the Health Insurance Portability and Accountability Act (HIPAA) in 1996. Among other actions, HIPAA set national standards, which could be modified within limits by the states, regarding what provisions could be included in health insurance policies. For example, under a group health policy—say, one that covers employees of a furniture manufacturer—coverage to individuals cannot be denied or limited, and employees cannot be required to pay more in premiums if they suffer from poor health.

HIPAA also limited insurers' ability to impose preexisting condition clauses and how long they could delay before beginning coverage. It allowed time credit for preexisting conditions under one plan to be counted toward a second plan should the employee change jobs, provided no break in coverage occurs. Under the Affordable Care Act (ACA), preexisting condition clauses are banned for health plans after 2014. (See section 3.8 for a discussion of the ACA; also see "For Your Consideration: Adverse Selection and Healthcare Reform.")

Finally, health insurance cannot be canceled if the policyholder becomes sick, and if a policyholder leaves the company, he has the right to purchase insurance (for a limited time) from the insurer that provided the company's group policy. All in all, the provisions of HIPAA and the ACA protect individuals against actions by insurers when their health status changes for the worse or when they leave the employer.

FOR YOUR CONSIDERATION
Adverse Selection and Healthcare Reform

When the cost of health insurance is relatively low, such as in an employer-subsidized plan, most people to whom it is made available will opt in (take the insurance). However, when the cost of health insurance is relatively high, the choice is not as easy to make. Often, those who opt in will be more likely to have immediate healthcare needs and hence be more expensive to insure than the population as a whole. Thus, as Kay Lazar wrote in a June 30, 2010, *Boston Globe* article titled "Short-Term Insurance Buyers Drive up Cost in Mass.," adverse selection is a factor in increased health insurance costs, and the higher the costs, the higher the premiums, which means even more individuals will do without coverage.

The traditional techniques used by insurers to mitigate adverse selection risk have included denying coverage to or charging higher premiums for individuals with pre-existing health conditions or excluding those conditions from the individual's policy. While supporting the healthcare insurance system's viability, these techniques were one major reason health insurance was viewed in a negative light by many consumers. Now, however, healthcare reform (discussed in section 3.8) has eliminated or limits most of the traditional adverse selection risk-management techniques. Instead, the legislation's aim is to maximize the number of healthy people who obtain coverage by offering subsidies to lower-income Americans and mandating penalties for those who refuse to take coverage. This "individual mandate" approach is intended to put almost everyone into the insurance pool, thereby eliminating adverse selection.

What do you think? Will the individual mandate eliminate adverse selection? What specific provisions are necessary for the mandate to work? Note that more than two dozen states, interest groups, and individuals sued the federal government, arguing that the individual mandate is unconstitutional. Ultimately, the US Supreme Court upheld the individual mandate in 2012.

CRITICAL CONCEPT
Moral Hazard

Moral hazard is the risk to an insurer that excess healthcare services are being consumed because individuals do not bear the full cost of the services provided. For example, a patient may be quick to agree to an expensive test, even though that test is not medically necessary, because most of the cost is covered by insurance.

Moral Hazard

The fact that insurance is based on the premise that payments are made only for random (unforeseen) losses creates the moral hazard problem (see "Critical Concept: Moral Hazard"). The most common illustration of moral hazard is the owner who deliberately sets a failing business on fire to collect the insurance.

Moral hazard is also present in health insurance, but its form typically is not so dramatic—not too many people are willing to sustain injury or illness voluntarily for the purpose of collecting health insurance benefits. However, undoubtedly some people do purposely use healthcare services that are not medically required. For example, some people who live alone might visit a physician or a walk-in clinic for the social value of human companionship rather than to address a medical necessity.

Insurers attempt to protect themselves from moral hazard claims by paying less than the full amount of healthcare costs. Forcing insured individuals to bear some of the cost lessens their tendency to consume unneeded services or engage in unhealthy behaviors. One way to make patients pay out of pocket is to require a **deductible**. Medical policies usually stipulate a dollar amount that must be satisfied before benefits are paid.

Deductible
The dollar amount that must be spent on healthcare services (e.g., $500 per year) before any benefits are paid by the insurer.

Although deductibles help offset the moral hazard problem, their primary purpose is to eliminate the need for an insurer to pay a small claim, if that is the only healthcare expense for the year. In such cases, the administrative cost of processing the claim may be larger than the amount of the claim itself. To illustrate, a policy may state that the first $500 (or more) of medical expenses incurred each year will be paid by the individual. Once the deductible is met, the insurer will pay all eligible medical expenses (less any copayments and coinsurance) for the remainder of the year.

Copayment
A fixed cost to the patient each time a service is rendered (e.g., $20 per outpatient visit).

The primary weapons that insurers have against the moral hazard problem are copayments and coinsurance. A **copayment** (or copay) is a fixed amount paid by the patient each time a service is rendered, such as $20 per office visit or $75 for each emergency department visit. **Coinsurance** is the sharing of costs between the patient and insurer, typically on a percentage basis. For example, the patient bears 20 percent of the costs of a hospital stay.

Coinsurance
A sharing of costs between the patient and the insurer (e.g., the patient pays 20 percent of the costs of hospitalization).

Copays and coinsurance serve two primary purposes. First, these payments discourage overutilization of healthcare services and hence reduce insurance benefits. By extension, by being forced to pay some of the costs, insured individuals will presumably seek fewer and more cost-effective treatments and embrace a healthier lifestyle than they would otherwise. Second, because insured individuals pay part of the cost, premiums can be reduced. Health insurance premiums (the cost of the policy to the subscriber) have risen rapidly in the past ten years and now exceed $15,000 annually for family coverage. Employers, on average, pay about 75 percent of the premium costs. Because of this alarming trend in health premium costs, employers are seeking ways to reduce them; one way is to pass more of the costs on to employees through copays and coinsurance.

Some health insurance policies contain out-of-pocket maximums, whereby the insurer pays all covered costs, including coinsurance, after the insured individual pays a certain amount of costs—say, $2,000. Finally, prior to 2010, most insurance policies had policy limits, for example, $1 million in total lifetime coverage, $1,500 per year for mental health benefits, or $100 for eyeglasses. These limits were designed to control excessive use of certain services and protect the insurer against catastrophic losses. The ACA banned lifetime limits and is phasing out annual limits on most health plans.

Before we move on, we should briefly mention a newer type of health insurance that is gaining popularity: **high-deductible health plans (HDHPs)**. An HDHP typically has a lower premium but has a higher annual deductible (more than $2,000 for family coverage) than traditional plans do. However, it allows individuals to set up savings accounts for the sole purpose of paying healthcare costs. Furthermore, contributions to such accounts are tax deductible (up to a set limit) and can roll over from year to year. HDHPs are popular with executives and other highly paid workers because of the tax shelter benefit, and many employers are offering a HDHP option to their employees to help control healthcare costs.

High-deductible health plan (HDHP)
A type of health insurance that requires high deductibles but allows insured individuals to set up tax-advantaged savings accounts to pay those deductibles.

? Self-Test Questions

1. Briefly explain the concept of health insurance.
2. What is adverse selection, and how do insurers deal with the problem?
3. What is moral hazard, and how do insurers handle it?

3.3 THIRD-PARTY PAYERS

As mentioned earlier, a large proportion of provider revenues does not come directly from patients (the users of healthcare services) but from insurers, known collectively as *third-party payers* (see “Critical Concept: Third-Party Payers”). Because a healthcare organization’s revenues are key to its financial viability, we first discuss the sources of most revenues in the healthcare sector. In section 3.5, we examine the types of reimbursement methods employed by these payers.

! CRITICAL CONCEPT
Third-Party Payers

Third-party payers are the insurers that reimburse health services organizations and hence are the major source of revenues for most providers. Third-party payers include private insurers, such as Blue Cross Blue Shield, and public (government) insurers, such as Medicare and Medicaid. Third-party payers use several reimbursement methods to pay providers, depending on the specific payer (e.g., the Blues vs. Medicare) and the type of service rendered (e.g., inpatient vs. outpatient).

Health insurance originated in Europe in the early 1800s when mutual benefit societies were formed to reduce the financial burden associated with illness or injury. Today, health insurers fall into two broad categories: private insurers and public programs.

Private Insurers

In the United States, the concept of public, or government, health insurance is relatively new, while private health insurance has been in existence since the early twentieth century. In this section, we discuss the major private insurers.

Blue Cross and Blue Shield

Blue Cross Blue Shield organizations trace their roots to the Great Depression, when both hospitals and physicians were concerned about their patients' abilities to pay healthcare bills. Blue Cross originated as a number of separate insurance programs offered by individual hospitals. At that time, many patients were unable to pay their hospital bills, but most people, except the poorest, could afford to pay small monthly premiums to purchase some type of hospitalization insurance. Thus, the programs were initially designed to benefit both patients and hospitals.

The programs were all similar in structure: Hospitals agreed to provide a certain number of services to program members who made periodic payments to the hospitals whether services were used or not. In a short time, these programs were expanded from single-hospital programs to community-wide, multihospital plans that were called hospital service plans. The American Hospital Association (AHA) recognized the benefits of such plans to hospitals, so a close relationship was formed between the AHA and the organizations that offered hospital service plans.

In the early years, several states ruled that the sale of hospital services by prepayment did not constitute insurance, so the plans were exempt from regulations governing insurance companies. However, the legal status of hospital service plans clearly would be subject to future scrutiny unless their status was formalized. Thus, the states, one by one, passed legislation that provided for the founding of not-for-profit hospital service corporations that were exempt both from taxes and from the capital requirements (reserves) mandated for other insurers. However, state insurance departments had (and continue to have) oversight of most aspects of the plans' operations. The Blue Cross name was officially adopted by most of these plans in 1939.

Blue Shield plans developed in a manner similar to that of the Blue Cross plans, except that the providers were physicians instead of hospitals and the professional organization involved was the American Medical Association instead of the AHA. Today, 36 Blue Cross Blue Shield (the Blues) organizations exist, some of which offer only one of the two plans (most offer both). The Blues are organized as independent corporations, but all belong to a single national association that sets the standards required for using the Blue

Cross Blue Shield name. Collectively, the Blues provide healthcare coverage for about 1 in 3 Americans across all 50 states, the District of Columbia, and Puerto Rico.

Historically, the Blues have been not-for-profit corporations that enjoyed the full benefits accorded to that status, including freedom from taxes. However, in 1986, Congress eliminated the Blues' tax exemption on the grounds that they engaged in commercial-type insurance activities. However, the plans were given special deductions, which resulted in taxes that are generally less than those paid by commercial insurers.

In spite of the 1986 change in tax status, the national association continued to require all Blues organizations to operate entirely as not-for-profit corporations, although they were allowed to establish for-profit subsidiaries. In 1994, the national association lifted its traditional ban on member plans becoming investor-owned companies, and several Blues have since converted to for-profit status.

Commercial Insurers

Commercial health insurance traditionally was issued by life insurance and casualty insurance (home and auto) companies. Today, however, most health insurance is provided by companies that exclusively write health insurance. Examples of commercial insurers include Aetna, Humana, and UnitedHealth Group. Most commercial insurance companies are shareholder owned, and all are taxable entities.

Commercial insurers moved strongly into health insurance following World War II. At that time, the United Auto Workers negotiated the first contract with employers in which fringe benefits were a major part of the contract. Like the Blues, the majority of individuals with commercial health insurance are covered under **group policies** with employee groups, professional and other associations, and labor unions.

Group policy
A single insurance policy that covers a common group of individuals, such as a company's employees or a professional group's members.

Self-Insurers

An argument can be made that all individuals who do not have some form of health insurance are self-insurers, but this statement is not accurate. Self-insurers make a conscious decision to bear the risks associated with healthcare costs and then set aside (or have available) funds to pay for costs they may incur in the future. Individuals, except the very wealthy, are not good candidates for self-insurance because, as discussed earlier, individuals who do not pool risks face much uncertainty in future healthcare costs.

On the other hand, large organizations, especially employers, are good candidates for self-insurance. In fact, most large companies, and many midsized companies, are self-insured. The advantages of self-insurance include the potential to reduce costs (cut out the middleman) and the opportunity to offer plans tailored to meet the unique characteristics of the organization's employees. Organizations that self-insure typically pay an insurance company to administer the plan. For example, employees of the State of North Carolina are covered by health insurance, the costs of which are paid directly by the state, but the plan is administered by Blue Cross Blue Shield of North Carolina.

Public Insurers

Government is both a major insurer and a direct provider of healthcare services. For example, the government provides healthcare services directly to qualifying individuals through Department of Veterans Affairs, Department of Defense, and Public Health Service medical facilities. In addition, it either provides or mandates a variety of insurance programs, such as workers' compensation and Tricare (health insurance for military members, their families, and uniformed services retirees). In this section, however, we focus on the two major government insurance programs—Medicare and Medicaid—that fund roughly one-third of all healthcare services provided in the United States.

Medicare

Medicare was established by Congress in 1965, primarily to provide medical benefits to individuals aged 65 or older (see "Critical Concept: Medicare"). According to the Centers for Medicare & Medicaid Services (CMS), about 54 million people have Medicare coverage, which pays for about 20 percent of all US healthcare expenditures.

Over the decades, Medicare has evolved to include four major types of coverage:

1. Part A provides hospital and some skilled nursing home coverage.
2. Part B covers physician services, ambulatory surgical services, outpatient services, and other miscellaneous services.
3. Part C is managed care coverage offered by private insurance companies. It can be selected in lieu of Parts A and B.
4. Part D covers prescription drugs.

CRITICAL CONCEPT
Medicare

Medicare is a federal health insurance program that primarily covers elderly individuals (those aged 65 or older). It consists of four major parts: Part A covers inpatient services, Part B covers outpatient services, Part C is managed care coverage that replaces Parts A and B, and Part D covers prescription drugs. Medicare is administered by CMS, which is an agency of the US Department of Health and Human Services (HHS).

In addition, Medicare covers healthcare costs associated with selected disabilities and illnesses (such as kidney failure) regardless of age.

Part A coverage is free to all individuals eligible for Social Security benefits. Individuals who are not eligible for Social Security benefits can obtain Part A medical benefits by paying monthly premiums. Part B is optional to all individuals who have

Part A coverage, and it requires a monthly premium from enrollees that varies with income level. According to the Kaiser Family Foundation's fact sheet on Medicare, about 93 percent of Part A participants purchase Part B coverage, while about 31 percent of Medicare enrollees elect to participate in Part C, also called **Medicare Advantage plans**, rather than Parts A and B. Part D offers prescription drug coverage through plans offered by private companies. Each Part D plan offers somewhat different coverage, so the cost of Part D coverage varies widely.

Medicare Advantage plan
Managed care plan coverage offered to Medicare beneficiaries that replaces Parts A and B coverage.

Because Parts A and B do not cover all costs of care and the remaining out-of-pocket costs can be significant, many Medicare participants purchase additional coverage from private insurers to help cover the gaps in Medicare coverage. Such coverage is called **Medigap insurance**.

Medigap insurance
Insurance taken out by Medicare beneficiaries that pays many of the costs not covered by Parts A and B. (Its purpose is to fill the gaps in coverage.)

The Medicare program falls under the purview of HHS, which writes the regulations (i.e., the specific rules of the program) based on enabling legislation passed by Congress. Medicare is administered by the **Centers for Medicare & Medicaid Services (CMS)**, which is an agency in HHS. CMS's eight regional offices oversee the Medicare and Medicaid programs and ensure that regulations are followed. Medicare payments to providers are not made directly by CMS but by contractors for 16 Medicare administrative contractor jurisdictions.

Centers for Medicare & Medicaid Services (CMS)
The federal agency in the US Department of Health and Human Services that administers the Medicare and Medicaid programs.

Medicaid

Medicaid began in 1965 as a modest program jointly funded and operated by the individual states and the federal government (see "Critical Concept: Medicaid"). The idea was to provide a medical safety net for low-income mothers and children and for elderly, blind, and disabled individuals.

Congress mandated that state programs, at a minimum, cover hospital and physician care but encouraged states to provide additional benefits either by increasing the range of benefits or extending the program to cover more people. States with large tax bases were quick to expand coverage to many groups, while states with limited revenues were forced to establish more restrictive programs. In addition to state expansions, a mandatory nursing home benefit was added in 1972. As a consequence, Medicaid is now the largest payer of long-term care benefits and the largest single budget item for many states. In total, Medicaid covers roughly 70 million individuals and pays for about 17 percent of all healthcare expenditures in the United States, according to Statista's information on Medicaid enrollment and CMS.

CRITICAL CONCEPT
Medicaid

Medicaid is a joint federal–state health insurance program that primarily covers low-income individuals and families. The federal government funds about half of the costs of the program, while the states fund the remainder. Although general guidelines are established by CMS, the program is administered by the individual states. Thus, each state, as long as it follows basic federal guidelines, can set its own rules regarding eligibility, benefits, and provider payments.

Over the years, Medicare and Medicaid have provided access to healthcare services for many low-income individuals who otherwise would have no health insurance coverage. Furthermore, these programs have become an important source of revenue for healthcare providers, especially for nursing homes and other providers that treat large numbers of low-income patients. However, Medicare and Medicaid expenditures have been growing at an alarming rate, forcing federal and state policymakers to search for more cost-effective ways to provide healthcare services.

Self-Test Questions

1. What are the different types of private insurers?
2. Briefly, what are the origins and purpose of Medicare?
3. What is Medicaid, and how is it administered?

3.4 MANAGED CARE ORGANIZATIONS

Managed care organizations (MCOs) strive to combine the provision of healthcare services and the insurance function into a single entity (see "Critical Concept: Managed Care Organizations: HMOs and PPOs"). Typically, MCOs are created by insurers that either directly own a provider network or create one through contractual arrangements with independent providers. Occasionally, however, MCOs are created by integrated delivery systems that establish their own insurance companies.

CRITICAL CONCEPT
Managed Care Organizations: HMOs and PPOs

Managed care organizations (MCOs) combine insurer and provider functions into a single administrative organization. The idea here is not only to pay for care but also to manage the care provided. MCOs come in different types, and their primary difference is in how tightly the care is managed. Health maintenance organizations (HMOs) tend to exercise the most control over the types and amount of care provided, while preferred provider organizations (PPOs) tend to be less controlling. In all managed care plans, the goal is to provide only services that are medically required in the lowest-cost setting.

Historically, the most common type of MCO was the health maintenance organization (HMO). HMOs were developed to thwart the perverse incentives created by traditional insurer–provider relationships whereby providers were rewarded for treating patients' illnesses but given little incentive to provide prevention and rehabilitation services. By combining the financing and delivery of healthcare services into a single system, HMOs theoretically have as strong an incentive to prevent as to treat illnesses. However, because their organizational structures, ownership, and financial incentives differ from plan to plan, HMOs can vary widely in cost and quality.

HMOs use a variety of methods to control costs. These include limiting patients to particular providers, called the **provider panel**, and using primary care physicians as **gatekeepers** who authorize all specialized and referral services. In general, services are not covered if beneficiaries bypass their gatekeeper physician or use providers that are not part of the HMO panel.

The federal Health Maintenance Act of 1973 encouraged the development of HMOs by providing federal funds for HMO operating grants and loans. In addition, the act required larger employers that offer healthcare benefits to their employees to include an HMO as one alternative, if one was available in the area, in addition to traditional insurance plans.

Although the number and sizes of HMOs grew rapidly during the 1980s and 1990s, since that time they have lost some of their luster because healthcare consumers have been unwilling to accept access limitations, even though such limitations might reduce costs. To address consumer concerns and falling enrollments, another type of MCO—the preferred provider organization (PPO)—was developed. These organizations do not wield as much control as HMOs but combine some of the cost-saving strategies of HMOs with features of traditional health insurance plans.

PPOs do not mandate that beneficiaries use specific providers. They do, however, offer financial incentives to encourage members to use providers that participate in the plan. That panel of providers typically negotiates discounted price contracts with the PPO. Furthermore, PPOs do not require plan members to use preselected gatekeeper physicians. Finally, PPOs are less likely than HMOs to provide preventive services, and they do not assume any responsibility for quality assurance because enrollees are not constrained to use only the PPO panel of providers.

In an effort to achieve the potential cost savings of MCOs, health insurers are now applying managed care strategies, such as preadmission certification, utilization review, and second surgical opinions, to their conventional plans. Thus, the term *managed care* now describes a continuum of plans that can vary significantly in their approaches to providing combined insurance and healthcare services. The common feature in MCOs is that the insurer has a mechanism to control, or at least influence, patients' consumption of healthcare services. Today, most employer-sponsored health coverage is provided by some type of MCO.

Provider panel
The group of providers—say, doctors and hospitals—designated as preferred by a managed care plan. Services delivered by providers outside of the panel may be only partially covered, or not covered at all, by the plan.

Gatekeeper
A primary care physician who controls specialist and ancillary service referrals. Some managed care plans only pay for referral services approved by the gatekeeper.

? SELF-TEST QUESTIONS

1. What is meant by the term *managed care organization* (MCO)?
2. What are two different types of MCOs?

3.5 ALTERNATIVE REIMBURSEMENT METHODS

Regardless of payer, only a limited number of payment methods are used to reimburse providers for healthcare services. Payment methods fall into two broad classifications:

CRITICAL CONCEPT
Fee-for-Service Reimbursement

Under fee-for-service reimbursement, health services organizations are paid on the basis of the amount of services provided. The term *service* can be defined several ways. For example, a physician may be paid for each procedure performed, such as conducting an office visit or reading a CT (computed tomography) scan. A hospital may be reimbursed for costs incurred, for each admission, or for each patient day; a clinical laboratory may be paid for each test performed. Regardless of the specific definition of a service, in fee-for-service reimbursement the greater the amount of services provided, the greater the revenues. Thus, the risk of utilization (volume of services) uncertainty is borne by the insurer rather than by the provider.

fee-for-service and capitation. In this section, we discuss the most frequently used reimbursement methods.

Fee-for-Service

In *fee-for-service* payment methods, of which many variations exist, the more services provided, the higher the reimbursement (see "Critical Concept: Fee-for-Service Reimbursement"). The three primary fee-for-service methods of reimbursement are cost based, charge based, and prospective payment.

Cost-Based Reimbursement

Under cost-based reimbursement, the payer agrees to reimburse the provider for the costs incurred in providing services to the insured population. Cost-based reimbursement is retrospective in the sense that reimbursement is based on what has happened in the past. This type of reimbursement is limited to allowable costs, usually defined as costs directly related to the provision of healthcare services. For all practical purposes, cost-based reimbursement guarantees that a provider's costs will be covered by revenues generated from the delivery of those services.

Charge-Based Reimbursement

Chargemaster
A provider's official list of charges (prices) for goods, supplies, and services rendered.

Under a charge-based reimbursement system, when payers pay billed charges, they pay according to a rate schedule, called a **chargemaster**, established by the provider. To a certain extent, this reimbursement system places payers at the mercy of providers, especially in markets where competition is limited. In the very early days of health insurance, all payers reimbursed providers on the basis of charges. Now, the trend is shifting toward other, less generous reimbursement methods, and the only payers expected to pay the full amount of charges are self-pay (private-pay) patients. Even among those consumers, low-income uninsured patients often are given discounts from charges or not required to pay at all.

Most insurers that still base reimbursement on charges now pay negotiated, or discounted, charges. Insurers that offer managed care plans, as well as conventional insurers, often hold bargaining power because they have the capacity to bring a large number of patients to a provider, which allows them to negotiate discounts that generally range from 20 percent to 50 percent (or more) of charges. The effect of these discounts is to create a system similar to hotel or airline pricing, whereby few people pay the listed rates (rack rates or full fares, respectively). Many people argue that chargemaster prices have become meaningless, and hence the entire concept should be abandoned. However, old habits die hard, and chargemaster prices still play a role in some reimbursement methods, so we expect they will be in use for some time.

Prospective Payment Reimbursement

In a **prospective payment** system, the rates paid by payers are determined by the payer before the services are provided. Furthermore, payments are not directly related to either costs or charges. Here are the common units of payment used in prospective payment systems:

Prospective payment
A reimbursement system meant to cover expected costs as opposed to historical (retrospective) costs.

- *Per procedure.* Under per-procedure reimbursement, a separate payment is made for each procedure performed on a patient. Because of the high administrative costs associated with this method when applied to complex diagnoses, per-procedure reimbursement is primarily used in outpatient settings.
- *Per diagnosis.* In the per-diagnosis reimbursement method, the provider is paid a rate that depends on the patient's diagnosis. Diagnoses that require higher use of resources, and hence are more costly to treat, have higher reimbursement rates. Medicare pioneered this basis of payment in its diagnosis-related group (DRG) system, which it first used for hospital inpatient reimbursement in 1983. (See "Healthcare in Practice: How Medicare Pays Providers" for examples of per-procedure and per-diagnosis reimbursement.)
- *Per diem* (per day). Some insurers reimburse institutional providers, such as hospitals and nursing homes, on a per diem (per day) basis. In this approach, the provider is paid a fixed amount for each day that service is provided. Often, per diem rates are stratified, which means that different rates are applied to different services. For example, a hospital may be paid one rate for a medical/surgical day, a higher rate for a critical care unit day, and yet a different rate for an obstetric day. Stratified per diems recognize that providers incur widely varied daily costs for providing different types of inpatient care.
- *Bundled (global) reimbursement.* Under bundled reimbursement, payers reimburse providers a single prospective payment that covers all services delivered in a single episode, whether the services are rendered by a single provider or by multiple providers. For example, a bundled price may be set for all obstetric services associated with a pregnancy provided by a single physician, including all prenatal and postnatal visits and the delivery. For another example, a bundled price may be paid for all physician and hospital

services associated with a cardiac bypass operation. Note that at the extreme, a bundled price could be set for all services provided to a single patient, which, in effect, is capitation reimbursement, as described in the next section.

HEALTHCARE IN PRACTICE
How Medicare Pays Providers

Medicare uses different reimbursement methods to pay for hospital services and physician services. In this box, we briefly describe the method for each. Understanding the basics of Medicare reimbursement is important to healthcare managers because many other third-party payers have adopted these or similar systems.

Hospitals

From its inception in 1965 until 1983, Medicare hospital payments for inpatients were based on a retrospective system that reimbursed hospitals for all reasonable costs. In 1983, in an attempt to curb Medicare spending, Congress established the inpatient prospective payment system (inpatient PPS or IPPS) for acute care hospitals. Under the IPPS, a single payment for each inpatient stay covers the cost of routine inpatient care, special care, and ancillary services. The amount of the prospective payment is based on the patient's DRG.

The starting point in determining the amount of reimbursement is the DRG itself. Potential patient diagnoses have been divided into 334 base DRGs (base diagnoses). These base diagnoses are split into subgroups (Medicare severity [MS]-DRGs) on the basis of complications or comorbidities. (A comorbidity is the presence of one or more diseases or disorders in addition to the primary diagnosis.) In all, Medicare has established approximately 760 total MS-DRGs.

To illustrate, consider the MS-DRGs for heart failure. DRG 293 is the base DRG (no complications or comorbidities [CC]), DRG 292 represents heart failure with CC, and DRG 291 is heart failure with major CC. Each MS-DRG is assigned a relative weight that represents the average resources consumed in treating that particular diagnosis relative to resources consumed in treating an average diagnosis. The greater the weight, the greater the reimbursement amount. The weights and sample payment amounts for the three heart failure DRGs are as follows:

MS-DRG	Weight	Payment
293	0.6737	$3,344
292	0.9707	4,818
291	1.4809	7,351

HEALTHCARE IN PRACTICE
How Medicare Pays Providers *(continued)*

The amount of resources required to treat an average inpatient is 1.0. As can be seen from the data, the DRG with no CC (293) has a lower weight than the DRG with CC (292), which, in turn, has a lower weight than that with major CC (291). In fact, the amount of hospital resources consumed to treat a patient with DRG 293 (basic heart failure) is less than that required to treat an average inpatient. An inpatient diagnosed with heart failure with CC (DRG 292) is about average in resource consumption, while a heart failure patient with major CC (DRG 291) uses roughly 53 percent more resources than the average inpatient.

The translation from DRG weight to payment amount (the actual dollar reimbursement) depends on several factors, such as hospital location and teaching status, and hence is somewhat complex. In essence, the DRG weight is multiplied by an adjusted base rate (dollar amount) that incorporates several factors unique to the hospital and its geographic location. In the table shown earlier in this section, see representative payment amounts calculated using an adjusted base rate of $4,964. For example, the reimbursement for a typical hospital for DRG 292 would be 0.9707 × $4,964 = $4,818. The bottom line is that the greater the amount of resources needed to treat the diagnosis, the greater the DRG weight and hence the reimbursement amount.

Note that the single DRG payment reimburses the hospital for all inpatient costs. To provide some cushion for the high costs associated with severely ill patients in each diagnosis, Medicare includes a provision for outlier payments. Such payments are designed to compensate hospitals for treating patients who consume resources that fall outside of normal bounds. Outliers are classified into two categories: length of stay (LOS) outliers and cost outliers. Medicare makes additional payments when a patient's LOS or cost exceeds established cutoff points.

Also, note that hospital outpatient visits are reimbursed on a prospective payment system that is similar in concept, but different in structure, to the inpatient MS-DRG system. The outpatient prospective payment system categorizes outpatient visits into groups called ambulatory payment classifications (APCs), which are clinically similar and tend to consume a similar amount of resources. As with MS-DRGs, Medicare multiplies each APC's weight by a hospital-specific payment rate to obtain the reimbursement amount.

Physicians

Through 1991, Medicare reimbursed physicians on the basis of the reasonable charge concept. In essence, Medicare defined a reasonable charge as the lowest of (1) the actual charge for the service performed, (2) the physician's customary charge, or (3) the prevailing charge for that service in the community.

(continued)

HEALTHCARE IN PRACTICE
How Medicare Pays Providers *(continued)*

Medicare changed its physician payment system in 1992 to a resource-based relative value scale (RBRVS) system. Under RBRVS, reimbursement is based on three resource components: physician work, practice (overhead) expense, and malpractice insurance expense. Each of roughly 8,000 procedure codes is assigned relative value units (RVUs) for the three resource components, which, after adjustment for geographic cost differentials, are summed to arrive at the total number of RVUs per procedure performed. The total RVUs are then multiplied by a conversion factor that equals the dollar value of one unit to obtain the dollar reimbursement amount.

For example, consider code 99213, which represents one category of office visit. The national average physician work RVU is 0.97, the practice expense RVU is 0.40, and the malpractice insurance RVU is 0.07. For a physician practicing in Marco Island, Florida, the adjusted RVU values are 0.97, 0.38, and 0.09, respectively. (The overhead costs associated with a practice in Marco Island are slightly less than the national average, but malpractice insurance is slightly more.) Assuming the 2016 Medicare conversion factor is \$35.80, the Medicare reimbursement amount for the Marco Island physician would be $(0.97 + 0.40 + 0.09) \times \$35.80 = 1.46 \times \$35.80 = \$52.27$.

Like Medicare's MS-DRG system for inpatients, the more complicated the patient treatment, the greater the reimbursement amount. However, because the codes used for physician reimbursement are specific to the services rendered, no provisions for outlier payments are given to physicians. In section 3.7 of this chapter, we explain medical coding, which provides the framework for most reimbursement methods.

Capitation

Capitation is an entirely different approach to reimbursement from fee-for-service (see "Critical Concept: Capitation"). Under capitated reimbursement, the provider is paid a fixed amount per covered life per period (usually a month), regardless of the amount of services provided. For example, a primary care physician might be paid \$15 per member per month to serve 100 members of a managed care plan. Capitation payment, which is used mostly by managed care organizations to reimburse primary care physicians, dramatically changes the financial environment of healthcare providers. Its implications are addressed in section 3.6 and as needed throughout the remainder of this book. (For additional information about capitation, see online chapter 15, which is available at ache.org/books/FinanceFundamentals3.)

Before closing our discussion of reimbursement, we should note that many insurers are now creating reimbursement systems that explicitly reward providers for achieving certain benchmarks. These reimbursement systems, which are really modified fee-for-service or capitation systems, are called **pay-for-performance (P4P)** systems.

> **CRITICAL CONCEPT**
> Capitation
>
> With capitation, providers are paid a set amount on the basis of the number of members (patients) assigned to that provider. Thus, the reimbursement amount is fixed on the basis of the population served, regardless of the amount of services provided to that population. In effect, the provider, rather than the insurer, faces utilization risk, because higher per-member utilization means higher provider costs with no additional revenues. Critics of capitation contend that it creates the incentive to withhold needed services, while proponents argue that it discourages unneeded services and hence reduces costs.

In most P4P reimbursement schemes, insurers pay providers an "extra" amount if certain standards, usually related to quality of care, are met. For example, a primary care practice may receive additional reimbursement if it meets specified goals, such as administering mammograms to 85 percent of female patients older than 50 or placing 90 percent of diabetic patients on appropriate medication and administering quarterly blood tests. A hospital may receive additional reimbursement if it falls in the lower 10 percent of hospitals experiencing medical errors and hospital-acquired infections.

The idea behind P4P is to create financial incentives for providing high-quality care, which may incur higher costs for insurers in the short run but will lead to lower overall medical costs in the long run. In some P4P plans, insurers reduce payments to poor performers and use the savings to increase payments to high performers, forcing some providers to bear the cost of the plan (see "For Your Consideration: Value-Based Purchasing").

Pay for performance (P4P)
A reimbursement system that rewards providers for meeting specific goals (e.g., 90 percent patient satisfaction).

> **FOR YOUR CONSIDERATION**
> Value-Based Purchasing
>
> Value-based purchasing, a form of pay-for-performance reimbursement, is founded on the concept that buyers of healthcare services should hold providers accountable for quality of care as well as costs. In April 2011, Medicare launched the Hospital Value-Based Purchasing program, which marked the beginning of a historic change in how Medicare pays healthcare providers. For the first time, 3,500 hospitals across the country were paid for inpatient acute care services based on care quality, not just the quantity of the services provided.
>
> "Changing the way we pay hospitals will improve the quality of care for seniors and save money for all of us," said HHS Secretary Kathleen Sebelius. "Under this initiative, Medicare will reward hospitals that provide high-quality care and keep their patients
>
> *(continued)*

FOR YOUR CONSIDERATION
Value-Based Purchasing *(continued)*

healthy. It's an important part of our work to improve the health of our nation and drive down costs. As hospitals work to improve quality, all patients—not just Medicare patients—will benefit." The measures to determine quality focus on how closely hospitals follow best clinical practices and how well hospitals enhance patients' care experiences. The better a hospital performs on its quality measures, the larger its reimbursement from Medicare. Hospitals are no longer paid solely on the quantity of services they provide. HHS set a goal of tying 90 percent of all Medicare fee-for-service to quality or value by 2018.

What do you think? Should providers be reimbursed on the basis of quality of care? How should quality be measured? Should the additional reimbursement to high-quality providers be obtained by reductions in reimbursement to low-quality providers?

SELF-TEST QUESTIONS

1. What is the major difference between fee-for-service reimbursement and capitation?
2. Briefly explain the following fee-for-service payment methods:
   - Cost-based reimbursement
   - Charge-based reimbursement and discounted charges
   - Per-procedure reimbursement
   - Per-diagnosis reimbursement
   - Per diem reimbursement
   - Bundled payment
3. What is pay-for-performance reimbursement?

3.6 THE IMPACT OF REIMBURSEMENT ON FINANCIAL INCENTIVES AND RISKS

Different methods of reimbursement create different incentives and risks for providers. In this section, we briefly discuss these issues.

PROVIDER INCENTIVES

Providers, like individuals or other businesses, react to the incentives created by the financial environment. For example, consider the experience of obtaining a loan from a bank.

Individuals can deduct mortgage interest from income for tax purposes, but they cannot deduct interest payments on personal loans. Loan companies responded to this tax code regulation by offering home equity loans to homeowners that function as a type of second mortgage for tax purposes. The intent is not for such loans to be used to finance home ownership, as the tax laws assumed, but for other expenditures, including paying for vacations and purchasing cars or appliances. In this instance, tax laws created incentives for consumers to carry mortgage debt rather than personal debt, and the mortgage loan industry responded accordingly to accommodate the consumers.

In the same vein, alternative reimbursement methods have an impact on provider behavior. Under cost-based reimbursement, providers are essentially issued a blank check to acquire facilities and equipment and incur operating costs. If payers reimburse providers for all service-related costs, the incentive is to incur such costs. Facilities will be lavish and conveniently located, and staff will be available to ensure that patients are given red-carpet treatment. Furthermore, services that are not required will be provided because more services lead to higher costs, which lead to higher revenues.

Under charge-based reimbursement, providers have the incentive to set high prices and offer more services. However, in competitive markets, prices will be constrained. Still, to the extent that insurers, rather than patients, are footing the bill, considerable leeway exists. Also, because reimbursement paid on the basis of charges is a fee-for-service type of reimbursement, a strong incentive exists to provide the highest possible amount of services. In essence, providers can increase utilization, and hence revenues, by creating more visits, ordering more tests, extending inpatient stays, and so on. Although charge-based reimbursement does encourage providers to contain costs, the incentive is weak because charges can more easily be increased than costs can be decreased. In recent years, the ability of providers to increase revenues by raising charges has been greatly offset by insurers through negotiated discounts or constrained reimbursement increases, which place additional pressure on profitability and hence sweeten the incentive for providers to reduce costs.

Under prospective payment reimbursement, provider incentives are altered. First, under per-procedure reimbursement, the profitability of individual procedures varies depending on the relationship between the actual costs incurred and the payment for that procedure. In other words, because of inconsistencies in reimbursement, some procedures are more profitable than others. Providers, typically physicians, have the incentive to perform procedures that have the highest profit potential. Furthermore, the more procedures performed, the better, because each procedure typically generates additional profit.

The incentives under per-diagnosis reimbursement are similar. Providers, usually hospitals, seek patients with diagnoses that have the greatest profit potential and discourage (or even discontinue) services that have the least potential. (Why, in recent years, have so many hospitals created cardiac care centers?)

In all prospective payment methods, providers have the incentive to reduce costs because the amount of reimbursement is fixed and independent of the costs actually incurred. For example, when hospitals are paid under per-diagnosis reimbursement, they have the incentive to reduce length of stay, which reduces overall costs. However, when per diem reimbursement is used, hospitals have an incentive to increase length of stay. Because the early days of a hospitalization typically are more costly than the later days, the later days are more profitable. However, as mentioned previously, hospitals have the incentive to reduce costs during each day of a patient stay regardless of the prospective payment method.

Bundled reimbursement
The payment of a single amount for several procedures. When reimbursement is unbundled, separate amounts are paid for each procedure.

Under **bundled reimbursement**, providers do not have the opportunity to be reimbursed for a series of separate services. For example, a physician's treatment of a fracture could be bundled and billed as one episode, or it could be unbundled, with separate bills submitted for making the diagnosis, taking the X-rays, setting the fracture, removing the cast, and so on. The rationale for unbundling is usually to provide more detailed records of treatments rendered, but often the result is higher total charges for the parts than would be charged for the entire package under bundled payment.

In addition, bundled reimbursement, when applied to multiple providers for a single episode of care, forces those providers (usually physicians and hospitals) to offer the most cost-effective treatment jointly. A multiprovider view of cost containment may be more effective than each participant separately attempting to minimize her treatment costs because the actions of one provider to lower costs could increase the costs of the others.

Finally, capitation reimbursement totally changes the playing field by reversing the actions that providers must take to ensure financial success. Under all fee-for-service methods, the key to provider success is to work harder, increase the amount of services provided (utilization), and hence maximize profits. Under capitation, the key to profitability is to work more thoughtfully and decrease utilization.

As with prospective payment, capitated providers have the incentive to lower the cost of the services provided, but now they also have the incentive to reduce the amount of services provided. Thus, only those procedures that are truly medically necessary should be performed, and treatment should take place in the lowest-cost setting that can provide the appropriate quality of care. Furthermore, providers have the incentive to promote health, rather than just treat illness and injury, because a healthier population consumes fewer healthcare services.

Provider Risks

One key issue providers contend with is the impact of various reimbursement methods on financial risk. Think of financial risk in terms of the effect that the reimbursement methods have on profit uncertainty—the greater the uncertainty in profitability (and hence the greater the chance of losing money), the higher the risk.

Cost- and charge-based reimbursements are the least risky methods for providers because payers more or less ensure that provider costs are covered, and hence profits will be earned. In cost-based systems, costs are automatically covered. In charge-based systems, providers typically can set charges high enough to ensure that costs are covered, although discounts introduce some uncertainty into the reimbursement process.

In all reimbursement methods, except cost-based payment, providers bear the cost-of-service risk in the sense that costs can exceed revenues. However, a primary difference among the reimbursement types is the ability of the provider to influence the revenue–cost relationship. If providers set charge rates for each type of service provided, they can most easily ensure that revenues exceed costs. Furthermore, if providers have the power to set rates above those that would exist in a truly competitive market, charge-based reimbursement could result in higher profits than cost-based reimbursement can realize.

Prospective payment creates additional risk for providers. In essence, payers are setting reimbursement rates on the basis of what they believe to be sufficient. If the payments are set too low, providers cannot make money on their services without sacrificing quality. Today, many hospitals and physicians believe that Medicare and Medicaid reimbursement rates are too low to compensate them adequately for providing healthcare services to those populations. Thus, the only way for these providers to survive is to recoup these losses from privately insured patients or stop treating government-insured patients, which for many providers would take away more than half of their revenues. Whether or not government reimbursement is too low is open to debate. Still, prospective payment can place significant financial risk on providers' operations.

Under capitation, providers assume utilization risk along with the risks assumed under the other reimbursement methods (see "Critical Concept: Utilization Risk"). The assumption of utilization risk has traditionally been an insurance, rather than a provider, function. In the traditional fee-for-service system, the financial risk of providing healthcare services is shared between providers and insurers: If costs are too high, providers suffer; if too many services are consumed, insurers suffer. Capitation, however, places both cost and utilization risk on providers.

When provider risk under different reimbursement methods is discussed in this descriptive fashion, an easy conclusion to make is that capitation is by far the riskiest reimbursement method to providers, while cost- and charge-based reimbursement are by far the least risky. Although this conclusion is not a bad starting point for analysis, financial risk is a complex subject, and we have just scratched its surface. For now, keep in mind that payers use different reimbursement methods. Thus, providers can face conflicting incentives and differing risk, depending on the predominant method of reimbursement.

In closing, note that all prospective payment methods create financial risk for providers.

CRITICAL CONCEPT
Utilization Risk

Utilization risk is the risk that patients, often members of a managed care plan, will use more healthcare services than initially assumed. For example, each employee of General Electric may be expected to make three visits per year to a primary care physician. However, the utilization risk is that each employee will actually make four visits. If the primary care physicians who treat the employees are paid on a fee-for-service basis, utilization risk is borne by the insurer (General Electric, because it is self-insured). The physicians will be paid for the actual number of visits, and, if employees visit more frequently than expected, the insurer must bear the added costs. However, if the physicians are capitated, they will be paid a fixed amount per employee based on the assumption of three visits. When employees make four visits, the primary care physicians bear the extra cost and hence the utilization risk.

This assumption of risk does not mean that providers should avoid such reimbursement methods; indeed, refusing to accept contracts with prospective payment provisions would be organizational suicide for most providers. However, providers must understand the risks involved in prospective payment arrangements, especially the impact on profitability, and make every effort to negotiate a level of payment that is consistent with the risk incurred.

Self-Test Questions

1. What provider incentives are created under (a) cost-based reimbursement, (b) prospective payment, and (c) capitation?
2. Which of the three payment methods listed in question 1 carries the least risk for providers? The most risk? Explain your answer.

3.7 MEDICAL CODING: THE FOUNDATION OF FEE-FOR-SERVICE REIMBURSEMENT

Medical coding, or medical classification, is the process of transforming descriptions of medical diagnoses and procedures into numerical codes that can be universally recognized and interpreted. The diagnoses and procedures are usually taken from a variety of sources in the medical record, such as doctors' notes, laboratory results, and radiological tests. In practice, the basis for most fee-for-service reimbursement is the patient's diagnosis (in the case of hospitals) or the procedures performed on the patient (in the case of outpatient settings). Thus, a brief background on medical coding will enhance your understanding of the reimbursement process,

Diagnosis Codes

The International Classification of Diseases (commonly known by the abbreviation ICD) is the standard resource for designating diseases and a wide variety of signs, symptoms, and external causes of injury. Published by the World Health Organization (WHO), **ICD codes** are used internationally to record many types of health events, including hospital inpatient stays and deaths. (ICD codes were first used in 1893 to report death statistics.)

ICD codes
International Classification of Diseases (ICD) codes are used by hospitals and other organizations to specify patient diagnoses.

WHO periodically revises the diagnostic codes in ICD, which is now in the tenth version (ICD-10). Conversion to ICD-10 codes in the United States was slated to occur in 2013; however, in April 2012 HHS proposed a one-year delay of the ICD-10 compliance date, to October 1, 2014. Another proposal delayed the ICD-10 further until it was officially launched on October 1, 2015. The conversion was time consuming and costly because ICD-10 contains more than five times as many individual codes as did the previous version, ICD-9. Of course, the information provided by the new code set is more detailed and complete.

The ICD-10 codes are three to seven characters. The first three characters denote the disease category, and additional characters further specify the patient's condition. For example, code I21 describes an acute myocardial infarction (heart attack), while code I21.0 is an attack involving the anterior wall of the heart.

In practice, the application of ICD codes to diagnoses is complicated and technical. Hospital coders must thoroughly understand the coding system as well as the medical terminology and abbreviations used by clinicians. The medical coding function is highly complex, and proper reimbursement from third-party payers depends on accurate coding; therefore, ICD coders require a great deal of training and experience.

Procedure Codes

While ICD codes are used to specify diseases, Current Procedural Terminology (CPT) codes are used to specify medical procedures (treatments). **CPT codes** were developed and are copyrighted by the American Medical Association.

CPT codes
Current Procedural Terminology (CPT) codes are used by clinicians to specify procedures performed on patients.

The purpose of CPT is to create a uniform set of descriptive terms and codes that accurately describe medical, surgical, and diagnostic procedures. CPT codes are revised periodically to reflect current trends in clinical treatments. To increase standardization and the use of electronic medical records, federal law requires that physicians and other clinical providers, including laboratory and diagnostic services, use CPT to code and transfer healthcare information. (The same law also requires that ICD-10-CM/PCS codes be used to document hospital inpatient services.)

The CPT code set includes ten codes for physician office visits: Five codes apply to new patients and five apply to established patients on repeat visits. The differences among the five codes in each category are based on the complexity of the visit, as indicated by three components: extent of patient history review, extent of examination, and difficulty of medical decision-making. For repeat patients, the least complex (typically shortest) office visit is coded 99211, while the most complex (typically longest) is coded 99215.

Because government payers (Medicare and Medicaid) and other insurers require additional information from providers beyond that contained in CPT codes, CMS developed an enhanced code set, the **Healthcare Common Procedure Coding System (HCPCS)** (commonly pronounced "hick picks"). This system expands the set of CPT codes to include nonphysician services, such as ambulance services, and durable medical equipment, such as prosthetic devices.

Healthcare Common Procedure Coding System (HCPCS)
A medical coding system that expands the CPT codes to include nonphysician services and durable medical equipment.

Although CPT and HCPCS codes are not as complex as the ICD codes, coders still must have a high level of training and experience to use them correctly. As in ICD coding, correct CPT coding ensures correct reimbursement. Medical coding is so important that many businesses offer services, such as books, software, education, and consulting, to hospitals and medical practices to improve coding efficiency.

SELF-TEST QUESTIONS

1. Briefly describe the coding system used in hospitals (ICD codes) and medical practices (CPT and HCPCS codes).
2. What is the link between coding and reimbursement?

3.8 HEALTHCARE REFORM

Healthcare reform is a generic term used to describe the actions taken by Congress in 2009 and 2010 to reform the healthcare system (see "Critical Concept: Healthcare Reform"). The messy legislative process was completed in early 2010, when President Barack Obama signed the ACA.

CRITICAL CONCEPT
Healthcare Reform

Healthcare reform is a generic term used to describe the actions taken by Congress in 2010 to transform the healthcare system. The legislation, titled the Patient Protection and Affordable Care Act (ACA), had as its primary purpose to help an additional 32 million Americans obtain health insurance. Most of the provisions affect the insurance side of healthcare, but provisions are also in place to increase the quality and decrease the costs of healthcare services.

Healthcare reform includes a large number of provisions that were expected to take effect over the next several years with the primary goal of helping an additional 32 million Americans obtain health insurance. The provisions included expanding Medicaid eligibility, subsidizing insurance premiums, providing incentives for businesses to provide healthcare benefits, prohibiting denial of coverage on the basis of preexisting conditions, establishing health insurance exchanges, and providing financial support for medical research. For the most part, reform focused on the insurance side of the healthcare sector as opposed to the provider side. Thus, many people believed that the legislation should be called *insurance reform* rather than *healthcare reform*.

In addition to those affecting the insurance segment of healthcare, some provisions were designed to offset the costs of reform by instituting a variety of taxes, fees, and cost-saving measures. Examples included new Medicare taxes for high-income earners, taxes on indoor tanning services, cuts to the Medicare Advantage (Part C) program, fees on medical devices and pharmaceutical companies, and tax penalties on citizens who do not obtain health insurance.

Finally, other provisions funded pilot programs to test various changes to provider systems and reimbursement methodologies (primarily Medicare) designed to increase quality and decrease costs. Provisions likely to have the greatest impact on providers and how they are reimbursed included the establishment of pilot programs to explore the feasibility of accountable care organizations (ACOs) (discussed later in the chapter), the effectiveness of payment bundling, and the potential quality gains from the medical home model (also discussed later).

Legislative changes may occur that could significantly alter some of the program's features or eliminate it altogether. All of these conditions create uncertainty for insurers and providers, but the good news is that the finance principles and concepts contained in this book remain valid regardless of the ultimate outcome of healthcare reform.

Accountable Care Organizations

Accountable care organizations, one of the cornerstone concepts of healthcare reform, integrate local physicians with other members of the healthcare community and reward them for controlling costs and improving quality. While ACOs are not radically different from other attempts to improve the delivery of healthcare services, their uniqueness lies in the flexibility of their structures and payment methodologies and their ability to assume risk while meeting quality targets. Similar to some MCOs and integrated healthcare systems such as the Mayo Clinic, ACOs are responsible for the health outcomes of the population served and are tasked with collaboratively improving care to reach cost and clinical quality targets set by Medicare.

Accountable care organization (ACO)
An organization that integrates physicians and other healthcare providers with the goal of controlling costs and improving quality.

To help achieve cost control and quality goals, ACOs can distribute bonuses when targets are met and sometimes impose penalties when targets are missed. To be effective, an ACO should include, at a minimum, primary care physicians, specialists, and a hospital, although some ACOs are being established solely by physician groups. In addition, it should have the managerial systems in place to administer payments, set benchmarks, measure performance, and distribute shared savings. A variety of federal, regional, state, and academic hospital initiatives are investigating how to implement ACOs. Although the concept shows potential, many legal and managerial hurdles must be overcome for ACOs to live up to their initial promise.

One feature of healthcare reform is a shared savings program in which Medicare pays a fixed (global) payment to ACOs that covers the full cost of care of an entire population. In this program, cost and quality targets are established. Any cost savings (costs that are below target) are shared between Medicare and the ACO as long as the ACO also meets its quality targets.

Medical home (patient-centered medical home)
A team-based model of care led by a personal physician who provides, or arranges with other qualified professionals to provide, continual and coordinated care throughout a patient's lifetime to maximize health outcomes.

Medical Home Model

A **medical home (patient-centered medical home)** is a team-based model of care led by a personal physician who works collaboratively with the team's other healthcare professionals to provide continual, coordinated, and integrated care throughout a patient's lifetime to maximize health outcomes. This responsibility includes the provision of preventive services, treatment of acute and chronic illnesses, and assistance with end-of-life issues.

The medical home model is independent of the ACO concept, but observers anticipate that ACOs will provide an organizational setting that facilitates implementation of the model. Supporters of the model claim that it will allow better access to healthcare, increase patient satisfaction, and improve health. Although the development and implementation of the medical home model are in their infancy, the model's key characteristics are shaping up as follows:

- *Personal physician.* Each patient will have an ongoing relationship with a personal physician trained to provide first contact and continual and comprehensive care.
- *Whole-person orientation.* The personal physician is responsible for providing for all of a patient's healthcare needs or for appropriately arranging care with other qualified professionals. In effect, the personal physician will lead a team of clinicians who collectively take responsibility for patient care.
- *Coordination and integration.* The personal physician will coordinate care across specialists, hospitals, home health agencies, nursing homes, and hospices.
- *Quality and safety.* Quality and patient safety are ensured by a care-planning process, evidence-based medicine, clinical decision–support tools, performance measurement, active participation of patients in decision-making, use of information technology, and quality improvement activities.
- *Enhanced access.* Medical care and information are available at all times through open scheduling, expanded hours of service, and new and innovative communication technologies.
- *Payment methodologies.* Payment methodologies recognize the added value provided to patients. Payments should reflect the value of work that falls outside of face-to-face visits, should support adoption and use of health information technology for quality improvement, and should recognize differences in the patient populations treated in the practice.

Several ongoing pilot projects are assessing the effectiveness of the medical home and ACO models, and a great deal of information is available online.

Theme Wrap-Up: Big Sky's Revenue Sources

Just hired as Big Sky's practice manager and now learning the workings of the practice, Jen decided to first focus on the practice's revenues. Specifically, she wanted to answer two questions to better identify the steps toward increasing revenues and reducing the riskiness associated with those revenues: where Big Sky's revenue comes from and what methods the payers use to determine the payment amount.

After reviewing Big Sky's revenue records, Jen found the following payer mix:

Commercial	
Fee-for-service	37%
Managed care	15
Total	52%
Government	
Medicare	29%
Medicaid	8
Total	37%
Miscellaneous	
Self-pay	6%
Other	5
Total	11%
Total	100%

The largest payer category for the practice is commercial insurance, with a total of 52 percent of revenues. (Note that commercial revenues include Blue Cross Blue Shield plans.) Of the commercial patients, 37 percent are enrolled in fee-for-service plans and 15 percent are enrolled in managed care plans. Next largest is government programs (Medicare and Medicaid), constituting 37 percent of Big Sky's payers, followed by self-pay with 6 percent and other sources at 5 percent. ("Other" sources consist of workers' compensation and other government programs, a small amount of charity care, and about 2 percent bad debt losses. Bad debt losses arise when patients who have the ability to pay fail to do so.) Although not shown in the earlier table, 5 percent of Big Sky's revenues come from capitated contracts, while the remaining 95 percent are paid on a fee-for-service basis.

This payer mix should present few problems for Big Sky. In general, commercial insurers are considered to be more generous than government programs, so the revenue stream should be adequate and not overly dependent on payments influenced by political decisions related to public funding. In addition, bad debt losses appear not to be a major concern for the practice.

Because Big Sky's revenue stream is mostly fee-for-service, its physicians have an overall incentive to increase production—that is, to perform more procedures and hence increase revenues. However, the incentive for capitated patients (who make up 5 percent of revenues) is to provide only the services that are absolutely needed. Do the physicians know which patients are fee-for-service and which are capitated? Absolutely. Although capitated revenues provide a steady stream of monthly payments to the practice, they bring with them utilization risk. However, with only a small percentage of capitated revenues, the practice faces minimal risk.

All in all, Big Sky's revenue stream appears sound, with no significant negative factors. This is the good news for Jen. The bad news is that now she must tackle an issue that is potentially more difficult to deal with—examining Big Sky's costs and balancing them against the revenue stream.

Key Concepts

This chapter explores the insurance function, the third-party payer system, and reimbursement methods. Here are the key concepts:

- Health insurance is widely used in the United States because individuals are risk averse and insurers can spread the financial risk over a large population.
- *Adverse selection* occurs when individuals most likely to have claims purchase insurance, while those least likely to have claims do not.
- *Moral hazard* occurs when an insured individual purposely sustains a loss, as opposed to a random loss. In a health insurance setting, moral hazard is more subtle, producing such behaviors as seeking more services than needed and engaging in unhealthy behavior because the potential costs are borne by someone else.
- Insurers are classified as either private or public (government). The major private insurers are Blue Cross Blue Shield, commercial insurers, and self-insurers.
- The government is a major insurer and direct provider of healthcare services. The two major forms of government health insurance are Medicare and Medicaid.
- When payers pay billed charges, they pay according to the schedule of charge rates established by the provider in its *chargemaster*.
- *Negotiated charges*, which are discounted from billed (chargemaster) charges, are often used by insurers in conjunction with managed care plans.
- Under a *retrospective cost system*, the payer agrees to pay the provider certain allowable costs that are incurred in providing services to the payer's enrollees.
- In a *prospective payment system*, the rates are determined in advance and are not tied directly to either reimbursable costs or billed charges. Typically, prospective payments are made on the basis of the following service definitions: (1) *per procedure*, (2) *per diagnosis*, (3) *per diem* (per day), or (4) *bundled reimbursement*.
- In 1983, the federal government adopted the *inpatient prospective payment system* (IPPS) for Medicare hospital inpatient reimbursement. Under this system, the amount of payment is fixed by the patient's diagnosis, as indicated by the diagnosis-related group (DRG).

- Physicians are reimbursed by Medicare using the *resource-based relative value scale* (RBRVS) system. Under RBRVS, reimbursement is paid on the basis of three resource components: (1) physician work, (2) practice (overhead) expenses, and (3) malpractice insurance.
- *Medical coding* is the foundation of fee-for-service reimbursement systems. In inpatient settings, ICD codes are used to designate diagnoses, while in outpatient settings, CPT codes are used to specify procedures.
- *Healthcare reform* is legislation signed into law in 2010 that is expected to have a significant impact on health insurers. However, its final form will not be known for a number of years.
- *Accountable care organizations (ACOs)* are a method of integrating physicians with other members of the healthcare community and rewarding them for controlling costs and improving quality.
- *A medical home (patient-centered medical home)* is a team-based model of care led by a personal physician who provides continual and coordinated care throughout a patient's lifetime to maximize health outcomes.

The information in this chapter plays a vital role in financial decision-making in health services organizations. Thus, we will use it over and over in the chapters that follow.

End-of-Chapter Questions

3.1 Briefly describe the major third-party payers.

3.2 a. What are the primary characteristics of managed care organizations (MCOs)?
b. Describe two different types of MCOs.

3.3 What is the difference between fee-for-service reimbursement and capitation?

3.4 What is pay-for-performance?

3.5 Describe provider incentives and risks under each of the following reimbursement methods:
a. Cost based
b. Charge based, including discounted charges
c. Prospective payment
d. Capitation

3.6 Briefly describe the coding systems for diseases (diagnoses) and procedures.

3.7 How does Medicare reimburse hospitals for inpatient stays?

3.8 How does Medicare reimburse physician services?

3.9 What are the key features of the ACA?

PART II

PLANNING, MANAGING, AND CONTROL

In part II, we begin our discussion of the actual practice of healthcare finance. Here, the major topics, which span four chapters, are planning for the future, managing current operations, and imposing controls to ensure that plans are met.

Chapter 4 addresses cost estimation, the foundation of managerial accounting. If an organization does not know its costs, its business decisions are doomed to failure.

Chapter 5 adds pricing and revenues to the cost picture. After both revenues and costs are estimated, managers can project future profits and, more important, understand the effect of changing assumptions about volume, costs, or prices on profits.

Chapter 6 covers the important subject of planning and budgeting. If healthcare businesses did not plan for the future, they would be operating at the whims of the economic environment. During the planning and budgeting processes, specific operational goals are set, along with a plan for meeting these goals.

Chapter 7 discusses several topics related to operational and financial management, with emphasis on how managers monitor operations to ensure that the goals set in the planning and budgeting process are met.

Taken together, the four chapters in part II provide you with the tools necessary to manage the financial aspects of your organization's performance more effectively.

CHAPTER 4

ESTIMATING COSTS

THEME SET-UP: COST STRUCTURE

As you know from chapter 3, Big Sky Dermatology Specialists is a small group practice located in Jackson, Wyoming. Jen Latimer, a recent health administration graduate and newly hired manager for the group, completed her review of Big Sky's revenue sources. Now she wants to take a closer look at Big Sky's cost structure—that is, the way Big Sky's total costs change as volume changes.

Jen remembers from her healthcare finance courses that a business's costs can be classified in several ways. The major classifications are (1) the relationship of the cost to the amount of services offered (does the cost increase as volume increases?) and (2) the relationship of the cost to the subunit being analyzed (does the cost go away if the subunit is abolished?).

As she thought about these classifications, she breathed a sigh of relief. Big Sky was not formally divided into departments (subunits), so she would not have to develop a system to allocate overhead costs, such as billing expenses, to separate departments in the practice. Still, she had to identify the costs that are unrelated to volume (fixed costs) and the costs that are tied to volume (variable costs). By identifying these two types of costs, Jen would be able to forecast Big Sky's profit potential under different assumptions about volume (number of visits).

By the end of this chapter, you will have an appreciation for the costs inherent to healthcare businesses and how those costs are classified. Then you, like Jen, will be able to apply this knowledge to estimate the cost structure of Big Sky Dermatology Specialists.

Learning Objectives

After studying this chapter, you will be able to do the following:

- Discuss the nature and purpose of managerial accounting.
- Explain how costs are classified according to their relationship with volume.
- Describe how costs are classified according to their relationship with the unit being analyzed.
- Explain why proper cost allocation is important to healthcare organizations.
- Define the terms *cost pool* and *cost driver*, and describe the characteristics of a good cost driver.
- List the three primary methods used to allocate overhead costs among revenue-producing (patient services) departments.
- Describe three methods used to cost individual services: the cost-to-charge ratio (CCR), relative value units (RVUs), and activity-based costing (ABC).
- Articulate the differences between traditional costing and ABC.

4.1 INTRODUCTION

Healthcare managers have many responsibilities. The more important ones include planning for the future, overseeing the day-to-day activities of line employees, and establishing policies that control the operations of the organization.

For example, the practice manager of a primary care practice must estimate future demand (volume) and see to it that the practice has the facilities, staff, and supplies necessary to meet this demand. He does so primarily by creating budgets that use forecasted future volume to estimate the resources needed to meet expected patient demand. As the future unfolds, the practice manager must monitor operations to see if the volume estimates were correct. If not, supplies and staffing requirements must be adjusted to reflect variations from forecasts. Finally, he must constantly review the resources used to ensure that they are being used appropriately and efficiently and are being acquired at the lowest possible costs.

All of these activities require information—a great deal of it. Furthermore, it has to be compiled in a format that facilitates analysis, interpretation, and decision-making. Without timely and relevant information, healthcare managers would be making decisions essentially in the dark. Of course, accurate information does not ensure good decision-making, but without it, the chances of making good decisions are almost nil.

The foundation of a good information system is the manager's ability to estimate costs with confidence. This task is not easy. You may be able to precisely estimate the cost of your college education—just add up the costs of tuition, books and supplies, room and board, and so on—but what about the costs of healthcare organizations? Their overall (total) costs can be measured with some precision, such as the total costs of running a hospital or a medical practice. However, what about the costs of running the emergency department, or the costs associated with Medicare patients, or the costs of treating patients who have had heart attacks? Estimating these costs with confidence is essential to sound management, yet many factors complicate the estimation process.

Although cost estimation comes with a multitude of problems, it is far too important to the financial well-being of healthcare providers to do in a sloppy way. Thus, organizations put a lot of time and effort into doing the best possible job.

4.2 THE BASICS OF MANAGERIAL ACCOUNTING

Cost estimation is an accounting function, so our coverage begins with some accounting basics. Accounting is split into two primary areas: managerial accounting and financial accounting. Whereas financial accounting (discussed in chapters 11 and 12) focuses on the reporting of operational and financial results to outsiders, managerial accounting focuses on the development of information used internally for managerial decision-making (see "Critical Concept: Managerial Accounting").

CRITICAL CONCEPT
Managerial Accounting

The accounting function in businesses is broken down into two major areas: managerial accounting and financial accounting. Financial accounting, which is covered later in the book, involves the creation of financial statements that report what has occurred at the organization. Managerial accounting concerns the creation and use of data needed to manage an organization's current and future operations. Thus, managerial accounting produces reports used at various levels in an organization, such as department operations, contract negotiations, or specific services delivery, to enhance financial performance.

Managerial accounting information is used in routine budgeting processes, to allocate managerial bonuses, and to make pricing and service decisions, all of which deal with subunits of an organization. In addition, managers can use managerial accounting data for special purposes, such as assessing alternative modes of delivery or projecting the profitability of a particular reimbursement contract.

Because managers are more concerned with what will happen in the future than with what has happened in the past, managerial accounting is for the most part forward-looking. However, because most of the future is unknown, compiling managerial accounting information requires making many assumptions about future events. For example, as managers create budgets, they often must make assumptions regarding utilization (volume), reimbursement rates, and costs.

Cost
A resource use associated with providing, or supporting, a specific service.

A critical part of managerial accounting is the measurement of costs. One issue that makes this task difficult is the fact that no single definition of the term **cost** exists. Rather, different costs exist for different purposes. As a general rule, for healthcare providers, a cost involves a resource use associated with providing, or supporting, a specific service. However, the cost per service identified for pricing purposes can differ from the cost per service used for management control purposes. Also, the cost per service used for long-range planning purposes may differ from the cost per service defined for short-term purposes. Thus, when dealing with costs, managers have to understand the context so that the correct cost is identified. To complicate matters further, costs do not necessarily reflect actual cash outflows.

Costs are classified in two primary ways: by their relationship to the volume (amount) of services provided and by their relationship to the unit (i.e., department) being analyzed. This chapter focuses on these two cost classifications. In chapter 5, we add revenues to the mix and show how to convert cost estimates into profit estimates.

SELF-TEST QUESTIONS

1. What is the primary purpose of managerial accounting information?
2. What is meant by the term *cost*?
3. What are the two primary ways that costs can be classified?

4.3 COST CLASSIFICATION 1: FIXED VERSUS VARIABLE COSTS

One way to classify costs is on the basis of their relationship to the amount of services provided, often referred to as **volume** or *utilization*. Future volume—the number of patient days, visits, enrollees, laboratory tests, and so on—is almost always uncertain.

Volume
The amount of services provided (e.g., number of visits, number of inpatient days). Also called *utilization*.

Volume may be forecasted in a number of ways. One way is to review historical trends, say, over the past five to ten years. In many situations, the past is a good predictor of the future. If the manager believes this to be the case, then she can apply statistical analysis (linear regression) to the historical data to predict future volumes. If past data are not available or if significant changes in the operating environment are taking place, then volume forecasting becomes more difficult. In that situation, the manager must evaluate population and disease trends in the service area, actions of competitors, pricing strategies, the impact of new contracts with insurers, and a whole host of additional factors that influence future volume.

If a provider's volume forecast turns out to be inaccurate, the consequences can be severe. First, if the market for any particular service expands more than expected and planned for, the provider will not be able to meet its patients' needs. Potential patients will go elsewhere, and the provider will lose market share and perhaps miss a major opportunity to maintain or increase its business. On the other hand, if projections are overly optimistic, the provider could end up with excess equipment, supplies, and staff, and hence costs that are higher than necessary.

In spite of the difficulties in forecasting volume with precision, managers typically have some idea of the potential range. For example, the manager of Northside Clinic, a small walk-in clinic, might estimate that the total number of patient visits for next year will likely range from 12,000 to 14,000 or from about 34 to 40 per day. If utilization is not likely to fall outside of these bounds, then the range of 12,000 to 14,000 annual visits defines the clinic's **relevant range**. Note that the relevant range pertains to a particular period—in this case, next year. For other periods, the relevant range might differ from this estimate.

Relevant range
The range of output (volume) for which the organization's cost structure holds.

Fixed Costs

Some costs, called *fixed costs*, are more or less known with certainty, regardless of the level of volume in the relevant range. For example, Northside Clinic's labor force would be increased or decreased only under unusual circumstances. Thus, as long as volume falls within the relevant range of 12,000 to 14,000 patient visits, labor costs at the clinic are fixed for the coming year. The actual number of visits might turn out to be 12,352 or 13,877, but labor costs will remain at their forecasted level as long as volume falls in the relevant range (see "For Your Consideration: Cost Structure and Relevant Range"). Other examples of the clinic's fixed costs include expenditures on facilities (e.g., rent, property taxes, utilities), diagnostic equipment, and information systems. After an organization has acquired these assets, it typically is locked into them for some period regardless of volume fluctuations, so these costs are known beforehand.

FOR YOUR CONSIDERATION
Cost Structure and Relevant Range

In general, an organization's underlying cost structure is defined for a specified relevant range. For example, assume that Atlanta Clinic's underlying cost structure is given as follows:

$$\text{Total costs} = \text{Fixed costs} + \text{Total variable costs}$$
$$= \$4{,}967{,}462 + (\$28.18 \times \text{Number of visits}).$$

Assume that the expected number of visits next year is 75,000 and the relevant range for this cost structure is 70,000 to 80,000 visits. Now, assume that a new payer makes a proposal to the clinic that would increase next year's volume by 10,000 visits, which would increase the expected number of visits to 85,000. The financial staff presents you, the CEO, with an analysis of the costs under the new proposal that was calculated as follows:

$$\text{Total costs} = \$4{,}967{,}462 + (\$28.18 \times 85{,}000)$$
$$= \$4{,}967{,}462 + \$2{,}395{,}300$$
$$= \$7{,}362{,}762.$$

What is your initial reaction to the analysis? Is it valid or must it be redone? What variable in the underlying cost structure is most likely to change at a volume of 85,000 visits?

Of course, no costs are fixed over the long run or over large volume changes. At some level of increasing volume, healthcare businesses must incur additional fixed costs for new facilities and equipment, additional staffing, and so on. Likewise, if volume decreases by a substantial amount, an organization likely would reduce fixed costs by shedding some of its facilities and parts of its equipment and labor base.

Variable Costs

Whereas some costs are fixed regardless of volume (within the relevant range), other resources are more or less consumed as volume dictates. Costs that are related to (depend on) volume are called *variable costs* (see "Critical Concept: Fixed Versus Variable Costs"). For example, the costs of the clinical supplies (e.g., rubber gloves, tongue depressors, hypodermics, bandages) used by Northside would be classified as variable costs. Also, some of the clinic's diagnostic equipment is leased on a per-use basis (a fixed payment each time the equipment is used), which converts the cost of the equipment from a fixed cost to a variable cost. Finally, some healthcare organizations pay their employees on the basis of the amount of work performed, which would convert labor costs from fixed to variable. The bottom line is that fixed costs are independent of the volume of services delivered (within the relevant range), while variable costs depend on volume.

CRITICAL CONCEPT
Fixed Versus Variable Costs

One way to classify costs is by their relationship to volume. Fixed costs are known and predictable regardless of volume (within some relevant range). Conversely, variable costs depend on the volume of services supplied. Consider a clinical laboratory. The costs of the building, equipment, and personnel to run the lab are known with some certainty for the coming year. Furthermore, these costs are independent of the number of tests actually conducted. Such costs are fixed. However, the annual costs of reagents and other test supplies depend on the number (and type) of tests conducted—the greater the number of tests, the greater these costs. Thus, the accounting system would classify these costs as variable.

Underlying Cost Structure

Healthcare managers are vitally interested in how costs are affected by changes in the amount of services supplied. The relationship between costs and volume, called *underlying cost structure* (or just cost structure), is used by managers in planning, control, and decision-making (see "Critical Concept: Underlying Cost Structure"). The primary reason for defining an organization's cost structure is to provide managers with a tool for forecasting costs (and ultimately profits) at different volume levels.

CRITICAL CONCEPT
Underlying Cost Structure

The underlying cost structure of a business defines the relationship between volume and costs. To illustrate, assume you plan to sell customized pens to your classmates to make some extra money. To get started, you pay someone $50 to design the logo for the pens. Then, you pay $1.75 for each pen. The cost structure of your pen business consists of $50 in fixed costs and a variable cost rate of $1.75. Thus, the cost structure of the business can be written as:

$$\text{Total costs} = \$50 + (\$1.75 \times \text{Volume}).$$

If you sell 100 pens, your total costs are $225:

$$\begin{aligned}\text{Total costs} &= \$50 + (\$1.75 \times \text{Volume})\\ &= \$50 + (\$1.75 \times 100)\\ &= \$50 + \$175\\ &= \$225.\end{aligned}$$

Variable cost rate
The added cost for each additional unit of service (e.g., the variable cost rate at a neighborhood walk-in clinic is $15 per patient visit).

Total variable costs
The variable cost rate multiplied by volume (e.g., if a walk-in clinic has a variable cost rate of $15 per visit and experiences 10,000 visits annually, total variable costs for the year equal $15 × 10,000 = $150,000).

To illustrate the concept, consider the hypothetical cost data presented in exhibit 4.1 for a hospital's clinical laboratory. The cost structure consists of both fixed and variable costs—that is, some of the costs are expected to be volume sensitive and some are not. This structure of both fixed and variable costs is typical in health services organizations as well as most other businesses (see "Healthcare in Practice: The Cost Structures of Medical Practices"). For illustrative purposes, let us assume the relevant range is from zero to 20,000 tests. (Of course, the actual relevant range might be from 15,000 to 20,000 tests.)

As noted in exhibit 4.1, the laboratory has $150,000 in fixed costs that consist primarily of labor, facilities, and equipment. (We have purposely kept the numbers unrealistically small for ease of illustration.) These costs will occur even if the laboratory does not perform one test. In addition to the fixed costs, each test, on average, requires $10 in laboratory supplies, such as glass slides, blood test tubes, and reagents.

The per-unit (per test, in this example) variable cost of $10 is defined as the **variable cost rate.** If laboratory volume doubles—for example, from 500 to 1,000 tests—total variable costs will double from $5,000 to $10,000. However, the variable cost rate of $10 per test remains the same whether the test is the first, the hundredth, or the thousandth. **Total variable costs**, therefore, increase or decrease proportionately as volume changes, but the variable cost rate remains constant.

EXHIBIT 4.1
Cost Structure Illustration

Variable Cost per Test		Fixed Costs per Year	
Laboratory supplies	$10	Labor	$100,000
		Other fixed costs	50,000
			$150,000

Volume	Fixed Costs	Total Variable Costs	Total Costs	Average Cost per Test
0	$150,000	$ 0	$150,000	—
1	150,000	10	150,010	$150,010.00
50	150,000	500	150,500	3,010.00
100	150,000	1,000	151,000	1,510.00
500	150,000	5,000	155,000	310.00
1,000	150,000	10,000	160,000	160.00
5,000	150,000	50,000	200,000	40.00
10,000	150,000	100,000	250,000	25.00
15,000	150,000	150,000	300,000	20.00
20,000	150,000	200,000	350,000	17.50

HEALTHCARE IN PRACTICE
The Cost Structures of Medical Practices

Different healthcare organizations have different cost structures. Even in the same type of organization, cost structure differences occur. For example, medical practices that are hospital based, such as some radiology groups, tend to have low fixed costs (the hospital pays those). Other practices, such as cardiology, can have a great deal of diagnostic equipment and hence high fixed costs. In addition, the size of a practice influences its underlying cost structure.

Still, by examining the costs associated with a typical practice, we can get some feel for the cost structures involved. We have chosen a primary care practice to represent a typical medical practice. Because the costs involved in the practice are a function of the number of physicians in the practice, most of the data presented here are on a per-physician basis.

In 2011, the most recent data available, the average primary care practice employed roughly five full-time equivalent (adjusted to account for part-time staff) physicians. In addition, each practice, on average, employed two nonphysician providers, such as physician assistants and nurse practitioners, and a support staff of about 20. Thus, if we count the nonphysician providers as support staff for the physicians, each physician had about 4.4 individuals working to support her patient services activities.

The total operating cost to support each physician was about $325,000, not including physician compensation. Of these costs, about $160,000 were labor costs, with the remaining costs devoted to facilities, equipment, malpractice insurance, and supplies. Thus, practice costs (again, excluding physician compensation) were about evenly split between labor and nonlabor components. Taking a closer look at support staff costs, about 47 percent of the labor costs were for clinical staff, 34 percent for front-office staff (e.g., receptionists), and 19 percent for business office staff (e.g., coding, billing, collections).

On average, each primary care physician handled about 2,300 patients, who represented about 5,300 encounters (visits), during which the physician performed about 11,000 procedures. Thus, if we use patient visit as the unit of output (volume), the operating cost per visit averages out to be roughly $325,000 ÷ 5,300 = $61 per visit. The data do not break out fixed versus variable costs.

However, variable costs, which consist mostly of administrative supplies (e.g., forms, letterhead) and medical supplies (e.g., rubber gloves, needles, vaccines, dressings), were relatively small, say, $10 per visit. Thus, the underlying cost structure for an average primary care physician looked something like the following:

$$\text{Total costs} = \$272{,}000 + (\$10 \times \text{Number of visits}),$$

(continued)

HEALTHCARE IN PRACTICE
The Cost Structures of Medical Practices *(continued)*

where the $272,000 represents the fixed costs of the practice (primarily facilities and labor) and the $10 represents the average cost of supplies consumed on each visit.

With this information, the support costs (on a per-physician basis) could be estimated for different volumes. For example, the total cost to support 4,500 visits was $317,000, while the cost to support 5,500 visits was $327,000:

$$\begin{aligned}\text{Total costs (4,500 visits)} &= \$272{,}000 + (\$10 \times 4{,}500)\\ &= \$272{,}000 + \$45{,}000\\ &= \$317{,}000\end{aligned}$$

$$\begin{aligned}\text{Total costs (5,500 visits)} &= \$272{,}000 + (\$10 \times 5{,}500)\\ &= \$272{,}000 + \$55{,}000\\ &= \$327{,}000.\end{aligned}$$

In the next chapter, we expand this industry practice discussion to include revenues.

Note: This Healthcare in Practice is based on information provided by the Medical Group Management Association, 2011, *Performance and Practices of Successful Medical Groups*, Englewood, CO: MGMA.

Total costs
The sum of fixed costs and total variable costs.

Average cost
Total costs divided by volume (e.g., if laboratory costs total $300,000 to conduct 15,000 tests, the average cost [per test] is $300,000 ÷ 15,000 = $20).

Fixed costs, in contrast to total variable costs, remain unchanged as the volume varies. When volume doubles from 500 to 1,000 tests, fixed costs remain at $150,000. Because all costs in this example are either fixed or variable, **total costs** are merely the sum of the two. For example, at 5,000 tests, total costs are Fixed costs + Total variable costs = $150,000 + (5,000 × $10) = $150,000 + $50,000 = $200,000. Because variable costs are tied to volume, total variable costs, and hence total costs, increase as the volume increases, even though fixed costs remain constant.

The rightmost column in exhibit 4.1 contains **average cost** per unit of volume, which in this example is average cost per test. It is calculated by dividing total costs by volume. For example, at 5,000 tests, with total costs of $200,000, the average cost per test is $200,000 ÷ 5,000 = $40. Because fixed costs are spread over more tests as volume increases, the average cost per test declines as volume increases. For example, when volume doubles from 5,000 to 10,000 tests, fixed costs remain at $150,000, but fixed cost per test declines from $150,000 ÷ 5,000 = $30 to $150,000 ÷ 10,000 = $15.

With fixed cost per test declining from \$30 to \$15, the average cost per test goes down from \$30 + \$10 = \$40 to \$15 + \$10 = \$25. The fact that higher volume reduces average fixed cost, and therefore average cost per unit of volume, has important implications for profitability related to volume changes. (In economics, the state of declining average cost as volume increases is called **economies of scale**.)

Economies of scale The business situation in which higher volume leads to lower per-unit cost.

The cost behavior presented in exhibit 4.1 in tabular format is presented in graphical format in exhibit 4.2. Here, costs are shown on the vertical (*y*) axis, and volume (number of tests) is shown on the horizontal (*x*) axis. Because fixed costs are independent of volume, they are shown as a horizontal dashed line at \$150,000. Total variable costs appear as an upward-sloping dotted line that starts at the origin (0 tests, \$0 costs) and rises at a rate of \$10 for each additional test. When fixed and total variable costs are combined to obtain total costs, the result is the upward-sloping solid line parallel to the total variable costs line but beginning at the *y*-axis at a value of \$150,000 (the fixed costs amount). In effect, the total costs line is nothing more than the total variable costs line shifted upward by the amount of fixed costs.

Note that exhibit 4.2 is not drawn to scale. Furthermore, the relevant range is unrealistically large. The intent here is to emphasize the general shape of a cost structure graph and not its exact position. Also, note that total variable costs plot as a straight line (linear), because the variable cost rate is assumed to be constant over the relevant range. We assume throughout the book that the variable cost rate is constant, and hence total variable costs are linear, at least within the relevant range. For most healthcare organizations in most situations, such an assumption is not unreasonable.

EXHIBIT 4.2 Cost Structure Graph

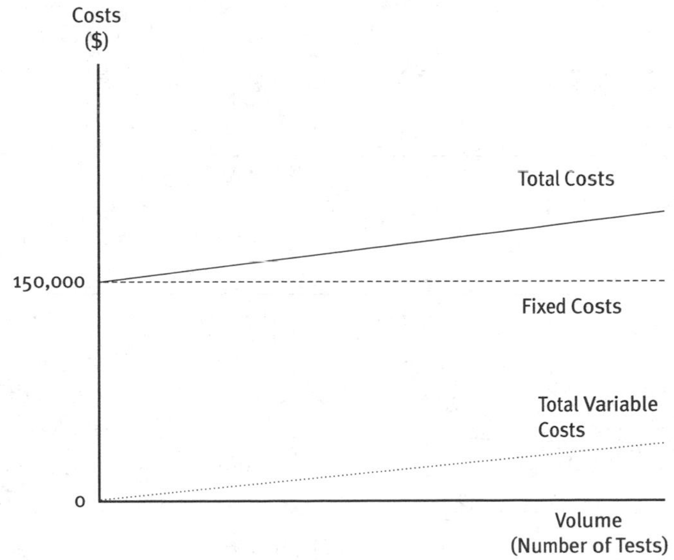

Before we leave this illustration of underlying cost structure, we should mention that fixed and variable costs represent two ends of the volume classification spectrum. Here, in the relevant range, the costs are either independent of volume (fixed) or directly related to volume (variable). A third classification, **semifixed costs**, falls between the two extremes. To illustrate, assume that the actual relevant range of volume for the clinical laboratory is 15,000 to 20,000 tests. However, the laboratory's current workforce can only handle up to 17,500 tests per year, so an additional technician, at an annual cost of $35,000, would be required if volume exceeds that level. Now, labor costs are fixed from 15,000 to 17,500 tests and again at a higher level from 17,500 to 20,000 tests, but they are not fixed at the same level throughout the entire relevant range of 15,000 to 20,000 tests. Semifixed costs are fixed within ranges of volume, but multiple ranges of semifixed costs occur within the relevant range. To keep the illustrations manageable, we do not include semifixed costs in our examples in this book.

Semifixed costs
Costs that are fixed, but not at a single amount throughout the entire relevant range.

SELF-TEST QUESTIONS

1. Define the term *relevant range*.
2. Explain the features and provide examples of fixed and variable costs.
3. How does period affect the definition of fixed costs?
4. What is meant by underlying cost structure?
5. Sketch and explain a simple cost structure diagram similar to exhibit 4.2.
6. What are semifixed costs?

4.4 COST CLASSIFICATION 2: DIRECT VERSUS INDIRECT (OVERHEAD) COSTS

The second major cost classification is by relationship to the unit being analyzed. Some costs—about 50 percent of a large healthcare organization's cost structure—are unique to the reporting subunit and hence usually can be identified with relative certainty. To illustrate, again think in terms of a hospital's clinical laboratory. Certain costs are unique to the laboratory, for example, the salaries and benefits for the technicians who work there and the costs of the equipment and supplies used to conduct the tests. These costs, which would not occur if the laboratory were closed, are classified as the *direct costs* of the department.

Direct costs constitute only a portion of the laboratory's total costs. The remaining resources used by the laboratory are *not* unique to the laboratory; the laboratory shares many resources of the hospital. For example, the laboratory shares the hospital's physical space as well as its infrastructure, which includes information systems, utilities, housekeeping, maintenance, medical records, and general administration. The costs not borne solely by the laboratory but shared by all of the hospital's departments are called *indirect (overhead) costs* (see "Critical Concept: Direct Versus Indirect [Overhead] Costs").

> **CRITICAL CONCEPT**
> Direct Versus Indirect (Overhead) Costs
>
> In addition to their relationship to volume, costs can be classified by their relationship to the unit being analyzed. Those costs that are unique to a department, and hence would disappear if the department were abolished, are called direct costs. Costs incurred from the use of resources shared across the organization are classified as indirect (overhead) costs. For example, the costs of the supplies used by a hospital's emergency department are direct costs; they would disappear if the department were closed. The costs of facilities (the space used) remain, so they represent overhead costs to the emergency department.

Indirect costs, in contrast to direct costs, are more difficult to measure at the department level because they arise from shared resources—that is, if the laboratory were closed, the indirect costs would not disappear. Perhaps some indirect costs could be reduced, but the hospital still requires a basic infrastructure to operate its remaining departments. Note that the direct or indirect classifications have relevance only at the subunit level. When the entire organization is considered, all costs are direct.

The two cost classifications (fixed or variable and direct or indirect) overlay one another. That is, fixed costs typically include both direct and indirect costs, while variable costs generally include only direct costs. For example, the fixed costs of a hospital laboratory include both salaried labor (direct) and facilities (overhead) costs, but the variable costs (reagents and other supplies) are all direct costs. Conversely, direct costs usually include fixed and variable costs, while indirect costs typically include only fixed costs.

Although this mixing of cost classifications can give anyone a headache, the good news is that the classifications typically are used independently of one another.

> **SELF-TEST QUESTIONS**
>
> 1. What is the difference between direct and indirect costs?
> 2. Give some examples of each type of cost for an emergency department.

4.5 COST ALLOCATION

A critical part of cost measurement at the department level is the assignment, or allocation, of overhead costs. **Cost allocation** is a process whereby managers allocate the costs of one department to other departments. Because this process does not occur in a marketplace setting, no observable prices exist for the transferred services. Thus, cost allocation must, to the extent possible, establish prices that mimic those that would be set under market conditions.

> ***Cost allocation***
> The assignment (allocation) of overhead costs, such as financial services costs, from a support department to the patient services departments.

What costs in a health services organization must be allocated? Typically, the costs associated with facilities and support personnel, such as land and buildings, administrators, financial staffs, and housekeeping and maintenance personnel, must be allocated to those departments that generate revenues for the organization (generally, patient services departments). The allocation of support costs to patient services departments is necessary because there would be no need for support costs if there were no patient services departments. Thus, decisions regarding pricing and service offerings by the patient services departments must be based on the **total (full) costs** associated with each service, including both direct and overhead costs. Clearly, the proper allocation of overhead costs is essential to good decision-making in healthcare organizations.

Total (full) costs
The sum of direct and indirect (overhead) costs. Thus, full costs include both direct and overhead costs.

The goal of cost allocation is to assign all of the costs of an organization to the activities that cause them to be incurred. Ideally, healthcare managers track and assign costs by individual patient, physician, diagnosis, reimbursement contract, and so on. With complete cost data available in the organization's managerial accounting system, managers can make informed decisions regarding how to control costs, what services to offer, and how to price those services. Of course, the more data needed, the higher the costs of developing, implementing, and operating the system. As in all situations, the benefits associated with more accurate cost data must be weighed against the costs required to develop such data.

Cost Pools

The first step in allocating costs is to identify the cost pools and the cost drivers. Typically, a cost pool consists of all the direct costs of one support department (see "Critical Concept: Cost Pool"). However, if the services of a single support department differ substantially, and if the patient services departments use the different services in varying proportions, the costs of that support department may need to be separated into multiple pools.

To illustrate multiple cost pools, suppose a hospital's Financial Services Department provides two significantly different services: patient billing and managerial budgeting. Furthermore, assume that the Routine Care Department uses proportionally more patient billing services than the Laboratory Department does, but Laboratory proportionally uses more budgeting services than Routine Care does. In this situation, it would be best to create two cost pools for one support department. The total costs of Financial Services

CRITICAL CONCEPT
Cost Pool

A cost pool is a group of overhead costs to be allocated to the patient services departments. Typically, a cost pool consists of all the direct costs of one overhead department. For example, the costs associated with the Housekeeping Department might constitute a cost pool. However, if an overhead department provides different types of support services, the direct costs of that department might be divided into several cost pools, one for each type of service supplied.

would be divided into a billing pool and a budgeting pool. Then, cost drivers would be chosen for each pool and the costs allocated to the patient services departments as described in the following sections.

> **CRITICAL CONCEPT**
> Cost Drivers
>
> A cost driver is the basis for allocating a cost pool. For example, if the cost pool consists of the direct costs of the Housekeeping Department, then the cost driver might be the amount of space occupied by each patient services department. The theory is that the greater the amount of square footage occupied by a patient services department, the greater the amount of housekeeping services required. Effective cost drivers have two important attributes: They are perceived by all involved as being fair, and they promote organizational cost reduction. Put another way, effective cost drivers allocate the greatest amount of overhead costs to those patient services departments that use the most overhead services and create incentives for department heads to use fewer overhead services.

Cost Drivers

One of the most important steps in the cost allocation process is the identification of proper cost drivers (see "Critical Concept: Cost Drivers"). The theoretical basis for identifying cost drivers is the extent to which the costs from a pool actually vary as the value of the driver changes. A good cost driver provides the most accurate cause-and-effect relationship between the use of services and the costs of the department providing those services, so that more costs are allocated to departments that create the greatest need for support department resources. For example, does a department with 10,000 square feet of space use twice the amount of housekeeping services as a department with only 5,000 square feet of space? The closer the relationship (correlation) between actual overhead resource expenditures at each patient services department and the value of the cost driver, the better the cost driver is and hence the better the resulting cost allocations.

Effective cost drivers possess two primary characteristics. The first is fairness—that is, do the cost drivers chosen result in an allocation that is equitable to the patient services departments? The second, and perhaps more important, characteristic is cost reduction—that is, do the cost drivers chosen create incentives for departments to use fewer overhead services? For example, inpatient department managers can do little to influence overhead cost allocations if the cost driver for administrative support is patient days. In fact, the action needed to reduce the overhead allocation—reduction in patient days—would likely lead to negative financial consequences for the organization. An effective cost driver encourages patient services department managers to take overhead cost reduction actions that do not have negative implications for the organization.

The Allocation Process

Exhibit 4.3 summarizes the steps involved in allocating overhead costs, illustrating how Prairie View Clinic allocated its housekeeping costs for the 2017 budget.

EXHIBIT 4.3
Prairie View Clinic: Allocation of Housekeeping Department Overhead to the Physical Therapy Department

Step One: Determine the cost pool. The departmental costs to be allocated are for the Housekeeping Department, which has total budgeted costs of $100,000.

Step Two: Determine the cost driver. The best cost driver was judged to be the number of hours of housekeeping services provided. An expected total of 10,000 hours of such services will be provided to those departments that will receive the allocation.

Step Three: Calculate the allocation rate. $100,000 ÷ 10,000 hours = $10 per hour of housekeeping services provided.

Step Four: Determine the allocation amount. The Physical Therapy Department uses 3,000 hours of housekeeping services, so its allocation of Housekeeping Department overhead is $10 × 3,000 = $30,000.

First, the cost pool must be established. In this case, the clinic is allocating housekeeping costs, so the cost pool is the projected total direct costs of the Housekeeping Department, $100,000.

Second, the most effective cost driver must be identified. After considerable investigation, Prairie View's managers conclude that the best cost driver for housekeeping costs is labor hours—that is, the number of hours of housekeeping services required by the clinic's departments is the measure most closely related to the actual cost of providing these services. The intent here, as explained earlier, is to pick the cost driver that (1) provides the most accurate cause-and-effect relationship between the use of housekeeping services and the costs of the Housekeeping Department and (2) creates an incentive to use fewer housekeeping services.

Third, the allocation rate must be calculated. For 2017, Prairie View's managers estimate that Housekeeping will provide a total of 10,000 hours of service to the departments that will receive the allocation. Now that the cost pool and cost driver have been defined and measured, the **allocation rate** is established by dividing the expected total overhead cost (the cost pool) by the expected total volume of the cost driver: $100,000 ÷ 10,000 hours = $10 per hour of services provided. (Note that different allocation methods can identify different departments as the ones that will receive the allocation. In the example here, the relevant departments [the patient services departments] receive 10,000 hours of housekeeping service. If we had included the Financial Services Department in the allocation, the total amount of service received might be 10,500 hours.)

Allocation rate
The numerical value used to allocate a cost pool to patient services departments (e.g., $40 per square foot of occupied space).

Fourth, the allocation must be made to each department. To illustrate the allocation, consider the Physical Therapy (PT) Department, one of Prairie View's patient services departments. For 2017, PT is expected to use 3,000 hours of housekeeping services, so the dollar amount of housekeeping overhead allocated is $10 × 3,000 = $30,000.

Other departments in the clinic will also use housekeeping services, and their allocations will be made in a similar manner (see "For Your Consideration: Hospitals and Housekeeping Cost Drivers"). The $10 allocation rate per hour of services used is multiplied

> **FOR YOUR CONSIDERATION**
> Hospitals and Housekeeping Cost Drivers
>
> Many hospitals use square footage to allocate housekeeping costs. The rationale, of course, is that one patient services department that is twice as big as another will require twice the expenditure of housekeeping resources. The advantage of this cost driver is that it is easy to measure and typically remains constant for a relatively long period (department space allotments do not change very often).
>
> The disadvantage of using square footage as the cost driver is that some patient services departments require more housekeeping support per square foot of occupied space because of the nature of the service that the department provides. For example, emergency departments require more intense housekeeping services than do neonatal care units, and surgical suites require more intense services than do routine care departments.
>
> What do you think? Is a more effective cost driver available for allocating housekeeping costs than square footage? If so, what is it? Describe how the suggested cost driver might work.

by the amount of each department's usage of housekeeping services to obtain the dollar allocation. When all patient services departments are considered, the entire clinic is projected to use 10,000 hours of housekeeping services, so the total amount allocated must be $10 × 10,000 = $100,000, which is the amount in the cost pool. For any department, the amount allocated depends on both the allocation rate and the amount of overhead services used.

Cost Allocation Methods

Mathematically, cost allocation can be accomplished in a variety of ways, and the method used is somewhat discretionary. No matter what method is chosen, all support department costs eventually must be allocated to the departments (primarily patient services departments) that create the need for those costs.

The key differences among the methods are how support services provided by one department are allocated to other support departments. Exhibit 4.4 summarizes the three primary allocation methods as applied to Prairie View Clinic. To simplify the illustration, the clinic has only three support departments (Human Resources, Housekeeping, and Administration) and two patient services departments (PT and Internal Medicine).

> ***Direct method***
> A cost allocation method that allocates overhead costs directly to patient services departments. This method does not recognize services provided by one support department to another.

Under the **direct method**, shown in the top section of exhibit 4.4, each support department's costs are allocated directly to the patient services departments that use the services. In the illustration, both PT and Internal Medicine use the services of all three support departments, so the costs of each support department are allocated to both patient

EXHIBIT 4.4
Prairie View Clinic: Alternative Cost Allocation Methods

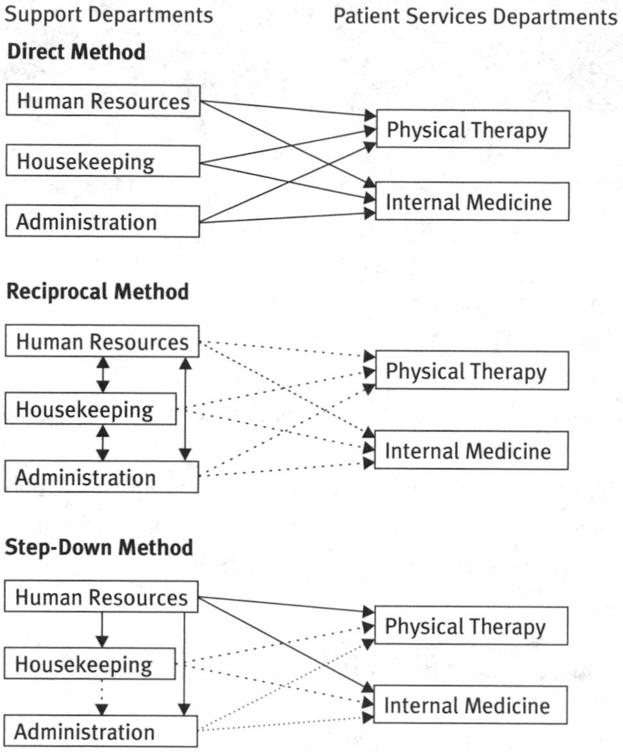

services departments. The key feature of the direct method, and the feature that makes it relatively simple to apply, is that none of the costs of providing support services are allocated to other support departments. In effect, under the direct method, only the direct costs of the support departments are allocated to the patient services departments because no indirect costs have been created by intra–support department allocations.

Reciprocal method
A cost allocation method that fully recognizes all services provided from each support department to other support departments.

As shown in the center section of exhibit 4.4, the **reciprocal method** recognizes the support department interdependencies among Human Resources, Housekeeping, and Administration, and hence the reciprocal method generally is considered more accurate and objective than the direct method. The reciprocal method derives its name from the fact that it recognizes all services that departments provide to and receive from other departments. The good news is that this method captures all of the intra–support department relationships, so no information is ignored and no biases are introduced into the cost allocation process. The bad news is that the reciprocal method relies on the simultaneous solution of a series of equations representing the use of intra–support department services. Thus, it is relatively complex, which makes explaining it to department heads difficult and implementing it costly.

Step-down method
A cost allocation method that partially recognizes services provided from support departments to other support departments.

The **step-down method**, which is shown in the lower section of exhibit 4.4, represents a compromise between the simplicity of the direct method and the complexity of the reciprocal method. It recognizes some of the intra–support department effects that the direct method ignores, but it does not recognize the full range of interdependencies. The step-down method derives its name from the sequential, stairstep pattern of the allocation process, which requires that the allocation take place in a specific sequence.

Here is how it works. First, all the direct costs of Human Resources are allocated to both the patient services departments and the other two support departments. Human Resources is then closed out because all its costs have been allocated. Next, Housekeeping costs, which now consist of both the direct costs of Housekeeping and indirect costs (the allocation from Human Resources), are allocated to the patient services departments and the remaining support department—Administration. Finally, the direct costs of Administration and the indirect costs (the allocations from Human Resources and Housekeeping) are allocated to the patient services departments. The final allocation includes Human Resources, Housekeeping, and Administration costs because a portion of these support costs has been "stepped down" to Administration.

The critical difference between the step-down and reciprocal methods is that after each allocation is made in the step-down method, a support department is removed from the process. Even though Housekeeping and Administration provide support services back to Human Resources, these indirect costs are not recognized because Human Resources is removed from the allocation process after the initial allocation. Such costs are recognized in the reciprocal method.

Self-Test Questions

1. What is the goal of cost allocation?
2. Under what conditions should a single overhead department be divided into multiple cost pools?
3. On what theoretical basis are cost drivers chosen?
4. What two characteristics make an effective cost driver?
5. What are the four steps in the cost allocation process?
6. What are the three primary methods of cost allocation? How do they differ?

4.6 SERVICE LINE COSTING

While cost measurement at the department level can help managers make decisions about pricing and service offerings, the holy grail of cost estimation is costing at the individual service or patient level. Understanding costs at the microlevel allows managers to focus on cost containment and to make better decisions when negotiating contracts with payers. Several methods are used to estimate costs at the service or patient level. We start this

Cost-to charge ratio (CCR)
A ratio used to estimate the overhead costs of individual services. Defined as the ratio of indirect (overhead) costs to charges (or alternatively, to service revenues).

Relative value unit (RVU)
A measure of the amount of resources consumed to provide a particular service.

Activity-based costing (ABC)
An upstream approach to costing that relies on the premise that all costs in an organization stem from activities in or across departments.

section by discussing two traditional costing methods: **cost-to-charge ratio (CCR)** and **relative value unit (RVU)**. Next, we discuss a bottom-up method called **activity-based costing (ABC)**.

The Setting

To illustrate costing at the service level, consider Tarheel Family Practice (TFP), a large physician group that provides multiple services to its patient population. TFP is organized into five departments, one of which is the Routine Services Department. For ease of discussion, we assume that the department provides only two services: X and Y. Data relevant to our illustrations are summarized in exhibit 4.5.

The department has 10,000 visits annually, split evenly between the two services (service X and service Y). The department's total annual costs come to $1,027,500. These costs include the following: $300,000 of department overhead (including both TFP overhead allocated to the department through a step-down cost allocation and department overhead that supports both services); $242,500 in direct costs of service X; and $485,000 in direct costs of service Y. The department's charges (based on chargemaster prices) total $2,100,000, while actual revenues (reimbursements) total $1,300,000, split between the two services, as shown in exhibit 4.5. Before we begin discussing the individual costing methods, we want to emphasize that this example is highly simplified. Its purpose is merely to give you a flavor of the alternative methods available for costing individual services.

Cost-to-Charge (CCR) Method

The cost-to-charge (CCR) method is the most basic of the three methods for costing individual services. The CCR method is based on two assumptions:

1. The indirect costs allocated to the services constitute a single cost that is proportional across all services provided. In other words, each service consumes indirect costs in the same proportion as the department as a whole.
2. Charges, or alternatively reimbursement rates, reflect the level of intensity of the service provided and hence the use of shared resources by each service, including both TFP and department overhead.

We will begin by focusing on charges. With indirect (overhead) costs of $300,000 supporting total charges of $2,100,000, the cost-to-charge ratio is CCR = Indirect costs ÷ Total charges = $300,000 ÷ $2,100,000 = 0.143 = 14.3%. Once the CCR has been calculated for the department, it is used to estimate the overhead costs for each individual service:

$$\text{Service overhead costs} = \text{CCR} \times \text{Service charges}.$$

EXHIBIT 4.5
Tarheel Family Practice: Selected Routine Services Department Data

	Service X	Service Y	Total
Annual volume (visits)	5,000	5,000	10,000
RVUs per service	10	18	
Annual costs:			
Direct	$ 242,500	$ 485,000	$ 727,500
Indirect (overhead)			300,000
Total costs			$1,027,500
Annual charges	$ 700,000	$1,400,000	$2,100,000
Annual revenues (reimbursements)	$ 400,000	$ 900,000	$1,300,000

Source: Reprinted from L. Gapenski and K. Reiter, *Healthcare Finance: An Introduction to Accounting and Financial Management*, 6th ed., Chicago: Health Administration Press.

Thus, the overhead cost allocation for service X is 0.143 × $700,000 = $100,100. Similarly, the overhead cost allocation for service Y is 0.143 × $1,400,000 = $200,200. The total amount of overhead allocated to the two services is $100,100 + $200,200 = $300,300, which, except for a rounding error, equals the $300,000 in total indirect costs for the department.

Finally, to obtain the full costs of each service line, merely add the direct costs to the amounts allocated for overhead:

Full (total) service costs = Direct cost + Indirect cost.

The full costs of service X are $242,500 + $100,100 = $342,600 and the cost per one visit for service X is $342,600 ÷ 5,000 visits = $68.52. The full costs of service Y are $485,000 + $200,200 = $685,200 and the cost per one visit for service Y is $685,200 ÷ 5,000 visits = $137.04. As a check, the full costs of both services total $342,600 + $685,200 = $1,027,800, which once again equals the total costs of the department, except for a rounding error.

Note that revenues can be used as an alternative to charges in the CCR method (see "For Your Consideration: Charges Versus Revenues in the CCR Method"). The procedure is the same as described earlier, but now revenues are used to calculate the CCR. With indirect (overhead) costs of $300,000 supporting total revenues (reimbursements) of $1,300,000, CCR = $300,000 ÷ $1,300,000 = 0.231 = 23.1%. Using this new value for the CCR, and revenues in lieu of charges, the overhead cost allocation for service X is 0.231 × $400,000 = $92,400. The overhead cost allocation for service Y is 0.231 × $900,000 = $207,900. Finally, to obtain the full costs of each service line, allocated overhead costs are added to the

> **FOR YOUR CONSIDERATION**
> **Charges Versus Revenues in the CCR Method**
>
> This chapter's illustration of the cost-to-charge ratio (CCR) method of costing at the service level presented two possible approaches: using charges as the basis of the allocation and using revenues (reimbursements) as the basis of the allocation.
>
> Healthcare providers using the CCR method—and many do—must make a choice. (For some Medicare calculations, the use of charges is required. However, for internal use, providers may use either charges or revenues.) In theory, the choice should reflect the metric (charges or revenues) that best mimics the relationship to the amount of overhead resources consumed. Is that metric charges or revenues? Charges supposedly reflect the underlying costs of the service—the higher the charges, the higher the costs. However, much anecdotal evidence indicates that charges are not a good reflection of costs (for example, a charge of $25 for an aspirin administered in the hospital). On the other hand, are revenues a better reflection of costs? Private insurers, Medicare, and Medicaid often have large differences in reimbursement amounts for the same service.
>
> What do you think? Should the CCR method use charges or revenues as the metric? What justification is there to support your answer?

direct costs of each service. The resulting full costs of service X are $242,500 + $92,400 = $334,900 and the full costs of service Y are $485,000 + $207,900 = $692,900. As a check, the full costs of both services total $334,900 + $692,900 = $1,027,800, and except for a rounding error, this once again equals the total costs of the department.

Relative Value Unit (RVU) Method

Relative value unit (RVU) method
A method for estimating the overhead costs of individual services based on the intensity of the service provided as measured by RVUs.

In contrast to the CCR method, which ties overhead resource consumption to charges (or revenues), the **relative value unit (RVU) method** ties the use of overhead resources to the complexity and time required for each service. In other words, this method uses the intensity of the service provided, as measured by RVUs, as the basis for allocating overhead. As we discussed in chapter 3 (in "Healthcare in Practice: How Medicare Pays Providers"), its use in healthcare pricing and reimbursement was influenced primarily by the resource-based relative value scale system, which uses RVUs to set Medicare payments for physician services.

To begin our illustration of the RVU method, assume that a study by the medical director of Tarheel Family Practice identified the number of RVUs required to perform each service. The result was the assignment of 10 RVUs for service X and 18 RVUs for service Y as shown in exhibit 4.5. (RVU estimates for many healthcare services are available from several sources including Medicare and professional associations.)

To calculate service-level costs using the RVU method, first, the RVUs for each service are multiplied by the annual volume for each service, and the products are summed to obtain the total RVUs for the department. For example, for service X, the total RVUs are 10 RVUs × 5,000 visits = 50,000 RVUs. Total RVUs for service Y are 18 RVUs × 5,000 visits = 90,000 RVUs. Total RVUs for the department = 50,000 + 90,000 = 140,000 RVUs.

Now with department overhead costs of $300,000 to support 140,000 RVUs, the overhead cost per RVU is $300,000 ÷ 140,000 = $2.143. The final step in the overhead cost allocation is to multiply the cost per RVU by the total number of RVUs of each service to obtain the overhead allocation. For example, the overhead allocated to service X is $2.143 × 50,000 = $107,150. The overhead allocated to Service Y is $2.143 × 90,000 = $192,870. As a check, the total allocated overhead equals $107,150 + $192,870 = $300,020, which, except for a rounding error, is equal to the total overhead of $300,000 shown in exhibit 4.5.

Now, the total costs of each service are merely the direct costs of the service plus the overhead allocation. The total (full) costs of service X are $242,500 + $107,150 = $349,650, and the total costs of service Y are $485,000 + $192,870 = $677,870. The cost per visit for service X is $349,650 ÷ 5,000 visits = $69.93 and the cost per visit for service Y is $677,870 ÷ 5,000 visits = $135.57. As a final check, note that the total costs of each service sum to $1,027,520, which, except for a small rounding error, equals the total costs of the department, $1,027,500.

The goal of RVU costing is to reflect the cost of the overhead resources used to provide the service. Of course, the key to the fairness of RVU costing is how well the number of RVUs assigned to each service matches the cost of the overhead resources consumed. Because of the difficulties involved in initially assigning RVU values to services, this method is used most often when RVU values have already been estimated, such as for procedures performed by physicians.

Activity-Based Costing

Our discussion thus far has focused on **traditional costing** methods. In essence, the traditional methods begin with aggregate costs, typically at the department level. Overhead costs are then allocated downstream, first to the patient services departments and then, using the CCR or RVU method, down to individual services. Thus, traditional methods can be thought of as top-down allocation. Although traditional costing works well for estimating full costs at the department level, its usefulness for estimating the costs of activities in or across departments—such as individual tests, services, or diagnoses—or by individual patients is limited.

Traditional costing
The top-down approach to costing that first identifies costs at the department level and then (potentially) assigns these costs to individual services.

> **CRITICAL CONCEPT**
> Activity-Based Costing
>
> Activity-based costing (ABC) is an alternative to traditional costing. Consider the costs associated with a particular service. To apply ABC costing, first identify the activities needed to provide the service. Next, estimate the cost of each activity. The sum of the activity costs, then, reflects the cost of providing that service. For example, the activities required to give a vaccination might include check-in, administration of the shot, recording the treatment, and checkout. In ABC, the cost of each activity would be estimated (including supplies and overhead costs) on a per-vaccination basis and then summed to estimate the cost of a vaccination visit.

ABC uses an upstream approach to cost allocation (see "Critical Concept: Activity-Based Costing"). Its premise is that all costs in an organization stem from activities, hence its name. In ABC, because activities are considered the basic building blocks of costs, costs can be more easily assigned to individual patients, individual physicians, particular diagnoses, reimbursement contracts, managed care populations, and so on than in traditional costing.

The steps required to implement ABC are as follows:

- Identify the relevant activities.
- Determine the cost of each activity, including equipment, supplies, and both direct and overhead costs.
- Determine the cost driver for each activity.
- Collect activity data for each service and calculate an allocation rate for each activity.
- Calculate the total cost of the service by aggregating activity costs.

To illustrate ABC, suppose that seven activities are performed by the Routine Services Department of Tarheel Family Practice: (1) patient check-in, including insurance verification; (2) preliminary assessment; (3) diagnosis; (4) treatment; (5) prescription writing; (6) patient checkout; and (7) third-party payer billing. Furthermore, assume that the clinic has 10,000 visits annually split evenly between the two services: X and Y. (Before we go further, note that this example is highly simplified. Its purpose is merely to give you a taste of how ABC works.)

Exhibit 4.6 contains the initial data and allocation rate calculations. For example, the annual costs of patient check-in, consisting of clerical labor and supplies (direct costs) plus space and other overhead (indirect costs), are $50,000 to support 10,000 total visits. Because the cost driver for patient check-in is visits, the allocation rate is $5 per visit, calculated as $50,000 ÷ 10,000 visits = $5. Also, the total (direct labor by a nurse and overhead) costs required to conduct the initial assessment is $75,000, spread over (5,000 visits × 5 minutes for X) + (5,000 visits × 10 minutes for Y) = 25,000 + 50,000 = 75,000 minutes annually, giving an allocation rate of $1 per minute calculated as $75,000 ÷ 75,000 minutes = $1.

Exhibit 4.6
ABC Illustration: Initial Data and Allocation Rate Calculation

Activity	Annual Costs	Cost Driver	Service X	Service Y	Total Units of the Cost Driver	Allocation Rate
Check-in	$ 50,000	Number of visits	5,000	5,000	10,000	$ 5.00
Assessment	75,000	Number of minutes per visit	5	10	75,000	1.00
Diagnosis	250,000	Number of minutes per visit	10	15	125,000	2.00
Treatment	450,000	Number of minutes per visit	10	20	150,000	3.00
Prescription	2,500	Number of drugs prescribed per visit	0.5	2.0	12,500	0.20
Checkout	50,000	Number of visits	5,000	5,000	10,000	5.00
Billing	150,000	Number of bills per visit	1.0	2.0	15,000	10.00
Total costs	$1,027,500					

As shown in exhibit 4.7, the final step is to aggregate the activity costs for each service. Note that this step is performed on a per-visit basis. For example, for service X, the cost of check-in is 1 visit × $5.00 per visit = $5.00, the cost of assessment is 5 minutes per visit × $1.00 per minute = $5.00, and the cost of diagnosis is 10 minutes per visit × $2.00 per minute = $20.00. Other activity costs for the two services are calculated in a similar manner.

The result of summing the individual activity costs associated with each service is a total cost of $75.10 per visit for service X and $130.40 per visit for service Y. The ability of the family practice to estimate the costs of its individual services allows the services to be priced properly (on the basis of costs). In addition, cost control is made easier because the activities, and hence resource expenditures, associated with each service have been clearly identified.

Note that the total annual costs of providing service X are 5,000 visits × $75.10 = $375,500, while the total costs for service Y are 5,000 visits × $130.40 = $652,000. Because we only have two services in this simple example, the total costs of the practice are $375,500 + $652,000 = $1,027,500, which equals the total cost amount identified in exhibit 4.6.

Exhibit 4.7
ABC Illustration: Final Aggregation of Activity Costs per Visit

			Service X		Service Y	
Activity	**Cost Driver**	**Rate**	**Consumption of Cost Driver**	**Cost**	**Consumption of Cost Driver**	**Cost**
Check-in	Number of visits	$ 5.00	1	$ 5.00	1	$ 5.00
Assessment	Number of minutes	1.00	5	5.00	10	10.00
Diagnosis	Number of minutes	2.00	10	20.00	15	30.00
Treatment	Number of minutes	3.00	10	30.00	20	60.00
Prescription	Number of drugs	0.20	0.5	0.10	2.0	0.40
Check out	Number of visits	5.00	1	5.00	1	5.00
Billing	Number of bills	10.00	1.0	10.00	2.0	20.00
Total cost per service				$75.10		$130.40

ABC allows managers to estimate the costs of individual services and hence provides managers with information that can be used in pricing and contract negotiations. However, the data and resource requirements to establish an ABC system far exceed those required for traditional costing. For this reason, traditional costing still dominates the healthcare arena, but ABC is becoming more prevalent as the need for better cost data increasingly becomes important and providers invest in newer and more powerful managerial accounting systems.

Self-Test Questions

1. What are the two traditional service line costing methods?
2. What two assumptions is the CCR method based on?
3. What is overhead allocation tied to in the RVU method?
4. What are the key differences between traditional and ABC?
5. Why does ABC hold so much promise for healthcare providers?

THEME WRAP-UP: COST STRUCTURE

What did Jen learn about the cost structure at Big Sky Dermatology Specialists? First, the good news: Because the practice is relatively small, with two dermatologists and a support staff, it does not have a departmental organization. To think of it another way, the entire practice is a single department. Thus, Jen does not have to grapple with allocating overhead costs from one department to another. Certainly, the practice has both patient services functions and overhead functions, but they all operate in a single organizational structure.

On the other hand, the practice does have both fixed and variable costs. (Finding a healthcare provider with either all fixed costs or all variable costs would be impossible, although, as shown in the next chapter, businesses can have an incentive to move their cost structures in one direction or the other.)

After some research, Jen concluded that Big Sky's cost structure (not including physician compensation) can be expressed as follows:

$$\begin{aligned}\text{Total costs} &= \text{Fixed costs} + \text{Total variable costs}\\ &= \text{Fixed costs} + (\text{Variable cost rate} \times \text{Volume})\\ &= \$850{,}000 + (\$15 \times 10{,}000 \text{ visits})\\ &= \$850{,}000 + \$150{,}000\\ &= \$1{,}000{,}000.\end{aligned}$$

Furthermore, the relevant range is 8,000 to 12,000 visits. Thus, if the number of visits were at the bottom of the range (8,000), total support costs would be

$$\begin{aligned}\text{Total costs} &= \$850{,}000 + (\$15 \times 8{,}000 \text{ visits})\\ &= \$850{,}000 + \$120{,}000\\ &= \$970{,}000.\end{aligned}$$

However, if the number of visits were at the top of the range (12,000), total support costs would equal

$$\begin{aligned}\text{Total costs} &= \$850{,}000 + (\$15 \times 12{,}000 \text{ visits})\\ &= \$850{,}000 + \$180{,}000\\ &= \$1{,}030{,}000.\end{aligned}$$

With this knowledge of Big Sky's cost structure, the next job that Jen must tackle is to combine the practice's cost structure with its revenues to examine the practice's expected profitability. We will help Jen with that task in the next chapter.

Key Concepts

This chapter points out that managers rely on managerial accounting information to plan for and control a business's operations. A critical part of this information is the measurement and allocation of costs. Here are the key concepts:

- Costs can be classified by their relationship to the amount of services provided. Variable costs are expected to increase and decrease with volume (patient days, number of visits, and so on), while fixed costs are expected to remain constant regardless of volume (within some relevant range).
- The relationship between cost and activity (volume) is called *underlying cost structure,* or just *cost structure*.
- Costs can also be classified according to their relationship to the unit being analyzed. *Direct costs* are the unique (exclusive) resources used only by one unit of an organization, such as a department, and therefore are fairly easy to measure. *Indirect (overhead) costs*, in contrast, are inherently difficult to measure at the unit level because they constitute a shared resource of the overall organization, such as administrative costs.
- Cost allocation is a critical part of the costing process because it addresses the issue of how to assign the costs of support activities to the revenue-producing (patient services) departments. The goal of cost allocation is to assign all costs of an organization to the activities that cause them to be incurred.
- A *cost pool* is the dollar amount of one type of overhead services to be allocated. In general, a cost pool consists of the total costs of one support department. However, under some circumstances, it may be better to divide the costs of a single support department into multiple cost pools.
- A *cost driver* is the basis for making allocations from a cost pool. Cost drivers are chosen on the basis of their positive correlation with the amount of overhead services used by the patient services departments.
- An effective cost driver is fair and will promote cost reduction in the organization.
- The three primary methods for cost allocation are *direct*, *reciprocal*, and *step down*. Regardless of the allocation method, all costs eventually end up being allocated to the patient services departments.
- The *direct method* recognizes no intra–support department services. Thus, support department costs are allocated exclusively to patient services departments.
- The *reciprocal method* recognizes all intra–support department services. However, the reciprocal method is the most difficult to understand and to implement.

- The *step-down method* represents a compromise between the direct and reciprocal methods that recognizes some intra–support department services.
- The primary methods for costing individual services are (1) *cost-to-charge ratio (CCR)*, (2) *relative value unit (RVU)*, and (3) *activity-based costing (ABC)*.
- Activity-based costing (ABC) allocates costs on the basis of the activities that create costs in the first place. Thus, ABC can estimate costs for individual services more precisely than traditional costing methods, and can even estimate costs for individual patients, diagnoses, physicians, reimbursement contracts, and so on. However, ABC requires a more sophisticated and costly managerial accounting information system than does traditional costing.

This chapter contains a great deal of detail, but the most important concept to remember is that a sound cost estimation system is required for making good managerial decisions. We extend the discussion in chapter 5, which covers pricing decisions and profit analysis.

End-of-Chapter Questions

4.1 Explain the difference between fixed and variable costs.

4.2 a. What is meant by a business's underlying cost structure?
b. Why is this information valuable to managers?

4.3 What cost structure creates economies of scale? Why?

4.4 What are the primary differences between direct and indirect (overhead) costs?

4.5 What is the goal of cost allocation?

4.6 a. What is a cost pool?
b. What is a cost driver?
c. How is the cost allocation rate determined?

4.7 Under what circumstances should an overhead department be divided into multiple cost pools?

4.8 Effective cost drivers, and hence the resulting allocation system, must have what two important attributes?

4.9 Briefly describe (illustrate) the cost allocation process.

4.10 a. What are the three primary methods of cost allocation?
b. What are the differences among them?

4.11 Which is the better cost driver for a hospital's Financial Services Department—patient services revenues or number of bills generated? Explain your rationale.

4.12 Describe the following methods used to estimate the cost of individual services:
   a. Cost-to-charge ratio (CCR) method
   b. Relative value unit (RVU) method
   c. Activity-based costing (ABC) method

4.13 How does ABC differ from traditional costing?

End-of-Chapter Problems

4.1 Assume that a radiology group practice has the following cost structure:

Fixed costs = $500,000 Variable cost per procedure = $25

Furthermore, assume that the group expects to perform 7,500 procedures in the coming year.
   a. What is the group's underlying cost structure?
   b. What are the group's expected total costs?
   c. What are the group's estimated total costs at 5,000 procedures? At 10,000 procedures?
   d. What is the average cost per procedure at 5,000, 7,500, and 10,000 procedures?

4.2 You are considering starting a walk-in clinic. Your financial projections for the first year of operations are as follows:

Number of visits	10,000	Utilities	$ 2,500
Wages and benefits	$220,000	Medical supplies	$50,000
Rent	$ 5,000	Administrative supplies	$ 10,000
Depreciation	$ 30,000		

Assume that all costs are fixed except supplies costs, which are variable.
   a. What is the clinic's underlying cost structure?
   b. What are the clinic's expected total costs?
   c. What are the clinic's estimated total costs at 7,500 visits? At 12,500 visits?
   d. What is the average cost per visit at 7,500, 10,000, and 12,500 visits?

4.3 General Hospital, a not-for-profit acute care facility, has estimated the following costs for its inpatient services:

Fixed costs $10,000,000 Variable cost per inpatient day $200

The hospital expects to have 15,000 inpatient days next year.

a. What is the hospital's underlying cost structure?
b. What are the hospital's expected total costs?
c. What are the hospital's estimated total costs at 12,500 inpatient days? At 17,500 inpatient days?
d. What is the average cost per inpatient day at 12,500, 15,000, and 17,500 inpatient days?

4.4 The Housekeeping Services Department of Ruger Clinic, a multispecialty practice in Toledo, Ohio, had $100,000 in direct costs during the year. These costs must be allocated to Ruger's three revenue-producing patient services departments using the direct method. Two cost drivers are under consideration: patient services revenue and hours of housekeeping services used. The patient services departments generated a total of $5 million in revenues during the year. To support these clinical activities, the departments used 5,000 total hours of housekeeping services.

a. What is the value of the cost pool?
b. What is the allocation rate if (1) patient services revenue is used as the cost driver and if (2) hours of housekeeping services are used as the cost driver?

4.5 Refer to problem 4.4. Assume that the three patient services departments are Adult Services, Pediatric Services, and Other Services. The patient services revenue and hours of housekeeping services for each department are as follows:

Department	Revenue	Housekeeping Hours
Adult Services	$3,000,000	1,500
Pediatric Services	1,500,000	3,000
Other Services	500,000	500
Total	$5,000,000	5,000

a. What is the dollar allocation to each patient services department if patient services revenue is used as the cost driver?
b. What is the dollar allocation to each patient services department if hours of housekeeping support are used as the cost driver?
c. What is the dollar difference in the amount allocated to each department between the two drivers?
d. Which of the two drivers is better? Why?

The following data pertain to problems 4.6 through 4.8.

St. Benedict's Hospital has three support departments and four patient services departments. The direct costs to each support department are:

General Administration	$2,000,000
Facilities	5,000,000
Financial Services	3,000,000

Selected data for the three support and four patient services departments are as follows:

Department	Patient Services Revenue	Space (Square Feet)	Housekeeping Labor Hours	Salary Dollars
Support				
General Administration		10,000	2,000	$ 1,500,000
Facilities		20,000	5,000	3,000,000
Financial Services		15,000	3,000	2,000,000
Total		45,000	10,000	$ 6,500,000
Patient services				
Routine Care	$30,000,000	400,000	150,000	$12,000,000
Intensive Care	4,000,000	40,000	30,000	5,000,000
Diagnostic Services	6,000,000	60,000	15,000	6,000,000
Other Services	10,000,000	100,000	25,000	7,000,000
Total	$50,000,000	600,000	220,000	$30,000,000
Grand total	$50,000,000	645,000	230,000	$36,500,000

4.6 Assume that the hospital uses the direct method for cost allocation. Furthermore, the cost driver for General Administration and Financial Services is patient services revenue, while the cost driver for Facilities is space usage.

a. What are the appropriate allocation rates?

b. Allocate the hospital's overhead costs to the patient services departments.

4.7 Assume that the hospital uses the direct method for cost allocation. Furthermore, salary is the cost driver for General Administration, housekeeping labor hours is the cost driver for Facilities, and patient services revenue is the cost driver for Financial Services. (The majority of the costs of the Facilities Department are devoted to housekeeping services.)
   a. What are the appropriate allocation rates?
   b. Allocate the hospital's overhead costs to the patient services departments.
   c. Compare the dollar allocations with those obtained in problem 4.6. Explain the differences.
   d. Which of the two cost-driver schemes is better? Explain your answer.

4.8 Now assume that $2 million of Financial Services costs are related to billing and managerial reporting and $1 million are related to payroll and personnel management activities.
   a. Devise and implement a direct method cost allocation scheme that recognizes that Financial Services has two widely different functions.
   b. What, if any, additional information would be useful in completing part a?
   c. What are the costs and benefits to St. Benedict's of creating two cost pools for Financial Services?

4.9 Consider the data for a clinical laboratory and then answer questions 4.9a–4.9c.
   a. Using ABC techniques, determine the allocation rate for each activity.
   b. Now, using this allocation rate, estimate the total cost of performing each test.
   c. Verify that the total annual costs aggregated from individual test costs equal the total annual costs of the laboratory given in the data.

			Activity Data			
Activity	**Annual Costs**	**Cost Driver**	**Test A**	**Test B**	**Test C**	**Test D**
Receive specimen	$ 10,000	No. of tests	2,000	1,500	1,000	500
Set up equipment	25,000	No. of mins. per test	5	5	10	10
Run test	100,000	No. of mins. per test	1	5	10	20
Record results	10,000	No. of mins. per test	2	2	2	4
Transmit results	5,000	No. of mins. per test	3	3	3	3
Total overhead costs	$150,000					

CHAPTER 5

PRICING DECISIONS AND PROFIT ANALYSIS

THEME SET-UP: PROFIT ANALYSIS

As you know from chapters 3 and 4, Jen Latimer is the new manager at Big Sky Dermatology Specialists, a small group practice in Jackson, Wyoming. After reviewing the practice's revenue sources and examining its cost structure, Jen was ready to combine Big Sky's cost and revenue structures to get a feel for next year's profit potential. (Jen was accounting for all costs, except for physician compensation, so the "profit" projection was, in reality, the compensation available for the two physicians.) Jen knew that the practice's profitability could be analyzed using a technique called profit analysis. (Accountants call this technique cost-volume-profit analysis.) She already identified the practice's cost structure. At an expected (base case) volume of 10,000 visits, total costs were forecasted to be $1,000,000:

$$\begin{aligned} \text{Total costs} &= \text{Fixed costs} + \text{Total variable costs} \\ &= \text{Fixed costs} + (\text{Variable cost rate} \times \text{Volume}) \\ &= \$850{,}000 + (\$15 \times 10{,}000 \text{ visits}) \\ &= \$850{,}000 + \$150{,}000 \\ &= \$1{,}000{,}000. \end{aligned}$$

Now, Jen must fold in the revenue structure of the practice. This process will allow her to analyze the impact of different volume assumptions on the practice's profitability. (In addition, she can analyze the impact of different revenue and cost assumptions.)

By the end of this chapter, you will have a better grasp of profit analysis and its benefit to healthcare managers. In addition, you, like Jen, will be able to examine Big Sky's profitability under varying assumptions of volume, costs, and revenues.

Learning Objectives

After studying this chapter, you will be able to do the following:

- Explain the difference between price setters and price takers.
- Differentiate full-cost pricing from marginal cost pricing.
- Describe how target costing is used.
- Conduct profit analyses to learn the impact of volume changes on profitability and to determine breakeven points.
- Discuss the primary differences in profit analyses between fee-for-service and capitation reimbursement.
- Explain how revenue and cost structures affect a healthcare organization's risk.

5.1 INTRODUCTION

One of the most important uses of managerial accounting data is to establish a price for a particular service or, given a price, to determine whether the service will be profitable. For example, in a charge-based environment, healthcare managers must set prices on the services their organizations offer. Managers also must determine whether to offer volume discounts to valued payer groups, such as managed care plans or business coalitions, and how large these discounts should be.

After prices are set, managers can estimate revenues on the basis of volume estimates. Furthermore, the business's revenue structure (volumes coupled with reimbursement rates) can be combined with its cost structure to forecast profits under a wide range of operating assumptions. Having some knowledge of future profitability requirements, and the prices (and hence revenues) for attaining profitability, is critical for good financial decision-making.

This chapter discusses pricing strategies and profit analysis. Along the way, it covers other important healthcare finance principles.

5.2 HEALTHCARE PROVIDERS AND THE POWER TO SET PRICES

A healthcare provider's power to set prices falls somewhere along a spectrum of two extremes. At one extreme, providers have no power whatsoever and must accept the prices (reimbursement amounts) set by the marketplace. At the other extreme, providers can set any prices desired (within reason), and payers must accept those prices. Clearly, few real-world markets for healthcare services support such extreme positions. Nevertheless, thinking in such terms can help healthcare managers understand the pricing decisions they face.

Providers as Price Takers

If a healthcare organization is one of many providers in a service area that has numerous purchasers (typically third-party payers), and if little distinguishes the services offered by the various providers, then economic theory suggests that the prices are set by local supply-and-demand conditions. Furthermore, the actions of a single participant—whether a provider or payer—cannot influence the prices set in the marketplace. In such a perfectly competitive market, healthcare providers are said to be **price takers** because they are constrained by (or must accept) the prices set in the marketplace.

Price taker
A provider that has no power to influence the prices set by the marketplace.

Few markets for healthcare services are perfectly competitive. But some payers—notably government payers and managed care plans with market power—can set reimbursement levels on a take-it-or-leave-it basis. In this situation, as in competitive markets, providers are price takers in the sense that they have very little influence over reimbursement rates. Because many markets either are somewhat competitive or are dominated by large payer groups, and because government payers cover a significant proportion of the population, most providers probably qualify as price takers for a large percentage of their revenue.

In general, providers that are price takers must take price as a given and concentrate managerial efforts on cost structure and utilization to ensure that their services are profitable. Thus, price takers are just as concerned about costs as are price setters (discussed in the next section).

From a purely financial perspective, a price-taking provider should offer all profitable services, even when the price is reduced by discounting or other market actions. Although this approach to service decisions is obviously simplistic, it does raise an important issue: What costs are relevant to the decision at hand? To ensure long-term sustainability, prices must cover full (all) costs. However, prices that do not cover full costs may be acceptable for short periods, and it might be in the provider's best interests to accept such prices.

Providers as Price Setters

Healthcare providers with market dominance enjoy large market shares and hence exercise some pricing power. Within limits, such providers can decide what prices to set on the services offered. Furthermore, if a provider's services can be differentiated from others on the basis of quality, convenience, or another characteristic, the provider also has the ability, again within limits, to set prices on the differentiated services. Healthcare providers that have such pricing power are called **price setters**.

Price setter
A provider that has the power (within reason) to set market prices for its services.

Accounting for market conditions when making forecasts or decisions about service offerings would be much easier for healthcare managers if a provider's status as a price taker or a price setter were fixed for all payers, for all services, for long periods. But the healthcare market is ever changing, and providers can quickly move from one status to the other. For example, the merger of two healthcare providers may create sufficient market power to change two price takers (as separate entities) into one price setter (as a combined entity). Furthermore, providers can be price takers for some services (or some third-party payers or some geographic markets) and price setters for others.

? Self-Test Questions

1. What is the difference between a price taker and a price setter?
2. Are healthcare providers generally either price takers or price setters exclusively? Explain your answer.

5.3 PRICE-SETTING STRATEGIES

When providers are price setters, alternative strategies can be used to price healthcare services. No single strategy is most appropriate in all situations. In this section, we discuss the two price-setting strategies most frequently used by healthcare organizations.

Full-Cost Pricing

> **CRITICAL CONCEPT**
> Full-Cost Pricing
>
> In full-cost pricing, prices are set to cover all costs associated with providing a particular service. Thus, the price must cover both direct and overhead costs. In addition, to truly cover all costs of doing business, including economic costs, the price must include a profit component. All providers, even not-for-profit ones, must earn a profit to ensure the ability to replace assets as needed, invest in new technologies, and expand facilities to meet growing community needs.

Full-cost pricing recognizes that to remain viable in the long run, healthcare organizations must set prices that recover all costs associated with operating the business (see "Critical Concept: Full-Cost Pricing"). Thus, the full cost of a service—whether a patient day in a hospital, a visit to a clinic, a laboratory test, or the treatment of a particular diagnosis—must include the following: (1) the direct variable costs of providing the service, (2) the direct fixed costs, and (3) the appropriate share of the overhead expenses of the organization.

Because allocating overhead costs is complicated (see chapter 4), the full costs of an individual service are difficult to determine with precision and hence have to be viewed as merely an estimate of the true costs. Nevertheless, in the aggregate, revenues must cover both direct and overhead costs, and hence prices in total must cover all costs of an organization.

Furthermore, all businesses need profits to survive in the long run. In not-for-profit businesses, prices must be set high enough to provide the profits needed to support asset replacement and to acquire new assets as needed to support volume growth and provide new technologies. For-profit providers, in addition to these support expenditures, must provide equity investors (owners) with a financial return on their investment. The bottom line is that full-cost pricing must cover all accounting costs plus a profit target.

Marginal Cost Pricing

> ***Marginal cost***
> The cost of one additional unit of output; in an outpatient setting, the cost (typically only for supplies) of one more patient visit on top of the existing volume.

In economics, the **marginal cost** of an item is the cost of providing one additional unit of output, whether that output is a product or service, beyond the current volume. For example, suppose that a 150-bed hospital currently provides 40,000 patient days of care. Its marginal cost, based on inpatient day as the unit of service, is the cost of providing the 40,001st day of care. When only one additional day is added to a current volume of 40,000 patient days, fixed costs likely will not increase, so the marginal cost consists solely of the variable costs associated with an additional one-day stay.

In most situations, no additional labor costs would be involved. The marginal cost, therefore, consists of expenses such as laundry, food and expendable supplies, and any additional utility services consumed during that day. Obviously, the marginal cost associated with one additional patient day is far less than the full cost of that patient day, which must include all direct fixed and overhead costs plus a profit component.

Should any prices be set on the basis of marginal costs? In theory, the answer is no. If all payers for a particular provider set reimbursement rates on the basis of marginal costs, the organization would not recover its full costs, including direct and overhead, and hence would ultimately fail. For prices to be equitable, all payers should pay their fair shares in covering providers' total costs. Furthermore, if marginal cost pricing should be adopted, which payer(s) should receive its benefits by being charged lower prices (see "Critical Concept: Marginal Cost Pricing")? Should it be the government because it is taxpayer funded, or should it be the last payer to contract with the provider? These questions do not have good answers. The easy solution, at least conceptually, is to require all payers to pay full costs and hence equitably share the burden of the organization's total costs.

> **CRITICAL CONCEPT**
> Marginal Cost Pricing
>
> In marginal cost pricing, prices are set to cover only the marginal cost of providing the service. In general, this means setting a price equal to variable costs. Marginal cost pricing is usually a temporary strategy, because it does not cover the full cost of providing services. Thus, it can be sustained over the long run only if the provider recoups the losses by charging more than full costs on other services.

However, as a practical matter, it may make sense for healthcare providers to occasionally use marginal cost pricing to attract a new patient group or to retain an existing group (gain or retain market share). To survive in the long run, though, businesses must earn revenues that cover their full costs (see "For Your Consideration: Hospitals, Captive Health Plans, and Price Setting"). Thus, marginal cost pricing must be a temporary measure, or the organization must overcharge other payers for services (compared to full cost) to make up for the losses on patients who are undercharged, called **price shifting** (or cross-subsidization).

> ***Price shifting***
> The act of charging more than full costs to one set of patients to compensate for charging less to another set. Also called *cross-subsidization*.

Historically, price shifting was used to support services that were not self-supporting, such as emergency care, teaching and research, and indigent care. Without using price-shifting strategies, many providers would not have been able to offer a full range of services. Payers were willing to accept price shifting because the additional burden was not excessive. Today, however, overall healthcare costs have risen to the point where the major purchasers of healthcare services are less willing to support the costs associated with providing services to others, and hence purchasers are demanding prices that cover only the true costs of the covered populations. Payers believe that they do not have the moral responsibility to fund healthcare services for others.

SELF-TEST QUESTIONS

1. Describe two common pricing strategies and their implications for financial survivability.
2. What is price shifting (cross-subsidization)?
3. Is cross-subsidization used as frequently today as it was in the past? If not, why?

FOR YOUR CONSIDERATION
Hospitals, Captive Health Plans, and Price Setting

Assume that you are the CEO of Gold Coast Healthcare, a large regional hospital serving a patient population of more than 300,000. The hospital has virtually no competition and hence has a strong position in the local inpatient services market. However, the local health insurance market is dominated by two large companies: one national in scope and the other a major statewide player. You fear that the purchasing clout of the two third-party payers will put so much pressure on prices that the hospital will have difficulty maintaining sufficient profitability to ensure financial soundness.

To counteract the market dominance of the payers, the hospital is starting its own managed care organization, beginning with a single managed care plan organized like a health maintenance organization (HMO). Once the managed care plan begins operations, it will send any of its covered patients who require hospitalization to Gold Coast. Thus, a decision must be made regarding the hospital's pricing policy for its self-operated managed care plan. Should the hospital price high (full-cost pricing) to maintain strong margins, or should it price low (marginal cost pricing) to help the fledgling managed care plan attract members?

What do you think? Which pricing approach makes more sense for Gold Coast? Is the optimal pricing strategy the same in the short run as in the long run?

5.4 TARGET COSTING

Target costing is a management strategy that helps providers offset the limitations imposed when they are price takers (see "Critical Concept: Target Costing"). Target costing assumes that the amount received for a service is fixed and subtracts the desired profit on that service to obtain the target cost level. If possible, management uses this strategy to reduce the full cost of the service to the target level, with a goal of continuous cost reduction, which eventually pushes costs below the target. Essentially, target costing backs into the cost at which a healthcare service must be provided in the long run to attain a given profitability target.

Perhaps the greatest value of target costing lies in the fact that it forces managers to take seriously the prices set by external forces; that is, it recognizes that the purchasers of healthcare services are not concerned about the underlying costs of the services provided. Thus, to ensure financial survival, providers must attain cost structures compatible with the revenue stream. Providers that cannot lower costs to the level required to make a profit ultimately fail.

CRITICAL CONCEPT
Target Costing

Target costing is a strategy used by price takers. In essence, the price (reimbursement rate) is assumed to be fixed, and the goal is to create a cost structure for that service that allows the provider to make a profit. Target costing forces managers to focus on costs, rather than prices, as the key to profitability. To achieve a profit using this strategy, managers examine factors that are within their control (costs) as opposed to factors that are, for the most part, uncontrollable (prices).

SELF-TEST QUESTIONS

1. What is target costing?
2. What is its greatest value?

5.5 PROFIT ANALYSIS

Profit analysis is a technique used to analyze the effects of volume changes on profit. (Accountants often refer to this technique as cost-volume-profit [CVP] analysis.) In addition, profit analysis can be used to examine the effects of alternative assumptions regarding costs and prices. Such information is useful as managers evaluate future courses of action regarding pricing and the introduction of new services (see "Critical Concept: Profit Analysis").

CRITICAL CONCEPT
Profit Analysis

Profit analysis combines data on costs, volume, and prices to estimate the profitability of organizations, departments, or services. Profit analysis is an important component in planning for the future because it allows managers to see how profitability is affected by changes in cost, volume, and price assumptions. In essence, profit analysis is used to conduct "what if" analyses—What if volume is lower than expected? What if prices are higher than anticipated? What if costs are higher than forecasted? And so on. The answers to these and similar questions provide managers with insights into the organization's financial future.

Basic Data

Base case
In profit analysis, the scenario (outcome) that is expected (most likely) to occur.

Exhibit 5.1 presents the estimated annual costs for Atlanta Clinic, a large primary care practice, for 2016. These costs are based on the clinic's best (most likely) estimate of volume: 75,000 visits. The most likely estimate often is called the **base case**, so the data in exhibit 5.1 represent the clinic's base case cost forecast. Expected total costs for 2016 are \$7,080,962. Because these costs support 75,000 visits, the forecasted base case average cost per visit is \$7,080,962 ÷ 75,000 = \$94.41.

Focusing solely on total costs does not provide the clinic's managers with much information regarding potential alternative financial outcomes for 2016. Total cost information is necessary and useful, but the detailed breakdown in exhibit 5.1 gives the clinic's managers more insight into the possible financial outcomes than can be obtained using a total cost focus.

Relevant range
The range of output (volume) for which the organization's cost structure holds.

Exhibit 5.1 categorizes the clinic's total costs of \$7,080,962 into two components: total variable costs of \$2,113,500 and total fixed costs of \$4,967,462. As you know, these cost amounts are fundamentally different. The total fixed costs of \$4,967,462 must be borne by the clinic regardless of actual volume, as long as it stays in the **relevant range** of 70,000–80,000 visits. However, total variable costs of \$2,113,500 apply only to a volume of 75,000 patient visits. If the actual number of visits realized in 2016 is less than or greater

Exhibit 5.1
Atlanta Clinic: Forecasted Cost Data for 2016 (Based on 75,000 Patient Visits)

	Variable Costs	Fixed Costs	Total Costs
Salaries and benefits			
Management and supervision	\$ 0	\$ 928,687	\$ 928,687
Coordinators	442,617	598,063	1,040,680
Specialists	0	38,600	38,600
Technicians	681,383	552,670	1,234,053
Clerical/administrative	71,182	58,240	129,422
Social Security taxes	89,622	163,188	252,810
Group health insurance	115,924	211,081	327,005
Professional fees	325,489	383,360	708,849
Supplies	313,283	231,184	544,467
Utilities	74,000	45,040	119,040
Allocated overhead costs	0	1,757,349	1,757,349
Total	\$2,113,500	\$4,967,462	\$7,080,962

than 75,000, total variable costs will be less than or greater than \$2,113,500. (Of course, this is the primary reason that costs are classified as fixed and variable in the first place.)

To conduct a profit analysis, it is necessary to express variable costs on a per-unit (variable cost rate) basis. For Atlanta Clinic, the implied variable cost rate is \$2,113,500 ÷ 75,000 visits = \$28.18 per visit. Thus, the clinic's total costs at any volume in the relevant range can be calculated as follows:

$$\begin{aligned}\text{Total costs} &= \text{Fixed costs} + \text{Total variable costs}\\ &= \$4{,}967{,}462 + (\$28.18 \times \text{Number of visits}).\end{aligned}$$

This equation, the clinic's **underlying cost structure** (first introduced in chapter 4), shows that total costs depend on volume. To illustrate use of this model, consider three potential volumes for 2016: 70,000, 75,000, and 80,000 patient visits:

Underlying cost structure
The relationship between volume and an organization's total costs. Often called *cost structure*.

Volume = 70,000:

$$\begin{aligned}\text{Total costs} &= \$4{,}967{,}462 + (\$28.18 \times 70{,}000)\\ &= \$4{,}967{,}462 + \$1{,}972{,}600 = \$6{,}940{,}062.\end{aligned}$$

Volume = 75,000:

$$\begin{aligned}\text{Total costs} &= \$4{,}967{,}462 + (\$28.18 \times 75{,}000)\\ &= \$4{,}967{,}462 + \$2{,}113{,}500 = \$7{,}080{,}962.\end{aligned}$$

Volume = 80,000:

$$\begin{aligned}\text{Total costs} &= \$4{,}967{,}462 + (\$28.18 \times 80{,}000)\\ &= \$4{,}967{,}462 + \$2{,}254{,}400 = \$7{,}221{,}862.\end{aligned}$$

When an organization's costs are expressed in this way, it is easy to see that higher volume leads to higher total costs.

Atlanta Clinic's cost structure is plotted in exhibit 5.2. (To simplify the graph, we assume that the relevant range extends to zero visits.) Fixed costs are shown as a horizontal dashed line, and total costs are shown as an upward-sloping solid line with a slope (rise over run) equal to the variable cost rate of \$28.18 per visit. Total variable costs are represented by the vertical distance between the total costs line and the fixed costs line.

Note that Atlanta Clinic's financial manager does not literally write out a check for \$28.18 for each visit, although examples of variable costs in which she does so may exist. Rather, the clinic's cost structure indicates that the clinic uses certain resources that its managers have defined as inherently variable, and the best estimate of the value of such resources, on average, is \$28.18 per visit.

To complete the profit analysis graph, a revenue component must be added to the cost structure. For 2016, the clinic expects revenues, on average, to be \$100 per patient

EXHIBIT 5.2
Atlanta Clinic: Profit Analysis Graph

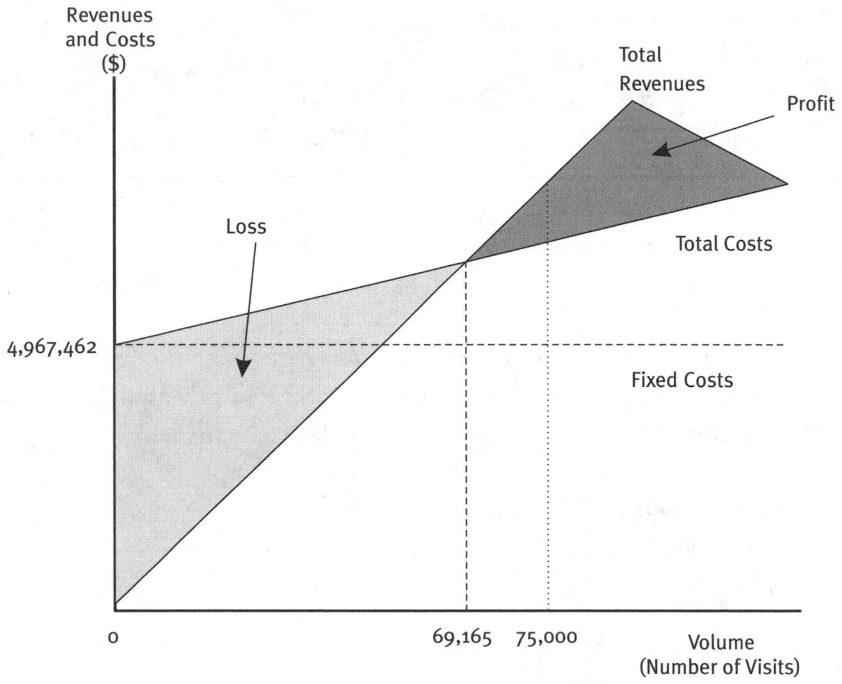

visit. Total revenues are plotted in exhibit 5.2 as an upward-sloping solid line starting at the origin and having a slope of $100 per visit. If no visits occurred, total revenues would be zero; at 1 visit, total revenues would be $100; at 10 visits, total revenues would be $1,000; at 75,000 visits, total revenues would be $7,500,000; and so on. Note that the vertical dashed line is drawn at the point where total revenues equal total costs and the vertical dotted line is drawn at the base case volume estimate, 75,000 visits. We examine the significance of these two vertical lines in later sections.

The Projected Profit and Loss Statement

To begin the profit analysis, Atlanta Clinic's managers forecast profit given the base case assumptions on costs, volume, and prices. Such a forecast is called a *profit and loss (P&L) statement.* P&L statements, as with all managerial accounting data, are developed for specific purposes and hence can be formatted to best fit the situation at hand (see "Critical Concept: Profit and Loss [P&L] Statement").

Atlanta Clinic's base case projected P&L statement is shown in exhibit 5.3. The bottom line projects Atlanta's 2016 profit using base case (most likely estimate) values for costs, volume, and prices. Note that the format of a P&L statement for CVP analysis

CRITICAL CONCEPT
Profit and Loss (P&L) Statement

A P&L (pronounced "P and L") statement is a listing of revenues, expenses, and profit (revenues minus expenses). P&L statements can be provided in numerous formats, depending on the specific purpose of the statement. For example, for use in profit analysis, costs must be broken out as fixed and variable. P&L statements can be constructed for the entire organization, a department, or a service. Also, they can contain historical data, which report what has happened in the past, or forecasted data, which express expectations about the future.

purposes distinguishes between variable and fixed costs, whereas that of a P&L statement for other purposes may not make this distinction. Also, note that the projected P&L statement contains a line labeled "total contribution margin." This concept is discussed in the next section.

The projected P&L statement used in profit analysis contains four variables; three of the variables are assumed and the fourth is calculated. In exhibit 5.3, the assumed variables are expected volume (75,000 visits), expected price ($100 per visit), and expected costs (as defined by the clinic's cost structure). Profit, the fourth variable, is calculated on the basis of the three assumed variables.

The base case projected P&L statement in exhibit 5.3 represents only one point on the graphical model in exhibit 5.2. This point is shown by the dotted vertical line at a volume of 75,000 patient visits. Moving up along this dotted line, the distance from the *x*-axis to the horizontal line represents the $4,967,462 in fixed costs. The distance from the fixed costs line to the total costs line represents the $2,113,500 in total variable costs. The distance between the total costs line and the total revenues line represents the $419,038 profit. Of

EXHIBIT 5.3
Atlanta Clinic: 2016 Base Case Projected P&L Statement (Based on 75,000 Patient Visits)

Total revenues ($100 × 75,000)	$7,500,000
Total variable costs ($28.18 × 75,000)	2,113,500
Total contribution margin ($71.82 × 75,000)	$5,386,500
Fixed costs	4,967,462
Profit	$ 419,038

course, the graph in exhibit 5.2 is not drawn to scale and hence cannot be used to develop numerical data. Rather, it provides the clinic's managers with a pictorial representation of the clinic's projected profitability.

Contribution Margin

The base case projected P&L statement in exhibit 5.3 introduces the concept of *contribution margin*, which is defined as the difference between per-unit revenue and per-unit variable cost (variable cost rate). In this illustration, the contribution margin is $100.00 – $28.18 = $71.82. What is the inherent meaning of this contribution margin value of $71.82? The contribution margin appears to be a type of "profit" because it is calculated as revenue minus costs.

However, because no fixed costs of providing service have been included in the calculation, it is not profit. Rather, because only variable costs have been stripped out, the contribution margin is the dollar amount of per-visit revenue available to cover Atlanta Clinic's fixed costs. Only after fixed costs are fully recovered does the contribution margin begin to contribute to profit.

With a contribution margin of $71.82 on each of the clinic's 75,000 visits, the projected base case total contribution margin for 2016 is $71.82 × 75,000 = $5,386,500, which is sufficient to cover the clinic's fixed costs of $4,967,462 and then provide a $5,386,500 – $4,967,462 = $419,038 profit (see "Critical Concept: Contribution Margin and Total Contribution Margin"). After fixed costs have been covered, any additional visits contribute to the clinic's profit at a rate of $71.82 per visit. Because many fixed costs cannot be changed quickly, contribution margin is often the measure managers look to when making short-term service decisions. For example, even if a service does not generate sufficient revenue to cover its full costs (including allocated overhead), the organization may be better off keeping the service than dropping it. A positive contribution margin will contribute to covering the fixed costs, many of which would likely remain even if the service were eliminated.

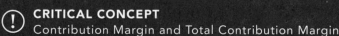

> **CRITICAL CONCEPT**
> Contribution Margin and Total Contribution Margin
>
> Contribution margin is the amount of per-unit revenue that is available to first cover fixed costs and then contribute to profitability. It is calculated as the revenue per unit of service minus the variable cost per unit of service (variable cost rate). The idea is that if we strip the variable costs out of revenue, we will be left with the amount available per unit of output to cover fixed costs. Once fixed costs are covered, any additional contribution margin amounts flow directly to profit.

CRITICAL CONCEPT
Contribution Margin and Total Contribution Margin *(continued)*

To illustrate, consider your custom pen business (which we set up in chapter 4). The pens cost you $1.75 each, but you had to pay $50 to design the logo. The contribution margin on each pen is Per-unit revenue – Variable cost rate. If you sell the pens for $3 each, the contribution margin is $3.00 – $1.75 = $1.25. Thus, each pen sold will contribute $1.25 to cover the $50 fixed costs. Once you sell 40 pens, you will have recouped the $50 fixed costs (40 × $1.25 = $50), so all sales after the first 40 create profits for your custom pen enterprise at a rate of $1.25 per pen sold.

Total contribution margin is the sum of the contribution margins of all units sold. Assume that you sell 50 pens. With a contribution margin of $1.25 per pen, the total contribution margin is 50 × $1.25 = $62.50. The first $50 of the total contribution margin is needed to cover your fixed costs of $50, so the remaining $12.50 flows to profit. Thus, at a volume of 60 pens, your profit is $12.50.

SELF-TEST QUESTIONS

1. Construct a simple P&L statement such as that shown in exhibit 5.3, and discuss its elements.
2. Sketch and explain a simple diagram to match your exhibit.
3. Define and explain the use of contribution margin and total contribution margin.

5.6 BREAKEVEN ANALYSIS

Breakeven analysis is a method used to determine the value of a given input variable (e.g., volume, costs, price) that is required to achieve some minimum desired profit, holding other variables constant (see "Critical Concept: Breakeven Analysis"). For example, a clinical laboratory might determine that, at a given volume of tests, it must charge $23 per test to break even on total costs (i.e., produce a profit of zero). This means that at a price of $23 per test, the reimbursement rate just equals the full cost of providing that test. Alternatively, the laboratory might determine that, given a reimbursement rate of $20 per test, it would need to perform at least 1,050 tests in order to break even on total costs. At that volume, given a price of $20, the laboratory's total revenues from the test equal the total costs of the test.

CRITICAL CONCEPT
Breakeven Analysis

Breakeven analysis has many applications in healthcare finance. In the context of profit analysis, breakeven analysis involves finding the value of an input variable that produces some desired profit, holding other variables constant. *Breakeven* can be defined in two ways: on the basis of accounting costs alone (where the target profit is zero) or on the basis of accounting costs plus a nonzero profit target. For example, given current reimbursement rates and the organization's cost structure, a nursing home might break even in an accounting sense when it has 45 residents, but may require 53 residents to reach a profit target of $50,000. Breakeven analysis can also be applied to variables other than volume. For example, a home health agency might break even if its per-visit costs are $70 or less, given reimbursement rates and expected volume. Or a radiology group might break even if its reimbursement averages $25 per reading, given expected volume and current costs.

Although the breakeven analysis discussed here is actually part of profit analysis, the concept is important enough to deserve its own section. For now, we use breakeven analysis to estimate the volume at which a business, department, or service becomes financially self-sufficient.

When considering breakeven volume, you should be familiar with both definitions of the term. **Accounting breakeven** is defined as the volume needed to produce zero profit. In other words, it is the volume that produces revenues equal to total accounting costs. **Economic breakeven** is defined as the volume needed to produce some target profit level. In other words, it is the volume that creates revenues equal to total accounting costs plus the desired profit amount.

Accounting breakeven
Accounting breakeven occurs when all accounting costs are covered (zero profitability).

Economic breakeven
Economic breakeven occurs when all accounting costs plus a profit target are covered.

As mentioned in the previous section, the P&L statement format used for profit analysis is a four-variable model. When the focus is profit (the calculated variable), the three assumed variables are costs, volume, and price. When the focus is volume breakeven, the same four variables are used, but profit is now assumed to be known while volume is the unknown (calculated) value (see "Critical Equation: Volume Breakeven").

To illustrate volume breakeven, the projected P&L statement presented in exhibit 5.3 can be expressed in equation form as shown here:

$$\text{Total revenues} - \text{Total variable costs} - \text{Fixed costs} = \text{Profit}$$
$$(\$100 \times \text{Volume}) - (\$28.18 \times \text{Volume}) - \$4{,}967{,}462 = \text{Profit.}$$

CRITICAL EQUATION
Volume Breakeven

Volume breakeven can be estimated using a very simple equation:

$$(\text{Contribution margin} \times \text{Volume}) - \text{Fixed costs} = \$0 \text{ (or some profit target).}$$

To illustrate, what is the accounting breakeven volume of your custom pen business? Remember that the pens cost $1.75 apiece, and you paid a $50 fee for the logo. Also, you plan to sell the pens for $3.00 each. Under these assumptions, the contribution margin is $3.00 – $1.75 = $1.25, and the breakeven point is 40 pens:

$$\begin{aligned}(\$1.25 \times \text{Volume}) - \$50 &= \$0\\ \$1.25 \times \text{Volume} &= \$50\\ \text{Volume} &= \$50 \div \$1.25\\ &= 40.\end{aligned}$$

As an alternative, breakeven could be defined as meeting some profit target. For example, assume you wanted to make $100 on your pen business. The breakeven volume now is 120 pens:

$$\begin{aligned}(\$1.25 \times \text{Volume}) - \$50 &= \$100\\ \$1.25 \times \text{Volume} &= \$150\\ \text{Volume} &= \$150 \div \$1.25\\ &= 120.\end{aligned}$$

At accounting breakeven, the clinic's profit equals zero, so the breakeven equation can be rewritten this way:

$$(\$100 \times \text{Volume}) - (\$28.18 \times \text{Volume}) - \$4{,}967{,}462 = \$0.$$

Rearranging so that only the terms related to volume appear on the left side produces this equation:

$$(\$100 \times \text{Volume}) - (\$28.18 \times \text{Volume}) = \$4{,}967{,}462.$$

Using basic algebra, the two terms on the left side can be combined because volume appears in both. The result is

$$(\$100 - \$28.18) \times \text{Volume} = \$4{,}967{,}462$$
$$\$71.82 \times \text{Volume} = \$4{,}967{,}462.$$

The left side of the breakeven equation now contains the contribution margin, $71.82, multiplied by volume. Thus, the clinic will break even when the total contribution margin equals fixed costs. Solving the equation for volume results in a breakeven point of $4,967,462 ÷ $71.82 = 69,165 visits. Any volume greater than 69,165 visits produces an accounting profit for the clinic, while any volume less than 69,165 results in a loss.

The logic behind the breakeven point is this: Each patient visit brings in $100, of which $28.18 is the variable cost to treat the patient. Once the variable cost is deducted, a $71.82 contribution margin results from each visit. If the clinic sets the contribution margin aside for the first 69,165 visits in 2016, it accumulates $4,967,430, which is enough (except for a small rounding difference) to cover its fixed costs. Once the clinic exceeds breakeven volume, each visit's contribution margin flows directly to profit. If the clinic achieves its base case volume estimate of 75,000 visits, the 5,835 visits above the breakeven point will result in a total profit of 5,835 × $71.82 = $419,070, which matches the profit (again except for a rounding difference) shown on the clinic's projected income statement in exhibit 5.3.

On a profit analysis graph such as exhibit 5.2, accounting breakeven occurs at the intersection of the total revenues line and total costs line. This point is indicated by a vertical dashed line drawn at a volume of 69,165 visits. Before even one patient walks in the door, the clinic has already committed to $4,967,462 in fixed costs. Because the total revenues line is steeper than the total variable costs line (and hence the total costs line), contribution margin is positive. Thus, as volume increases, total revenues eventually catch up to the clinic's cost structure. Any volume to the right of the breakeven point, which is shown as a dark-shaded area, produces a profit; any volume to the left, which is shown as a light-shaded area, results in a loss.

This breakeven analysis contains three important assumptions:

1. The price, or set of prices, for different types of patients and different payers is independent of volume. In other words, volume increases are not attained by lowering prices, and price increases are not met with volume declines.
2. Costs can be reasonably subdivided into fixed and variable components.
3. The breakeven volume is contained within the relevant range.

Breakeven analysis is often performed in an iterative manner. After the breakeven volume is calculated, managers must determine whether the resulting volume can realistically be achieved at the price assumed in the analysis. If the price appears to be unreasonable for the breakeven volume, a new price has to be estimated and the breakeven analysis repeated. Likewise, if the cost structure used for the calculation appears to be unrealistic at the breakeven volume, operational and cost assumptions should be changed and the analysis repeated.

Instead of asking how many visits are needed for accounting breakeven, Atlanta Clinic's managers may ask how many visits are needed to achieve a \$100,000 profit (or any other profit level the clinic targets). By building a profit target into the breakeven analysis, the focus is now on economic breakeven. The clinic will have a \$419,038 profit if it receives 75,000 visits, and it will have no profit if it receives 69,165 visits. Thus, the number of visits required to achieve a \$100,000 profit target (economic breakeven) is somewhere between 69,165 and 75,000—in fact, the number is 70,558:

$$\begin{aligned}
(\text{Contribution margin} \times \text{Volume}) - \text{Fixed costs} &= \text{Profit target} \\
(\$71.82 \times \text{Volume}) - \$4{,}967{,}462 &= \$100{,}000 \\
\$71.82 \times \text{Volume} &= \$5{,}067{,}462 \\
\text{Volume} &= \$5{,}067{,}462 \div \$71.82 \\
\text{Volume} &= 70{,}558.
\end{aligned}$$

? SELF-TEST QUESTIONS

1. What is the purpose of breakeven analysis?
2. What is the equation for volume breakeven?
3. Why is breakeven analysis often conducted in an iterative manner?
4. What is the difference between accounting breakeven and economic breakeven?

5.7 MARGINAL ANALYSIS

Now assume that a new payer, Peachtree Managed Care Company (PMCC), makes a proposal to Atlanta Clinic's managers. PMCC would like the clinic to provide primary healthcare services to its 1,500 enrollees. The best estimate is that these individuals would add 5,000 visits to the clinic's base case forecast of 75,000. However, PMCC wants a discount of 40 percent from current pricing. Thus, the net price (and revenue) for the clinic's new patients would be, on average, \$60 per visit instead of the undiscounted \$100 that is received on current patients. If the clinic refuses, PMCC will take its business elsewhere.

At first blush, PMCC's proposal appears to be unacceptable. Most important, \$60 is less than the full cost of providing service, which was determined previously to be \$94.41 per visit at a volume of 75,000. Thus, Atlanta would lose roughly \$94.41 – \$60 = \$34.41

> **CRITICAL CONCEPT**
> Marginal Analysis
>
> Marginal analysis is used to analyze the impact of adding volume to an existing base. For example, assume you have sold 40 of your pens at $3.00 each, but now a classmate offers to buy 20 more at $2.00 apiece. The total cost of 60 pens, based on a $1.75 cost of each pen and a $50 up-front charge, is (60 × $1.75) + $50 = $155. Thus, the average cost per pen is $155 ÷ 60 = $2.58, so you might be inclined to say no to the offer, which is only $2.00 per pen. On the other hand, the $50 charge has already been covered by past sales, so the marginal cost to you of each additional pen is only the variable cost rate of $1.75. Thus, the contribution margin on each of the additional 20 pens is $2.00 – $1.75 = $0.25, so each pen sold would contribute that amount to your bottom line. Unless other issues are at play and need to be considered, you should take your classmate's offer.

per visit on PMCC's patients. (This estimate is rough, because the average cost per visit decreases as the number of patient visits increases.) However, before the clinic's managers reject PMCC's proposal, they must examine it in more detail using a technique called *marginal analysis* (see "Critical Concept: Marginal Analysis").

Although each new (marginal) visit from the contract brings in only $60, compared with $100 on the clinic's other contracts, the marginal cost of each new visit is the variable cost rate of $28.18. (Remember that marginal cost is the cost of the next unit sold.) The clinic's $4,967,462 in fixed costs will be incurred whether PMCC's offer is accepted or rejected, so these costs are not relevant to the decision. Because the contribution margin on the new contract is $60 – $28.18 = $31.82 per visit (a positive amount), each visit will contribute to the clinic's recovery of fixed costs and ultimately flow to profit. Thus, the offer must be seriously considered. Note that this conclusion is based on the assumption that the relevant range of volume is from 70,000 to 80,000 visits, and hence the current level of fixed costs can support the added volume of 5,000 visits. However, if the contract were expected to add 10,000 visits, the conclusion might be different because the new volume extends beyond the relevant range. In that case, it might be necessary to add fixed costs to accommodate the 5,000 "excess" visits. If so, the marginal cost of each visit would be the $28.18 variable cost rate plus an additional per-visit fixed cost, which would change the numbers used in the analysis.

To verify the positive impact of the proposal, consider the P&L statement in exhibit 5.4. Here, we have combined the existing 75,000 patient visits with the additional 5,000 visits, for a total of 80,000. The revenues had to be split between the two patient groups because of the price difference. However, the cost structure is assumed to hold, so it is the same, except for the fact that 80,000 visits are now expected. The result is that the clinic's profit is now expected to be $578,138 instead of the $419,038 shown in exhibit 5.3 for the base case (75,000 visits).

Note that the additional profit expected from the new contract is $578,138 – $419,038 = $159,100. We could have arrived at this result more easily by merely noting that

EXHIBIT 5.4
Atlanta Clinic: 2016 Projected P&L Statement (Based on 75,000 Visits at $100 and 5,000 Visits at $60)

Undiscounted revenue ($100 × 75,000)	$7,500,000
Discounted revenue ($60 × 5,000)	300,000
Total revenues	$7,800,000
Total variable costs ($28.18 × 80,000)	2,254,400
Total contribution margin	$5,545,600
Fixed costs	4,967,462
Profit	$ 578,138

each of the 5,000 new visits has a contribution margin of $31.82, so the total contribution margin is expected to be 5,000 × $31.82 = $159,100. Because the existing 75,000 patient visits are more than sufficient to cover fixed costs, the entire amount of the additional contribution margin flows to profit.

What should the clinic's managers do? If PMCC's proposal is accepted, the clinic is expected to make an additional $159,100 in profit, so it appears to be a no-brainer. However, acceptance may have unintended consequences.

For example, the clinic's other payers will undoubtedly learn about the new contract with reduced payments and will want to renegotiate their own contracts to achieve the same, or an even greater, discount. Such a reaction could result in discounts being offered to current payers, which could result in the clinic losing more money on current patients than it gains on new patients. If that outcome were anticipated, the clinic's managers would be better off saying no to the offer.

Perhaps Atlanta Clinic can negotiate with PMCC and reach a compromise on the size of the discount. The quantitative analysis required to make the decision is relatively easy, but the qualitative issues are more complex—such is the nature of most financial decision-making (see "Healthcare in Practice: Costs and Revenues of Medical Practices").

? SELF-TEST QUESTIONS

1. What is the impact of a discounted contract on revenues, fixed costs, total variable costs, and the breakeven point?
2. Describe marginal analysis.
3. Can qualitative issues come into play in marginal analysis? Give an example.

HEALTHCARE IN PRACTICE
Costs and Revenues of Medical Practices

The Healthcare in Practice box in chapter 4 discusses the cost structure of an average primary care practice. Because practice costs (and revenues) are a function of the number of physicians in the practice, the data presented here are on a per-physician basis.

On average, each physician handles about 2,300 patients, who make about 5,300 encounters (visits) during which the physician performs about 11,000 procedures. In addition, each physician requires $325,000 in operating (support) costs. If we use patient visits as the unit of output (volume), the operating cost per visit averages out to be about $325,000 ÷ 5,300 = roughly $61 per visit.

However, the data do not break out fixed versus variable costs. Variable costs, which consist mostly of administrative supplies (e.g., forms, letterhead) and medical supplies (e.g., rubber gloves, needles, vaccines, dressings) are relatively small, say, $10 per visit. Following this assumption, the underlying cost structure for an average primary care practice looks like this:

Total costs = $272,000 + ($10 × Number of visits).

On average, primary care physicians generate roughly $603,000 of revenues per physician. Thus, the per-physician P&L statement, assuming 5,300 visits, can be expressed as follows:

Total revenues	$603,000
Total variable costs ($10 × 5,300)	53,000
Total contribution margin	$550,000
Fixed costs	272,000
Profit	$278,000

Of course, the $278,000 "profit" here represents the amount available for reinvestment in the practice as well as the primary care physician's compensation.

To convert the average per-physician P&L statement to an equation format, note that the average revenue per visit is $603,000 ÷ 5,300 = $113.77. Thus,

Total revenues − Total variable costs − Fixed costs = Profit
($113.77 × Volume) − ($10 × Volume) − $272,000 = Profit.

HEALTHCARE IN PRACTICE
Costs and Revenues of Medical Practices *(continued)*

So, at 5,300 visits, the profit per physician is

$$(\$113.77 \times 5{,}300) - (\$10 \times 5{,}300) - \$272{,}000 = \text{Profit}$$
$$\$603{,}000 - \$53{,}000 - \$272{,}000 = \$278{,}000.$$

Of course, this profit amount is the same as that calculated in the P&L statement. The advantage of the equation format is that we can now estimate profit at different volume levels. For example, assume that the volume is only 5,000 visits per physician, instead of the 5,300 visits forecasted. With fewer visits, the profit (and hence physician compensation) falls to $246,850:

$$(\$113.77 \times 5{,}000) - (\$10 \times 5{,}000) - \$272{,}000 = \text{Profit}$$
$$\$568{,}850 - \$50{,}000 - \$272{,}000 = \$246{,}850.$$

But with more visits (say, 5,600), the profit rises to $309,112:

$$(\$113.77 \times 5{,}600) - (\$10 \times 5{,}600) - \$272{,}000 = \text{Profit}$$
$$\$637{,}112 - \$56{,}000 - \$272{,}000 = \$309{,}112.$$

This analysis confirms that fee-for-service reimbursement creates a powerful incentive for clinicians to see as many patients as possible.

Note. This Healthcare in Practice is based on information provided by the Medical Group Management Association, 2011, *Performance and Practices of Successful Medical Groups*, Englewood, CO: MGMA.

5.8 PROFIT ANALYSIS IN A CAPITATED ENVIRONMENT

Thus far, the discussion of profit analysis has assumed fee-for-service reimbursement. However, it is important to consider how the analysis changes when a provider operates in a capitated environment. A discussion of capitation provides an excellent review of profit analysis and highlights the basic differences between capitation and fee-for-service reimbursement methods.

To begin, assume that Atlanta Clinic's current payer is the Alliance, a local business coalition. The Alliance is paying the clinic $7,500,000 to provide services for an expected 75,000 visits, but the amount is capitated. Although the clinic's projected total revenues remain the same (see exhibit 5.3), the situation is actually quite different. The $7,500,000 that the Alliance is paying is not explicitly tied to the amount of services provided by the clinic. Rather, it is tied to the size of the employee group (covered population).

Under capitation, the clinic is taking on the additional risk associated with the amount of services provided (utilization risk). If the total costs of services delivered by the clinic exceed the premium revenue (paid monthly on a per-member basis), the clinic will suffer the financial consequences. However, if the clinic can efficiently manage the healthcare of the population served, it will be the economic beneficiary.

How might Atlanta Clinic's managers evaluate whether the $7,500,000 revenue attached to the contract is adequate? To conduct the analysis, the managers need two critical pieces of information: cost and utilization. The clinic already has the cost information—the full cost per visit is expected to be $94.41 (at a volume of 75,000 visits), with an underlying cost structure of $28.18 per visit in variable costs and $4,967,462 in fixed costs. For its **actuarial information**, the managers estimate that the Alliance will have a covered population of 18,750 members, with an expected (average) utilization rate of four visits per member per year. Thus, the total number of visits expected is 18,750 × 4 = 75,000.

Actuarial information
Data (including utilization data for the covered population) regarding the financial risks associated with insurance programs.

The revenues expected from this contract—$7,500,000—exceed the expected costs of serving this population, which are 75,000 visits multiplied by $94.41 per visit, or $7,080,750. Thus, this contract is expected to generate a profit of $419,250, which, not surprisingly, is the same as the original base case fee-for-service result (except for a rounding difference); see exhibit 5.3.

Graphical View Based on Utilization

Exhibit 5.5 contains a graphical profit analysis for the capitation contract that is constructed similarly to the fee-for-service graph shown in exhibit 5.2—that is, the horizontal axis shows volume as measured by number of visits, while the vertical axis shows revenues and costs. Also shown is the same underlying cost structure of $4,967,462 in fixed costs, coupled with a variable cost rate of $28.18. One significant difference exists, however. Instead of being upward sloping, the total revenues line is horizontal, which shows that total revenue is $7,500,000 regardless of volume as measured by the number of visits.

The flat revenue line in exhibit 5.5 tells managers that revenue is being driven by a factor other than the volume of services provided. Under capitation, revenue is driven by the per-member premium payment and number of **enrollees**.

Enrollee
A member of a managed care plan. Or, more generally, an individual who has (is enrolled in) a health insurance plan.

Also, note the difference between the revenue and fixed cost lines. Atlanta Clinic has a constant spread of $7,500,000 – $4,967,462 = $2,532,538 to work with in providing for the healthcare of this population for the period of the contract. If total variable costs

Exhibit 5.5
Atlanta Clinic: Profit Analysis Based on Number of Visits

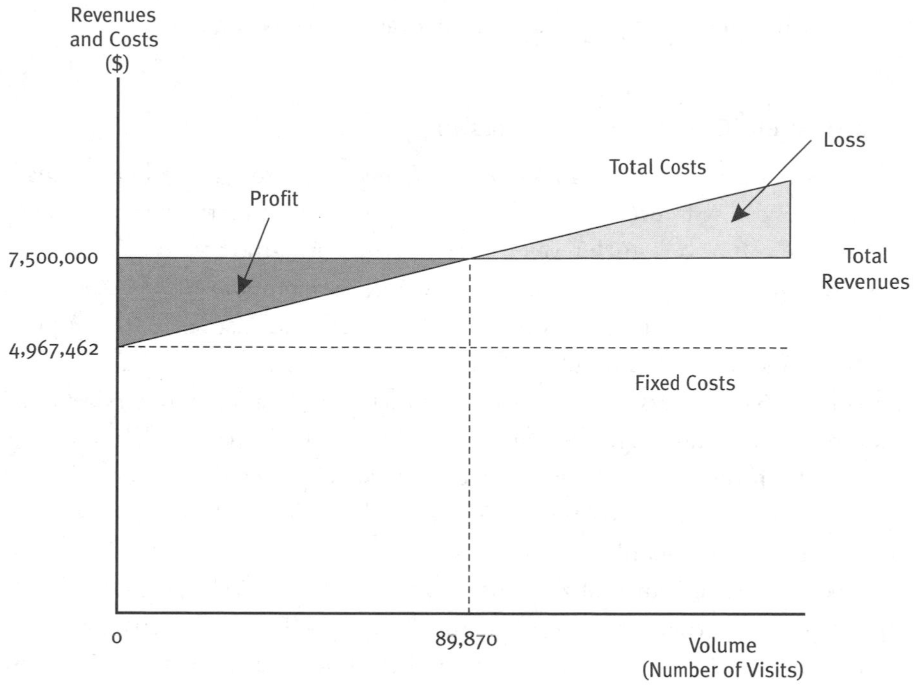

equal $2,532,538, the clinic breaks even; if total variable costs exceed $2,532,538, the clinic loses money. Thus, to make a profit, the number of visits must be less than $2,532,538 ÷ $28.18 = 89,870. If everyone at the clinic does not understand the inherent utilization risk under capitation, the clinic could find itself in serious financial trouble. On the other hand, if all of the clinic's managers and clinicians understand and manage this utilization risk, a handsome reward may result.

The key feature of capitation is the reversal of the profit and loss portions of the graph. To see this shift, compare exhibit 5.2 with exhibit 5.5. The fact that profits occur at lower volumes under capitation differs from what will happen under the fee-for-service environment. This fact can be verified by examining the per-visit contribution margin under capitation: Revenue per visit – Variable cost per visit = $0 – $28.18 = –$28.18. With a negative contribution margin, each additional visit increases costs by $28.18 without bringing in additional revenue.

From a purely financial perspective, the obvious response to capitation is to provide minimal services (reduce utilization) because doing so generates the greatest profit, at least in the short run. Of course, the clinic would have trouble renewing the contract in subsequent years, and patients may become more ill (and costly to the practice) if only minimal service is provided, so this course of action is neither appropriate nor feasible. Still, its implications are at the heart of concerns expressed by critics of managed care about the incentives to withhold patient care inherent in a capitated environment.

Graphical View Based on Membership

Exhibit 5.5 is like Alice (of *Alice in Wonderland*) peering through the looking glass and finding that everything is reversed. The key to this problem is that the horizontal axis does not measure the volume to which revenues are related; that is, the horizontal axis in exhibit 5.5 measures number of visits, just as if Atlanta Clinic were reimbursed on a fee-for-service basis. Because it is now selling both healthcare services and insurance, the appropriate horizontal axis measure is the number of members (enrollees).

Exhibit 5.6 recognizes that membership, rather than the amount of services provided, drives revenues. With number of members on the horizontal axis, the total revenues line is no longer flat; revenues only look flat when they are considered relative to the number of visits. The revenue earned by the clinic is actually $7,500,000 ÷ 18,750 = $400 per member; as membership increases, so do revenues.

The cost structure can easily be expressed on a membership basis as well. Fixed costs are no problem in the relevant range; they are inherently volume insensitive, whether volume is measured by number of visits or by number of members. Thus, exhibit 5.6 shows

Exhibit 5.6
Atlanta Clinic: Profit Analysis Based on Number of Members

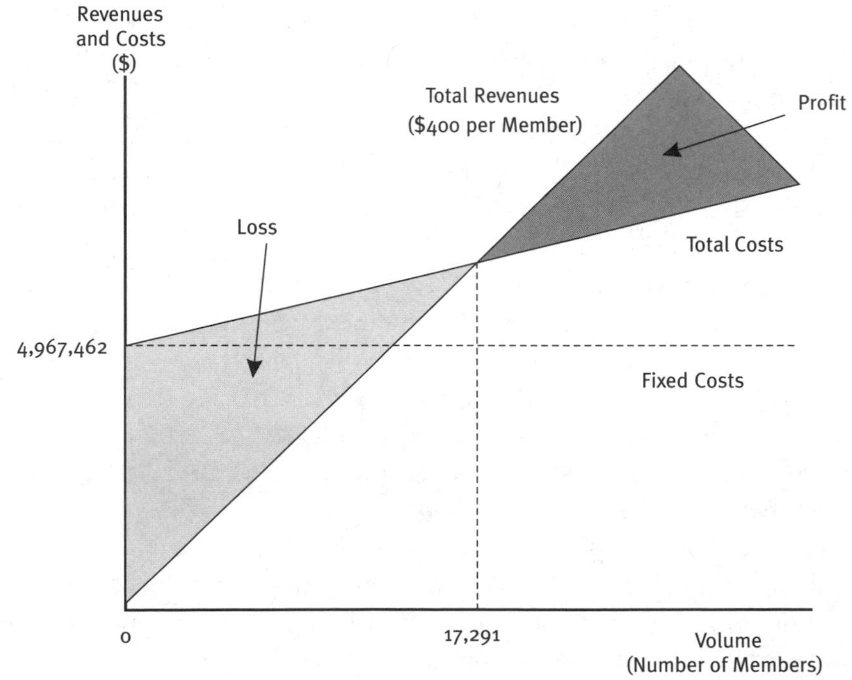

fixed costs as the same flat, dashed line as before. However, the variable cost rate based on number of enrollees is not the same as the variable cost rate based on number of visits. Per-member variable cost must be estimated from two factors: the variable cost rate of $28.18 per visit and the expected utilization of four visits per year. The combination of the two is 4 × $28.18 = $112.72, which is the clinic's expected variable cost per member.

Expressed on a per-member basis, the contribution margin is now Revenue per member – Variable cost per member = $400 – $112.72 = $287.28, rather than the –$28.18 when volume is measured by the number of visits. With a positive contribution margin, additional members translate to additional profitability.

Note that under capitation, utilization volume is a component of the variable cost rate and hence total variable costs. Thus, utilization management becomes an important cost-control tool. Furthermore, if both utilization and per-visit costs can be reduced, the clinic can reap greater benefits (profits) than is possible under fee-for-service reimbursement. Of course, control of fixed costs is always financially prudent, regardless of the type of reimbursement.

Also note that capitated revenues are driven by the number of members rather than the amount of services provided. Thus, capitation contracts must bring in a large number of enrollees. A large number of enrollees both increases revenues to providers and reduces risk. Risk reduction occurs because only a few high-utilization enrollees can create costs that exceed total capitated revenues if the number of patients is small.

? SELF-TEST QUESTIONS

1. Under capitation, what is the difference between a CVP graph with the number of visits on the *x*-axis and one with the number of members on the *x*-axis?
2. What is unique about the per-visit contribution margin under capitation? How would you convert this to a per-member contribution margin?
3. Why is utilization management so important in a capitated environment?
4. Why is the number of members important in a capitated environment?

5.9 THE IMPACT OF COST STRUCTURE ON FINANCIAL RISK

The financial risk of a healthcare provider, at least in theory, is minimized by having a cost structure that "matches" its revenue structure. To illustrate, consider a clinic with all payers using fee-for-service reimbursement, which means revenues are directly related to volume. If the clinic's cost structure consisted of all variable costs (no fixed costs), then each visit would incur costs but also create revenues. Assuming that the per-visit revenue amount exceeds the variable cost rate (the per-visit cost), the clinic would lock in a profit on each visit. The total profitability of the clinic would be uncertain, as it is tied to volume, but the ability of the clinic to generate a profit would be guaranteed.

To illustrate, if Atlanta Clinic's costs were all variable, then its variable cost rate at 75,000 visits would be $94.41. Thus, the contribution margin would be $100 – $94.41 = $5.59, and because there are no fixed costs to cover, that amount would flow directly to profit on every visit (even the first one). Of course, the amount of profit would be uncertain as it depends on volume, but the clinic would not lose money.

At the other extreme, consider a clinic that is totally capitated. In this situation, assuming a fixed number of covered lives, the clinic's revenue stream is fixed regardless of visit volume. Now, to match the revenue and cost structures, the clinic must have all fixed (no variable) costs. If the annual capitated (fixed) revenue exceeds annual fixed costs, the clinic has a guaranteed profit at the end of the year, assuming that visit volume does not increase beyond the relevant range.

Applying this concept to Atlanta Clinic, if its $7,080,962 in total costs at 75,000 visits were all fixed, and it received $7,500,000 in capitated revenues, it would lock in a profit of $419,038. Volume could be higher or lower than 75,000 visits, but the profit would remain the same as long as visit volume did not exceed the relevant range, requiring the clinic to increase fixed costs.

In both illustrations, the key to minimizing risk (ensuring a predictable profit) is to create a cost structure that matches the revenue structure: variable costs for fee-for-service revenues and fixed costs for capitated revenues. Of course, real-world problems occur when a provider tries to implement a cost structure that matches its revenue structure. First, few providers are reimbursed solely on a fee-for-service or capitated basis; most providers encounter a mix of reimbursement methods. Still, most providers are either predominantly fee-for-service or predominantly capitated.

Second, providers do not have complete control over their cost structures. Providers cannot create cost structures with all variable or all fixed costs. Nevertheless, a manager can take actions to make the existing cost structure compatible with the revenue structure so that it carries less risk. For example, assume a medical group practice is reimbursed almost exclusively on a per-procedure basis. To minimize financial risk, the practice can pay physicians on a per-procedure basis and use per-procedure leases for diagnostic equipment. The greater the proportion of variable costs in the practice's cost structure, the lower its financial risk (see "For Your Consideration: Matching Cost and Revenue Structures").

FOR YOUR CONSIDERATION
Matching Cost and Revenue Structures

Healthcare providers can lower their financial risk by matching the cost structure to the revenue structure. For example, providers that are primarily reimbursed on a fee-for-service basis can lower risk by converting as many fixed costs as possible to variable costs. Conversely, providers that are primarily reimbursed on a capitated basis can lower risk by converting variable costs to fixed costs.

Assume that you are the business manager of a large cardiology group practice. Virtually all of the practice's revenues are paid on a fee-for-service basis. However, the practice's two largest cost categories (labor and diagnostic equipment) are predominantly fixed. You are concerned about the potential for falling volumes in the future and want to take some actions to reduce the financial risk of the practice.

What cost structure (fixed vs. variable costs) is optimal for the practice? How can labor costs be adjusted to improve the cost structure? How can equipment costs be adjusted? Suppose the change in cost structure will increase overall practice costs at next year's expected volume. Does this fact influence your risk reduction actions?

Self-Test Questions

1. Explain this statement: To minimize financial risk, match the cost structure to the revenue structure.
2. What cost structure would minimize risk if a provider had all fee-for-service reimbursement? If it were entirely capitated?
3. What are the real-world constraints on creating matching cost structures?

Theme Wrap-Up: Profit Analysis

Jen concluded that Big Sky's cost structure (not including physician compensation) could be expressed as follows:

$$\begin{aligned}\text{Total costs} &= \text{Fixed costs} + \text{Total variable costs}\\ &= \text{Fixed costs} + (\text{Variable cost rate} \times \text{Volume})\\ &= \$850{,}000 + (\$15 \times 10{,}000 \text{ visits})\\ &= \$850{,}000 + \$150{,}000\\ &= \$1{,}000{,}000.\end{aligned}$$

By analyzing the practice's revenues, she determined that each patient visit brings in, on average, $160. Thus, the base case P&L statement looks like this:

Total revenues ($160 × 10,000)	$1,600,000
Total variable costs ($15 × 10,000)	150,000
Total contribution margin	$1,450,000
Fixed costs	850,000
Profit	$ 600,000

Here, the profit represents the amount available for compensation to the two dermatologist owners, less any funds that must be reinvested in the practice. Such reinvestments might be needed to update facilities or purchase new equipment, or they might be used to create a reserve fund to meet future requirements.

The profit analysis for Big Sky can also be expressed in this equation format:

$$\text{Total revenues} - \text{Total variable costs} - \text{Fixed costs} = \text{Profit}$$
$$(\$160 \times \text{Volume}) - (\$15 \times \text{Volume}) - \$850{,}000 = \text{Profit.}$$

Solving this equation permits Jen to analyze profitability under different assumptions. For example, at 9,000, 10,000 (base case), and 11,000 visits:

$$(\$160 \times 9{,}000) - (\$15 \times 9{,}000) - \$850{,}000 = \text{Profit}$$
$$\$1{,}440{,}000 - \$135{,}000 - \$850{,}000 = \$455{,}000.$$

$$(\$160 \times 10{,}000) - (\$15 \times 10{,}000) - \$850{,}000 = \text{Profit}$$
$$\$1{,}600{,}000 - \$150{,}000 - \$850{,}000 = \$600{,}000.$$

$$(\$160 \times 11{,}000) - (\$15 \times 11{,}000) - \$850{,}000 = \text{Profit}$$
$$\$1{,}760{,}000 - \$165{,}000 - \$850{,}000 = \$745{,}000.$$

The higher the volume, the greater the amount available for physician compensation and reinvestment in the practice.

Profit analysis also allows Jen to vary inputs other than volume. Suppose the variable cost rate is actually $20 rather than $15. Under that assumption, and assuming the base case volume of 10,000 visits, profit falls from $600,000 to $550,000.

$$(\$160 \times 10{,}000) - (\$20 \times 10{,}000) - \$850{,}000 = \text{Profit}$$
$$\$1{,}600{,}000 - \$200{,}000 - \$850{,}000 = \$550{,}000.$$

It should be obvious to you, and Jen, that she now has an important tool to help plan for and manage Big Sky's future.

KEY CONCEPTS

This chapter explains how managers rely on managerial accounting information to help make pricing decisions and to conduct profit analyses. Here are the key concepts:

- *Price takers* have to accept, more or less, the prices set in the marketplace for their services, including the prices set by government payers.
- *Price setters* provide services that can be differentiated from others, by either market share, quality, or other differences, such that they have the ability to set the prices on some or all of their services.
- *Full-cost pricing permits* businesses to recover all costs, including both fixed and variable and direct and indirect, while marginal cost pricing typically recovers only variable costs.
- *Target costing* is a concept that takes the prices paid for healthcare services as a given and then determines the cost structure necessary for financial success given the prices set.
- *Profit analysis*, sometimes called *cost-volume-profit (CVP) analysis*, is an analytical technique to determine the effects of volume changes on revenues, costs, and profit.
- A *projected profit and loss (P&L) statement* is a profit forecast that uses estimated values for volume, price, and costs.
- *Breakeven analysis* is used to estimate the volume needed (or the value of some other variable) for the organization to achieve a profit goal.
- *Accounting breakeven* occurs when revenues equal accounting costs (profit equals zero), while *economic breakeven* occurs when revenues equal accounting costs plus some profit target.
- *Contribution margin* is the difference between per unit price and the variable cost rate, or per-unit revenue minus per-unit variable cost. Thus, contribution margin is the per-unit dollar amount available to first cover an organization's fixed costs and then to contribute to profits.
- In marginal analysis, the focus is on the incremental (marginal) profitability associated with increasing (or decreasing) volume.
- A capitated environment dramatically changes the situation for providers vis-à-vis a fee-for-service environment. In essence, a capitated provider takes on the insurance function and hence bears utilization risk.
- The keys to provider success in a capitated environment are to (1) manage (reduce) utilization and (2) increase the number of members covered.

- To minimize financial risk, a provider should strive to attain a cost structure that matches its revenue structure.

Our coverage of managerial accounting continues in chapter 6 with a discussion of planning and budgeting.

End-of-Chapter Questions

5.1 a. Using a hospital to illustrate your answer, explain the difference between a price setter and a price taker.
  b. Can most providers be classified strictly as price setters or price takers?

5.2 Explain the essential differences between full-cost pricing and marginal cost pricing strategies.

5.3 What would happen financially to a healthcare organization over time if its prices were set at full costs? At marginal costs?

5.4 What is price shifiting (cross-subsidization)?

5.5 a. What is target costing?
  b. Suppose a hospital were offered a capitation rate for a covered population of $40 per member per month. Briefly explain how target costing would be applied in this situation.

5.6 a. What is profit cost-volume-profit (CVP) analysis?
  b. Why is it so useful to healthcare managers?
  c. What is a profit and loss (P&L) statement?

5.7 a. Define *contribution margin*.
  b. What is its economic meaning?

5.8 a. Write out and explain the equation for volume breakeven.
  b. What is the difference between accounting breakeven and economic breakeven?

5.9 What are the critical differences in profit analysis when conducted in a capitated environment versus a fee-for-service environment?

5.10 How does a provider's incentive differ when it moves from a fee-for-service to a capitated environment?

5.11 a. What cost structure is best when a provider is capitated? Explain.
  b. What cost structure is best when a provider is reimbursed primarily by fee-for-service payers? Explain.

END-OF-CHAPTER PROBLEMS

5.1 Assume that the managers of Fort Winston Hospital are setting the price on a new outpatient service. Here are the relevant data estimates:

Variable cost per visit	$5.00
Annual direct fixed costs	$500,000
Annual overhead allocation	$50,000
Expected annual utilization	10,000 visits

a. What per-visit price must be set for the service to break even? To earn an annual profit of $100,000?
b. Repeat part a, but assume that the variable cost per visit is $10.
c. Return to the data given in the problem. Again repeat part a, but assume that direct fixed costs are $1,000,000.
d. Repeat part a assuming both a $10 variable cost and $1,000,000 in direct fixed costs.

5.2 The Audiology Department at Randall Clinic offers many services to the clinic's patients. The three most common, along with cost and utilization data, are as follows:

Service	Variable Cost per Service	Annual Direct Fixed Costs	Annual Number of Visits
Basic examination	$ 5	$50,000	3,000
Advanced examination	7	30,000	1,500
Therapy session	10	40,000	500

a. What is the fee schedule for these services, assuming that the goal is to cover only variable and direct fixed costs?
b. Assume that the Audiology Department is allocated $100,000 in total overhead by the clinic, and the department director has allocated $50,000 of this amount to the three services listed earlier. What is the fee schedule, assuming that these overhead costs must be covered in addition to the variable and direct fixed costs? (To answer this question, assume that the allocation of the $50,000 in overhead costs to each of the three services is made on the basis of the number of visits.)
c. Assume that these three services must make a combined profit of $25,000. Now, what is the fee schedule? (To answer this question, assume that the profit requirement is allocated to each of the three services in the same way as overhead costs.)

5.3 Allied Laboratories is combining some of its most common tests into one-price packages. One such package will contain three tests that have the following variable costs:

	Test A	Test B	Test C
Disposable syringe	$3.00	$3.00	$3.00
Blood vial	0.50	0.50	0.50
Forms	0.15	0.15	0.15
Reagents	0.80	0.60	1.20
Sterile bandage	0.10	0.10	0.10
Breakage/losses	0.05	0.05	0.05

When the tests are combined, only one syringe, form, and sterile bandage will be used per patient. Furthermore, only one charge for breakage or losses will apply. Two blood vials are required, and reagent costs will remain the same (reagents are required for all three tests).

a. As a starting point, what is the price of the combined test assuming marginal cost pricing?
b. Assume that Allied wants a contribution margin of $10 per test. What price must be set to achieve this goal?
c. Allied estimates that 2,000 of the combined tests will be conducted during the first year. The annual direct fixed and allocated overhead costs total $40,000. What price must be set to cover full costs? What price must be set to produce a profit of $20,000 on the combined test?

5.4 Consider the CVP graphs below for two providers operating in a fee-for-service environment:

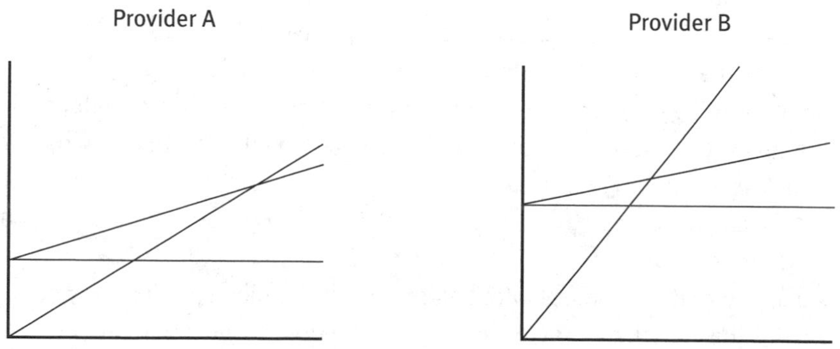

a. Assuming the graphs are drawn to the same scale, which provider has the greater fixed costs? The greater variable cost rate? The greater per-unit revenue?
b. Which provider has the greater contribution margin?
c. Which provider needs the higher volume to break even?
d. How would the graphs change if the providers were operating in a discounted fee-for-service environment? In a capitated environment?

5.5 Consider the data in the following exhibit for three independent healthcare organizations:

	Revenues	Total Variable Costs	Fixed Costs	Total Costs	Profit
a.	$2,000	$1,400	?	$2,000	?
b.	?	1,000	?	1,600	$2,400
c.	4,000	?	$600	?	400

Fill in the missing data indicated by question marks.

5.6 Assume that a radiology group practice has the following cost structure:

Fixed costs	$500,000
Variable cost per procedure	25
Charge (revenue) per procedure	100

Furthermore, assume that the group expects to perform 7,500 procedures in the coming year.

a. Construct the group's base case projected P&L statement.
b. What is the group's contribution margin? What is its breakeven point (in number of procedures)?
c. What volume is required to provide a pretax profit of $100,000? A pretax profit of $200,000?
d. Sketch out a CVP analysis graph depicting the base case situation.
e. Now, assume that the practice contracts with one HMO for all 7,500 procedures and the plan proposes a 20 percent discount from charges. Answer questions a, b, c, and d again under these conditions.

5.7 General Hospital, a not-for-profit acute care facility, has the following cost structure for its inpatient services:

Fixed costs	$10,000,000
Variable cost per inpatient day	200
Charge (revenue) per inpatient day	1,000

The hospital expects to have a patient load of 15,000 inpatient days next year.

a. Construct the hospital's base case projected P&L statement.
b. What is the hospital's breakeven point (in number of inpatient days)?
c. What volume is required to provide a profit of $1,000,000? A profit of $500,000?
d. Now, assume that 20 percent of the hospital's inpatient days come from a managed care plan that requests a 25 percent discount from charges. Should the hospital agree to the discount proposal? Assume that the managed care plan will contract with a different provider if the hospital does not agree to the discount (i.e., the hospital will lose the inpatient days associated with the contract).

5.8 You are considering starting a walk-in clinic. Your financial projections for the first year of operations are as follows:

Revenues (10,000 visits)	$400,000
Wages and benefits	220,000
Rent	5,000
Depreciation	30,000
Utilities	2,500
Medical supplies	50,000
Administrative supplies	10,000

Assume that all costs are fixed except supply costs, which are variable. Furthermore, assume that the clinic must pay taxes at a 30 percent rate.

a. Construct the clinic's projected P&L statement.
b. What number of visits is required to break even?
c. What number of visits is required to provide you with an after-tax profit of $100,000?

5.9 Grandview Clinic has fixed costs of $2 million and an average variable cost rate of $15 per visit. Its sole payer, an HMO, has proposed an annual capitation payment of $150 for each of its 20,000 members. Past experience indicates that the population served will average two visits per year.

a. Construct the base case projected P&L statement on the contract.
b. Sketch two CVP analysis graphs for the clinic—one with number of visits on the *x*-axis, and one with number of members on the *x*-axis. Compare and contrast these graphs with the one in problem 5.6, part d.
c. What is the clinic's per-visit contribution margin on the contract? How does this value compare with the value in problem 5.6, part b?
d. What profit gain can be realized if the clinic can lower per-member utilization to 1.8 visits?

CHAPTER 6

PLANNING AND BUDGETING

THEME SET-UP: ACTUAL VERSUS EXPECTED RESULTS

The Sumter County Organization for Rural Needs (SCORN) delivers low-cost healthcare services to residents of the county's rural areas. SCORN relies on volunteers to offer high-quality healthcare to people without health insurance and those who have insurance but find the organization's location and patient-friendly approach more attractive than other alternatives. In 2016, more than 50 physicians, dentists, nurse practitioners, and other clinical professionals volunteered their services, providing patient care worth more than $1.5 million.

One part of SCORN's operations is the dental clinic, whose services include pediatric dentistry, extractions, fillings, crowns, and dentures. Although the dentists are all volunteers, the support staff consists of volunteers as well as paid part-time staff; partially paid workers; and one full-time, paid employee.

At the end of 2015, Mark Mason, SCORN's director, created the following budget for the dental clinic's 2016 annual and first-quarter expenses:

	Annual 2016	First Quarter 2016
Coordinator's compensation	$ 53,334	$13,334
Hygienists' compensation	28,164	7,041
Assistants' compensation	103,877	25,969
Office staff compensation	38,047	9,512
Clinical supplies	40,000	10,000
Office supplies	2,000	500
Equipment maintenance	5,000	1,250
Utilities	6,000	1,500
Telephone	3,600	900
Total	$280,022	$70,006

In early April 2016, SCORN's accountant provided Mark with the actual expenses for the dental clinic for the first quarter (January–March):

Coordinator's compensation	$12,855
Hygienists' compensation	8,614
Assistants' compensation	27,443
Office staff compensation	8,470
Clinical supplies	9,344
Office supplies	529
Equipment maintenance	1,250
Utilities	1,355
Telephone	793
Total	$70,653

Mark must compare what has happened in the first quarter with what was expected to happen. Then, he must determine problem areas and take action to ensure that, at the close of 2016, actual expenses are in line with (or less than) those projected at the beginning of the year.

By the end of this chapter, you will have knowledge about the planning and budgeting process. In addition, you, like Mark, will be able to judge how well the dental clinic is sticking to its expense budget.

Learning Objectives

After studying this chapter, you will be able to do the following:

- Describe the overall planning process and the key components of the financial plan.
- Discuss briefly the format and use of several types of budgets.
- Differentiate between a simple budget and a flexible budget.
- Create a simple operating budget.
- Explain how variance analysis is used in the budgeting process.

6.1 INTRODUCTION

Planning and budgeting play a critical role in the finance function of all health services organizations. In fact, one could argue (and usually win the argument) that planning and budgeting are the most important of all finance-related tasks.

Planning encompasses the overall process of preparing for the future. Because of its importance to organizational success, most healthcare managers, especially at large organizations, spend a great deal of time on activities related to planning.

Budgeting
The creation and use of financial forecasts to plan for and control a business's operations.

Budgeting is one part of the planning process. Managers use a set of budgets (financial forecasts) to tie together planning and control functions. In general, organizational plans focus on the long-term big picture, whereas budgets address the details of both planning for the immediate future and, through the control process, ensuring that current performance is consistent with organizational goals.

This chapter explores the planning process and the way budgets are used in healthcare organizations. In particular, we focus on how managers can use variance analysis (comparing what has happened to what was expected to happen) to exercise control over current operations.

6.2 STRATEGIC PLANNING

Financial plans and budgets are developed within the framework of the organization's overall strategic plan (see "Critical Concept: Strategic Plan"). Thus, we begin our discussion with an overview of strategic planning.

Mission statement
A statement that defines the overall purpose of the organization.

Mission Statement

The **mission statement**, which is the guiding light for the strategic plan, defines the organization's overall purpose and reason for existence. The mission may be defined either specifically or generally, but it must describe what the organization does and for whom. For example, an investor-owned diagnostic imaging center might state that its mission is "to provide our patients with state-of-the-art diagnostic services at the lowest possible cost, which will also maximize benefits to our owners and employees."

CRITICAL CONCEPT
Strategic Plan

A business's strategic plan is a statement of where the business is now, where it wants to be in the future, and how it intends to get there. A comprehensive strategic plan contains many elements, including the mission, values, and vision statements, as well as goals and objectives. One way to think of a strategic plan is See-Think-Develop. In other words, *see* the current situation, *think* about where the organization wants to be, and *develop* plans to get there.

Normally, mission statements for not-for-profit businesses are stated in different terms than for-profit mission statements. The reality of competition in the healthcare field, however, forces all businesses, regardless of ownership status, to operate in a manner consistent with financial viability. To illustrate a not-for-profit mission statement, consider the following statement of Bayside Memorial Hospital:

The mission of Bayside Memorial Hospital is to

- provide comprehensive, state-of-the-art patient services;
- emphasize caring and other human values in the treatment of patients and in relations with employees, medical staff, and community; and
- provide employees and medical staff with maximum opportunities to achieve their personal and professional goals.

Values Statement

The **values statement** represents the core beliefs that define the organization. In general, this statement contains a brief list of the basic tenets that underlie the culture of the organization. For example, here is Bayside's statement:

Values statement
A statement of the core beliefs that underlie the culture of the organization.

Bayside Memorial Hospital believes in the following values:

- Treat everyone with respect and dignity.
- Be compassionate in comfort and care.
- Do the right thing at the right time for the right reason.
- Achieve excellence and ensure quality.

You can get a good feel for Bayside's organizational culture from this list, which, along with the mission statement, plays an important role in constructing the remainder of the strategic plan.

Vision Statement

The **vision statement** usually is a single-sentence description of the organization's desired position at a future point in time—say, ten years. The intent is to provide a single goal that motivates managers, employees, and the medical staff. Bayside's vision statement is "to be the regional leader in providing state-of-the-art, compassionate care in a humanistic environment."

Vision statement
A statement that describes the desired position of the business at a future point in time.

In addition to providing basic guidance regarding management and employee behavior at Bayside, the mission, values, and vision statements provide managers with a framework for establishing specific goals and objectives.

Organizational Goals

Organizational goals
Specified goals, including financial, that an organization strives to attain. Generally, organizational goals are qualitative in nature.

Although the mission, values, and vision statements articulate the general philosophy and approach of the organization, they do not provide managers with specific goals. **Organizational goals** set forth the outcomes from operations, usually qualitative, that management strives to attain. These goals should be changed over time as conditions change, and they should be challenging yet realistically achievable. Organizational goals occasionally conflict with each other, and when they do, senior managers have to make judgments regarding which ones should take precedence.

Bayside divides its organizational goals into the following five major areas:

1. Quality and customer satisfaction
   - Make quality performance the goal of each employee.
   - Be recognized by our patients as the provider of choice in our market area.
   - Rapidly identify and resolve areas of patient dissatisfaction.
2. Medical staff relations
   - Identify and develop timely channels of communication among all members of the medical staff, management, and board of directors.
   - Respond in a timely manner to all medical staff concerns brought to the attention of management.
   - Make Bayside Memorial Hospital a more desirable location to practice medicine.
   - Develop strategies to enhance the mutual commitment of the medical staff, administration, and board of directors for the benefit of the hospital's stakeholders.
   - Provide the highest-quality, most cost-effective medical care through a collaborative effort among the medical staff, administration, and board of directors.
3. Human resource management
   - Be recognized as the customer service leader in our market area.
   - Develop and manage human resources to make Bayside Memorial Hospital the most attractive location to work in our market area.
4. Financial performance
   - Maintain a financial condition that permits us to be highly competitive in our market area.
   - Develop the systems necessary to identify inpatient and outpatient costs by unit of service.
5. Health systems management
   - Be a leader in applied technology based on patient needs.
   - Establish new services and programs in response to patient needs.
   - Be at the forefront of electronic medical records technology.

Organizational Objectives

Once an organization has defined its organizational goals, it must develop **organizational objectives** to help achieve those goals. Organizational objectives generally are quantitative in nature, such as specifying a target market share, a target volume-growth rate, or a target profitability measure. Thus, organizational objectives set specific benchmarks (targets) that managers must strive to achieve. Furthermore, the extent to which organizational objectives are met is commonly the basis of managers' performance compensation (bonuses and the like).

Organizational objectives
Quantitative targets that an organization sets to meet its organizational goals.

To illustrate, consider Bayside's financial performance goal of maintaining a financial condition that permits the hospital to be highly competitive in its market area. The following objectives are tied to that goal (the financial measures listed here are explained in detail in chapter 13):

- Maintain or exceed the hospital's current 4.3 percent operating margin.
- Maintain the hospital's debt ratio in the range of 35–40 percent.
- Maintain the hospital's liquidity at a minimum of 2.0 as measured by the current ratio.
- Increase the use of fixed assets, as measured by the fixed-asset turnover ratio, to 1.5.

The keys to setting good organizational objectives are that they must (1) support the business's organizational goals and (2) be challenging yet attainable within a realistic period.

Self-Test Questions

1. Briefly describe the nature and use of the following corporate planning tools:
   a. Mission statement
   b. Values statement
   c. Vision statement
   d. Organizational goals
   e. Organizational objectives
2. Why do managers at all levels need to be familiar with the organization's strategic plan?

6.3 OPERATIONAL PLANNING

Operational planning provides a road map for executing the organization's strategic plan. The key document in this process is the operating plan, which contains detailed guidelines for meeting

> **CRITICAL CONCEPT**
> Operating Plan
>
> An operating plan is a schedule of events and a list of responsibilities for meeting the goals and objectives laid out in the strategic plan. The operating plan ensures that everyone in the organization knows what needs to get done by when, and it provides a means to coordinate and track progress. Operating plans are more detailed than strategic plans are. In fact, too much detail in the strategic plan can obscure the overall vision of the organization. Often, operating plans are constructed to cover a five-year period, so they are also called *five-year plans*. Typically, the plans for the first year are laid out in great detail, while the plans for the following years are increasingly less specific.

organizational objectives (see "Critical Concept: Operating Plan"). In other words, the operating plan provides the "how-to," or perhaps the "how we expect to," portion of an organization's overall plan for the future.

Operating plans can be developed for any time horizon, but most firms use a five-year horizon. Thus, the term *five-year plan* is often used in place of *operating plan*. In a five-year plan, the plans are most detailed for the first year, with each succeeding year's plan becoming less specific.

Exhibit 6.1 outlines the key elements of Bayside Memorial Hospital's five-year plan, divided into chapters, with an expanded section for the financial plan ("chapter 7," part C of the exhibit). A full five-year plan outline requires several pages, but the one in exhibit 6.1 provides insights into such a plan's format and contents. Note that the first two chapters of the operating plan are drawn from Bayside's strategic plan.

For Bayside, much of the financial planning function takes place at the department level, with technical assistance from the marketing, planning, and financial staffs. Large organizations undertake the planning process at the divisional level. Each division has its own mission and goals, as well as objectives and budgets designed to support the goals. When consolidated, division-level plans constitute the overall organizational plan.

> ***Financial plan***
> The portion of the operating plan that focuses on the finance function.

Section 1 of the **financial plan** (see part C in the "chapter 7" section of the operating plan shown in exhibit 6.1) is the analysis of current financial condition, which in turn provides the basis, or starting point, for the remaining sections of the financial plan. (Insights into financial condition analysis are presented in chapter 13.)

Section 2 lists planned investments in land, buildings, and equipment (the capital budget) along with how these investments will be financed. (Capital investment decisions are discussed in chapters 9 and 10, and business financing is covered in chapter 8.)

Section 3 provides overall guidance on day-to-day financial operations. (Many aspects of financial operations are discussed in chapter 7.)

Section 4 focuses on budgeting and control, laying out financial goals at the microlevel (e.g., by division, contract, diagnosis) and the mechanisms used to manage operations through frequent comparisons with actual results. In essence, this section contains the budgets that provide the benchmarks that line managers should be striving to attain throughout the year.

Much of the information from the first four sections feeds into the forecasted financial statements contained in section 5. (Financial statements are covered in chapters 11 and 12.) The forecasted statements allow managers to see the financial implications of executing the five-year plan. If the financial statements do not meet managerial goals for financial performance, then the initial operating plan must be modified to create the desired financial results.

EXHIBIT 6.1
Bayside Memorial Hospital: Five-Year Plan Outline

Chapter 1	Organizational mission, values, vision, and goals
Chapter 2	Organizational objectives
Chapter 3	Projected business environment
Chapter 4	Organizational strategies
Chapter 5	Summary of projected business results
Chapter 6	Service line plans
Chapter 7	Functional area plans

A. Marketing
B. Operations
C. Finance
   1. Current financial condition analysis
   2. Capital investments and financing
      a. Capital budget
      b. Financing plan
   3. Financial operations
      a. Overall policy
      b. Cash budget
      c. Cash and marketable securities management
      d. Inventory management
      e. Revenue cycle management
      f. Short-term financing
   4. Budgeting and control (first year only)
      a. Revenue budget
      b. Expense budget
      c. Operating budget
      d. Control procedures
   5. Future financial condition analysis

? SELF-TEST QUESTIONS

1. What is the primary difference between strategic and operating plans?
2. What is the most common time horizon for operating plans?
3. Briefly describe the contents of a typical financial plan.
4. What is the primary difference between sections 2 and 3 of the financial plan?

6.4 INTRODUCTION TO BUDGETING

Budgeting entails the entire process of constructing and using budgets, which are detailed plans for obtaining and using resources during a specified period (see "Critical Concept: Budgeting"). In general, budgets rely heavily on revenue and cost estimates, so the budgeting process applies many of the concepts presented in chapters 4 and 5.

> **CRITICAL CONCEPT**
> Budgeting
>
> *Budgeting* can be defined simply as planning for how much money you have and how it is spent. The purpose of budgeting for large businesses is essentially the same as budgeting for families (or individuals). However, the complexities in large organizations with many subunits make the budgeting process difficult and time consuming. Budgeting plays an important role in all organizations because it is the primary tool for senior managers both to establish performance goals and to monitor operations to ensure that those goals are met.

Managers must think of budgets not as accounting tools but as managerial tools. Budgets are more important to managers than to accountants because budgets provide the means to plan and communicate operational expectations within an organization. Every manager must be aware of the plans made by other managers and by the organization as a whole, and budgets help communicate these plans. The budgeting process and the resultant final budget allow senior managers to allocate financial resources.

Planning, communication, and resource allocation are major purposes of the budgeting process, but perhaps the greatest value of budgeting is that it establishes financial benchmarks for control. Comparing budgets to actual results provides managers with feedback about the financial performance of a department, a service, a contract, or the organization as a whole. Such comparisons help managers evaluate the performance of individuals, departments, product lines, reimbursement contracts, and so on.

Finally, budgets inform managers about what needs to be done to improve performance. When actual results fall short of those specified in the budget, managers must identify the areas that caused the subpar performance. In this way, managerial resources can be brought to bear on those areas of operations that offer the most promise for financial improvement.

The information developed by comparing actual results with expected (planned) results (the control process) is useful in improving the overall accuracy of the planning process. Managers want to meet budget targets, and hence most managers will think long and hard as they develop those targets.

> **SELF-TEST QUESTIONS**
>
> 1. What is budgeting?
> 2. What are its primary purposes and benefits?

6.5 BUDGETING DECISIONS

Managers must make several decisions regarding the budgeting process, including the three most important determinations: general approach to the process, timing of the budget(s), and basis of the forecast.

General Approach

Because budgets affect virtually everyone in the organization, and individuals' reactions to the budgeting process can have considerable influence on an organization's overall effectiveness, it is wise to plot with care how the budgeting process takes place.

In the **bottom-up approach**, budgets are developed first by department or program managers. Presumably, such individuals are most knowledgeable about the needs of their respective departments or programs. Next, the department budgets are submitted to the finance department for review and incorporation into the organizational budget, which then must be approved by senior management. Sometimes, the aggregation of department budgets results in an organizational budget that is not financially feasible. In such cases, the department budgets are sent back to the initial preparers (managers) for revision. This revision stage starts a negotiation process aimed at creating a budget that is acceptable to all parties, or at least to as many parties as possible.

Bottom-up approach
A budgeting system whereby budgets originate at the department or program level and then are aggregated and approved by senior managers.

A more authoritarian approach to budgeting is the **top-down approach**, in which the budget is developed by the finance staff and then, after approval by senior management, sent to department managers for implementation. Department managers may have some input into the process, but not nearly as much as in the bottom-up approach, because little negotiation takes place between department and senior managers.

Top-down approach
A budgeting system whereby the finance staff prepares the budget for senior management approval, after which it is sent to department and program heads for implementation.

The top-down approach has the advantages of being relatively expeditious and reflecting top management's perspective from the start. However, because it limits involvement and communication, the top-down approach often results in less commitment among department managers and employees to adhere to the budget than does the bottom-up approach. Most people perform better and make greater attempts to achieve budgetary goals if they have played a prominent role in setting those goals (see "For Your Consideration: Middle-Out Budgeting"). The idea of participatory budgeting is to involve as many managers, and even other employees, as possible in the budgeting process.

FOR YOUR CONSIDERATION
Middle-Out Budgeting

As you know, organizations may follow one of two primary approaches to start the budgeting process. In the top-down approach, budgets are established by senior management, perhaps the executive committee or board of directors (or trustees). In essence, senior management dictates the financial resources to be allocated to the department level. In the bottom-up approach, department heads create their own budgets, which are submitted up the chain for approval. Although the bottom-up approach has many

(continued)

FOR YOUR CONSIDERATION
Middle-Out Budgeting *(continued)*

virtues, in large organizations it often is impractical to have that many people directly involved in the budget process.

Some organizations are now experimenting with a hybrid budgeting approach called *middle-out budgeting*. Here, budgets are prepared at the divisional (or services) level, for example, a hospital's inpatient, outpatient, clinical support, and administrative support divisions. The budgets are sent to both senior and junior (department) managers for review and ultimate approval. In essence, middle managers—who presumably are in the best position to understand both sides and thus can create a budget that is adequate yet not excessive—act as go-betweens.

What do you think? Is there any merit to middle-out budgeting? Which approach is best for a small organization, such as a three-doctor medical practice? What about a 600-bed hospital?

Timing

Virtually all healthcare organizations have annual budgets, which set the standards for the coming year. The problem with an annual cycle is that it does not allow managers to detect adverse trends quickly. Thus, most organizations also have quarterly budgets, and many have monthly or even weekly budgets (see "For Your Consideration: Rolling Budgets").

FOR YOUR CONSIDERATION
Rolling Budgets

A rolling budget, also called a *continuous budget*, is constantly updated as time passes. In essence, a rolling budget is kept current by adding a period to the budget each time a period ends. For example, assume an annual budget is created for January–December 2016. When January 2016 ends, the budget is revised for the period February 2016–January 2017. Thus, the budget remains annual, but the year is rolled forward by adding an additional month as each month passes. Alternatively, the annual budget could be rolled forward by quarter, in which case it would be extended every three months as each quarter passes.

A rolling budget allows managers to incorporate new information into the organizational budget in a timely manner and get a feel for how that information affects

FOR YOUR CONSIDERATION
Rolling Budgets *(continued)*

annual (but not necessarily fiscal year) results. Thus, forecasts can be revised and the results of managerial actions can be incorporated monthly or quarterly, with results still forecasted on an annual basis.

What do you think? Are rolling budgets a valuable addition to the planning process? What information do rolling budgets provide that is not available in traditional quarterly and annual budgets?

Not all budget types or subunits in an organization have to use the same timing pattern. In addition, many organizations prepare budgets for one or more **out years**, which are more closely aligned with financial planning than with operational control.

Out year
A future year beyond the next budget year.

Forecast Basis

Traditionally, healthcare organizations have used the conventional (incremental) approach to budgeting as the forecast basis. In this approach, the previous budget is used as the starting point for creating the new budget. Each line in the old budget is examined, and then adjustments are made to reflect changes in circumstances (see "Critical Concept: Conventional Versus Zero-Based Budgeting").

CRITICAL CONCEPT
Conventional Versus Zero-Based Budgeting

Conventional (incremental) budgeting assumes that the previous year's budget accurately reflects the true (minimum) costs and (maximum) revenues of the organization. Thus, relatively minor changes are made to the current year's budget to reflect any changes in circumstances, such as increased labor rates. In zero-based budgeting, each budget unit starts with a clean slate, and all costs and revenues must be justified and created from scratch. Conventional budgeting is less costly to perform, but any inaccuracies and inefficiencies existing in such a budget tend to recur year after year. It follows that zero-based budgeting is more time consuming and hence more costly, but usually this approach produces a more realistic, and hence effective, budget than does conventional budgeting.

Under conventional budgeting, many budget changes are applied more or less equally across departments and programs. For example, wages and salaries might be assumed to increase at the same inflation rate for all departments and programs in an organization. In essence, conventional budgeting assumes that prior budgets are valid (make sound economic sense), so it focuses on determining the adjustments (typically minor) that must be made to account for changes in the operating environment.

As its name implies, zero-based budgeting starts with a clean slate. Thus, departments begin with a budget of zero. Department managers must fully justify every line item (e.g., employees, equipment used, amount of space allocated, inventories) on the basis of expected volume. In effect, departments and programs must justify their contribution (positive or negative) to the organization's financial condition each budget period. In some situations, department and program managers must create budgets that show the impact of alternative funding levels. Senior management can then use this information to make rational decisions about where cuts could be made in the event of financial constraints.

Conceptually, zero-based budgeting is superior to conventional budgeting, but the managerial resources required for zero-based budgeting far exceed those required for conventional budgeting. Zero-based budgeting is most useful at organizations facing reimbursement constraints, because such providers are forced to implement cost-control efforts on a more or less continuous basis.

As a compromise with bearing the higher costs of zero-based budgeting, some healthcare organizations use conventional budgeting annually but adopt a zero-based budget on a less-frequent basis—say, every five years. An alternative way to reduce zero-based budgeting costs is to use the conventional approach on 80 percent of the budget each year and the zero-based approach on 20 percent, rotating the areas that undergo zero-based budgeting. Then, over every five-year period, the entire organization will be subjected to zero-based budgeting. This approach takes advantage of the benefits of zero-based budgeting without allowing it to consume more resources than it is worth.

? Self-Test Questions

1. What are the three most important decisions managers must make regarding the budgeting process?
2. What is the primary difference between conventional budgeting and zero-based budgeting?
3. What strategies do companies use to limit the cost of zero-based budgeting?

6.6 BUDGET TYPES

Although an organization's immediate financial expectations are expressed in a document called the budget (or master budget), in most organizations "the budget" is actually made up of several components whose contents and format are dictated by the organization's structure and managerial preferences. That said, several types of budgets are used either formally or informally at virtually all healthcare organizations.

Revenue Budget

The starting point for the budgeting process is the volume forecast. However, volume forecasting can be difficult and complex (see "Healthcare in Practice: Volume Forecasting"). Detailed information from the volume estimate feeds into the **revenue budget**, which combines volume and reimbursement data to develop revenue forecasts. Planners at Bayside Memorial Hospital consider the hospital's pricing strategy for managed care plans, conventional fee-for-service contracts, and private-pay patients, as well as trends in inflation and third-party payer reimbursement, all of which affect operating (patient services) revenues.

Revenue budget A listing of the expected revenues (including both operating and nonoperating) of an organization, usually on a monthly, quarterly, and annual basis and broken out by department, service, and payer.

HEALTHCARE IN PRACTICE
Volume Forecasting

To get a feel for the complexities of volume forecasting, consider the procedures followed by Bayside Memorial Hospital.

First, Bayside's managers divide the demand for services into four major groups: inpatient, outpatient, ancillary, and other services. Second, they plot volume trends in each of these areas over the past five years, and they make a first approximation forecast, assuming a continuation of past trends. Third, the managers forecast the level of population growth and disease trends. For example, how much will the senior citizen population in the hospital's service area grow? These forecasts are used to develop volume by major diagnoses and to differentiate between normal services and critical care services.

Fourth, Bayside's managers analyze the competitive environment. Consideration is given to such factors as the hospital's inpatient and outpatient capacities, its competitors' capacities, and new services or service improvements that either Bayside or its competitors might institute. Fifth, they consider the effect of the hospital's planned pricing actions on volume. For example, does the hospital have plans to raise outpatient

(continued)

HEALTHCARE IN PRACTICE
Volume Forecasting *(continued)*

charges to boost profit margins or to lower charges to gain market share and use excess capacity? If such actions are expected to affect volume forecasts, these forecasts must be revised to reflect the expected impact. Marketing campaigns and changes in managed care plan contracts also affect volume, so probable developments in these areas must be considered.

The consequences can be serious if the hospital's volume forecast is off the mark. If the market for any particular service expands more than Bayside has expected and planned for, the hospital will not be able to meet its patients' needs. Potential patients will go to competitors, and Bayside may suffer reputational consequences and perhaps miss a major opportunity to gain visibility and market share. However, if Bayside's projections are overly optimistic, it could end up with too much capacity, which results in higher-than-necessary costs because of excess facilities and staff.

It may be interesting for readers to note that Bayside recently revised its entire budgeting process. Previously, the process was spreadsheet driven and took more than five months to complete. Departments were preoccupied with constant concern that the paper budget would not be completed in time to be presented at the September board of trustees meeting, which was the traditional approval date. Once the annual budget was approved, six more weeks were required to break down the budget into monthly and quarterly budgets and to distribute the reports to department managers.

Bayside currently uses proprietary software that creates the budget electronically. This system reduced the budget cycle by two months, or about 40 percent. The budget now is integrated with the hospital's financial reporting system, which means feedback (and hence control) is available on a continuous basis. The result is more efficiency in budget preparation, more confidence in the budget process, and streamlined reporting with easy online access for both department and senior managers.

The result is a compilation of operating revenue forecasts by service, both in the aggregate—for example, inpatient revenue—and on an individual diagnosis or procedure basis. The individual diagnosis and procedure forecasts are summed and then compared with the aggregate service group forecasts. Differences are reconciled, and the outcome is an operating revenue forecast for the hospital as a whole, but with breakdowns by service categories and by individual diagnoses and procedures.

In addition to operating revenues, other revenues (e.g., contributions, interest income on investments, rental receipts on medical office buildings) must be forecasted. Note that in all revenue forecasts, timing is important. Thus, the revenue budget must forecast not only the amount of revenue but also the time it is expected to occur—typically by month, quarter, and year.

Expense Budget

Like the revenue budget, the **expense budget** is driven by the volume of services provided. This budget focuses on the costs of providing services. Like the revenue budget, the expense budget is a compilation of expense forecasts by department, service, and individual diagnosis or procedure.

The expense budget typically is divided into labor and nonlabor components. Labor expenses include salaries; wages; and fringe benefits, including travel and education. Nonlabor components include expenses associated with depreciation, leases, utilities, and administrative and medical supplies. Expenses normally are broken down into fixed and variable components. (As discussed later in this chapter, cost structure information is required if an organization uses flexible budgeting techniques.)

Expense budget
A listing of the expected expenses of an organization, usually by department and service, and further broken down into components such as facilities, labor, and supplies.

Operating Budget

For large organizations, the operating budget is a combination of the revenue and expense budgets (see "Critical Concept: Operating Budget"). Small organizations may not prepare formal revenue and expense budgets at all, but rather use the data directly to prepare a single operating budget. Because the operating budget focuses on revenues and expenses, and hence profits, it can be thought of as a forecasted profit and loss (P&L) statement. Operating budgets can be, and are, prepared at multiple levels in organizations. Thus, operating budgets are prepared for entire organizations, departments, service lines, payers, and any other level that makes sense for managerial monitoring and control. In addition, they are prepared for different periods, usually annually, quarterly, and, at some organizations, monthly.

For budgeting purposes, departments often are classified as cost centers or profit centers. **Cost centers** are organizational subunits, typically departments, that incur costs but do not directly generate revenues. For example, the overhead units in a hospital, such as facilities and finance departments, are cost centers. Managers of cost centers are held responsible only for the costs of running their departments.

Cost center
A subunit in an organization that incurs costs but generates no revenues.

CRITICAL CONCEPT
Operating Budget

An operating budget uses underlying data, such as volume, reimbursements, and labor requirements, to forecast revenues, expenses (costs), and profits. They are prepared at multiple levels and for specific services and contracts. These budgets typically are prepared on a monthly and annual basis. For most organizations, operating budgets are the primary focus of the budgeting process because they focus on a key financial indicator—profitability.

Profit (revenue) center
A subunit in an organization that both generates revenues and incurs costs, hence creating profits.

Profit (revenue) centers are organizational subunits that generate revenues as well as costs, so their managers can be held accountable for profitability. Note, however, that profit center managers typically have more control over costs than over revenues. (In reality, their ability to control indirect, or overhead, costs also is limited. See chapter 4 for a discussion of overhead cost allocation.) In a hospital, examples of revenue centers include routine care, outpatient, and emergency departments.

SELF-TEST QUESTIONS

1. What are some budget types used in healthcare organizations?
2. What is the difference between a cost center and a profit center? Give examples of each in a hospital setting.

Exhibit 6.2 contains the 2016 operating budget for Carroll Clinic, a small primary care practice. Most operating budgets are more complex than this illustration, which has purposely been kept simple for ease of discussion.

Developed in late 2015, the starting point for this operating budget, as with most financial forecasts in healthcare organizations, is patient volume. A volume projection gives managers a starting point for developing revenue and cost estimates. Part I of exhibit 6.2 shows that Carroll Clinic's expected patient volume for 2016 comes from two sources: payer A and payer B. In total, the clinic's patient base is expected to produce 9,000 + 12,000 = 21,000 visits.

Part II contains reimbursement data. The clinic's net collection for each visit averages $100 from payer A and $90 from payer B. (Both payers reimburse the clinic on a fee-for-service basis.) Of course, some visits will generate greater revenues, and some will generate lesser revenues. The patients who visit the clinic are essentially the same in demographics, diagnoses, and treatment, regardless of payer. However, payer B has been more aggressive in negotiating discounts from charges, and hence it pays, on average, $10 less per visit than does payer A.

Part III focuses on costs. Supplies expense, the bulk of which is inherently variable in nature, is expected to total $315,000 for the year. Examples include forms, rubber gloves, syringes, medications, bandage materials, and a host of other medical expendables. Because these supplies will support 21,000 visits, their average cost per visit is $315,000 ÷ 21,000 = $15.

To support the forecasted 21,000 visits, the clinic is expected to incur labor costs of $1,035,000. Thus, labor costs are expected to average $1,035,000 ÷ 21,000 = $49.29 per visit. However, labor costs are predominantly fixed costs, so the per-visit amount is not as meaningful as the $15 per-visit supplies cost. Finally, the clinic is expected to incur

Exhibit 6.2
Carroll Clinic: 2016 Operating Budget

I. Volume (Number of Visits)		
Payer A		9,000
Payer B		12,000
Total		21,000
II. Reimbursement (per Visit)		
Payer A	$	100
Payer B	$	90
III. Costs		
Variable costs:		
Supplies		$ 315,000
Fixed costs:		
Labor		$1,035,000
Overhead		500,000
Total		$1,535,000
IV. Forecasted P&L Statement		
Revenues:		
Payer A		$ 900,000
Payer B		1,080,000
Total revenues		$1,980,000
Variable costs		$ 315,000
Fixed costs		1,535,000
Total costs		$1,850,000
Profit		$ 130,000

$500,000 of overhead costs in 2016, primarily for contract support (e.g., accounting, billing, collections) and facilities expenses (e.g., rent, housekeeping, utilities).

Part IV contains the budgeted (forecasted) 2016 P&L statement, the heart of the operating budget. Total revenues for the clinic are forecasted to be ($100 × Number of payer A visits) + ($90 × Number of payer B visits) = ($100 × 9,000) + ($90 × 12,000) = $900,000 + $1,080,000 = $1,980,000. If the actual number of visits is more or less than 21,000 in 2016, the resulting revenues will be different from the $1,980,000 forecast. The difference between the projected revenues of $1,980,000 and projected total costs of $315,000 + $1,535,000 = $1,850,000 produces a budgeted profit of $130,000.

The true purpose of the operating budget is to set financial goals for the clinic. In effect, the operating budget can be thought of as a contract between the organization and its managers and employees. Thus, the $130,000 profit forecast becomes the overall profit benchmark for Carroll Clinic in 2016, and the clinic's managers and employees will be held accountable for achieving the revenue and expense levels needed to meet the budget.

6.7 VARIANCE ANALYSIS

Variance
In accounting, the difference between what actually happened and what was expected to happen.

In accounting, a **variance** is the difference between an actual, or realized, value and the budgeted value. (Note that the accounting definition of variance is not the same as the statistical definition, although both meanings connote a difference from some base value.) Thus, variance analysis is an examination and interpretation of what has actually happened versus what was expected to happen (see "Critical Concept: Variance Analysis"). If the budget is based on realistic expectations, variance analysis can provide managers with useful information. Variance analysis does not provide all the answers, but it does help managers ask the right questions.

Variance analysis is essential to the managerial control process. Actions taken in response to variance analysis often have the potential to improve the operations and financial performance of the organization dramatically. Because many variances are more or less controllable by managerial actions, managers can take steps to avoid unfavorable variances in the future.

The primary goal of variance analysis should not be to assign blame for unfavorable results. Rather, it should be to uncover the cause of operational problems so that they can be avoided, or at least minimized, in the future. Even if the variances are beyond managerial control, their identification is still important to the well-being of the organization. For example, it may be necessary to tighten controllable costs to offset unfavorable variances in areas that are beyond managerial control.

Here we consider two approaches to variance analysis: simple variance analysis and flexible variance analysis.

CRITICAL CONCEPT
Variance Analysis

Variance analysis involves comparing what actually happened with what was expected to happen. A budget yields no value if it is not used as a benchmark for financial performance. If budget benchmarks are not met, managers must identify the shortcomings and, more important, take actions to ensure that the shortcomings are corrected and hence do not occur in future budgets. Furthermore, variance analysis of monthly and quarterly budgets should lead to operational changes that will help the organization meet annual goals when short-term performance lags behind expectations.

Simple Variance Analysis

Consider exhibit 6.3. In it, we combined Carroll Clinic's 2016 operating budget (shown in exhibit 6.2) with the actual results for 2016. Then, we calculated both dollar (or visit) and percentage variances.

As explained earlier, variance analysis involves comparing two amounts, with the variance being the difference between the values. For example, if at the beginning of the year, a hospital expected to make a profit of $2 million, but its actual profit was $2.2 million, the variance would be a positive $0.2 million, or $200,000.

Exhibit 6.3
Carroll Clinic: 2016 Simple Budget Variance Analysis

	Simple Budget	Actual Results	Variance: Dollar or Visit	Variance: %
I. Volume (Number of Visits)				
Payer A	9,000	10,000	1,000	11.1%
Payer B	12,000	11,500	(500)	(4.2)
Total	21,000	21,500	500	2.4
II. Reimbursement (per Visit)				
Payer A	$100	$105	$5	5.0%
Payer B	$90	$85	($5)	(5.6)
III. Costs				
Variable costs:				
Supplies	$ 315,000	$ 320,000	($ 5,000)	(1.6%)
Fixed Costs:				
Labor	$1,035,000	$1,050,000	($ 15,000)	(1.4)
Overhead	500,000	550,000	(50,000)	(10.0)
Total	$1,535,000	$1,600,000	($ 65,000)	(4.2)
IV. Forecasted P&L Statement				
Revenues:				
Payer A	$ 900,000	$1,050,000	$150,000	16.7%
Payer B	1,080,000	977,500	(102,500)	(9.5)
Total revenues	$1,980,000	$2,027,500	$ 47,500	2.4
Variable costs	$ 315,000	$ 320,000	($ 5,000)	(1.6)
Fixed costs	1,535,000	1,600,000	(65,000)	(4.2)
Total costs	$1,850,000	$1,920,000	($ 70,000)	(3.8)
Profit	$ 130,000	$ 107,500	($ 22,500)	(17.3)

Variance / Simple budget = %

The budgeted value, in this case $2 million of profits, is often called the **standard**, because that is the profit goal of the hospital (the standard to be reached) as expressed in the budget. In general, variances are calculated so that positive amounts signify "good" or desirable results, while negative amounts are "bad" results. As discussed in the following paragraphs, all variances are calculated in more or less the same way.

Standard
In variance analysis, the budgeted (expected) value established at the beginning of the budget period.

To begin a simple variance analysis on Carroll Clinic, consider the profit reported in part IV of exhibit 6.3. We start here because this is the most important single line on the operating budget. The profit variance was –$22,500, calculated as Actual value – Budgeted value = $107,500 – $130,000 = –$22,500. In other words, the clinic's 2016 profitability was $22,500 below standard, or $22,500 less than expected. Although this negative variance should generate concern, a more detailed analysis is required to determine the underlying causes.

Perhaps the first question that the clinic's management would want answered is this: Is the loss (relative to expectations) caused by a revenue shortfall, cost overruns, or both? To answer this question, we must examine the revenue and cost variances. The total revenues variance was Actual value – Budgeted value = $2,027,500 – $1,980,000 = $47,500, meaning that revenues were $47,500 greater than budgeted. Thus, all else the same, profits should be $47,500 greater than standard.

However, the total cost variance was a negative $70,000, so costs were $70,000 greater than budgeted: Budgeted value – Actual value = $1,850,000 – $1,920,000 = –$70,000. Note that we had to reverse the calculation to show that higher-than-budgeted costs are bad, and hence create a negative variance.

With revenues $47,500 greater than budgeted and costs $70,000 greater than budgeted, the net result is a profit shortfall of $47,500 + (–$70,000) = –$22,500, which, of course, is the profit variance reported in exhibit 6.3. However, once we break down the profit variance into its revenue and cost components, we readily see that the major cause of the clinic's poor financial performance in 2016 was related to costs rather than revenues.

In fact, we can go further in the analysis. Volume variance is a positive 500, meaning that volume exceeded expectations by 500 visits. Because the clinic's two payers use fee-for-service reimbursement, increased volume would lead to higher revenues, all else the same. However, in Carroll Clinic's case, payer A had higher-than-expected per-visit reimbursement (a positive $5 variance), while payer B had lower-than-expected reimbursement (a negative $5 variance). Payer A, with higher-than-expected average reimbursement, saw its volume increase, while payer B, with lower-than-expected average reimbursement, saw its visits decrease. The net result is total revenues that were higher than budgeted.

Finally, note that all cost categories (supplies, labor, overhead) had negative variances, meaning that all costs were greater than planned. However, the clinic's volume was greater than expected (by 500 visits), and higher volume typically leads to higher costs. The real question here is whether the higher costs were justified by the higher volume. To answer this question, we must construct another budget—the flexible budget.

Flexible Variance Analysis

Simple budget
The original budget, unadjusted for actual volume.

To be of maximum use, variance analysis must be approached systematically. The starting point is the initial approved budget unadjusted for differences between planned and actual volumes, which we have called a **simple budget**. However, at the end of a budget period, actual volume will rarely equal budgeted volume, so it would be useful to know whether the calculated variances are caused by volume forecast errors or some other factors.

A better examination of what is driving the variances calculated in exhibit 6.3 can be obtained by using a flexible budget in lieu of a simple budget (see "Critical Concept: Flexible Budget"). A flexible budget is merely the initial budget adjusted to reflect the actual volume achieved in the budget period. Essentially, a flexible budget is an after-the-fact device that tells managers what the results would have been under the volume level actually attained, assuming all other simple (initial) budget assumptions are held constant. A flexible budget permits a more detailed analysis than is possible in a simple budget variance analysis. However, a flexible budget requires the identification of fixed costs and variable costs and hence places a larger burden on the organization's managerial accounting system.

> **CRITICAL CONCEPT**
> Flexible Budget
>
> A flexible budget is one that is created after the budget period has elapsed. It is based on all of the assumptions, except volume, inherent in the simple budget. In other words, the flexible budget reflects the actual volume coupled with all other original assumptions. For example, assume that one of a hospital's payers is expected to provide 1,000 patient days at a per diem reimbursement rate of $900. Thus, the simple budget would show 1,000 × $900 = $900,000 in revenues from this payer. However, when the year is over, this payer actually had 1,100 patient days at a per diem reimbursement rate of $925, for actual revenues of 1,100 × $925 = $1,017,500. The flexible budget would show revenues from this payer as 1,100 × $900 = $990,000, because the flexible budget reflects the actual volume along with all other original assumptions. By creating a flexible budget, managers are able to identify whether variances stemmed from factors considered to be under line managers' control or from volume forecast errors.

To illustrate flexible variance analysis, consider Carroll Clinic's 2016 simple budget, contained in exhibit 6.3. The profit projection—$130,000—is predicated on specific volume assumptions: 9,000 visits from payer A and 12,000 visits from payer B. At the end of the year, the clinic's managers will compare actual profits with budgeted profits. The problem is that actual profits are not likely to be based on 21,000 visits.

Exhibit 6.4 is similar to exhibit 6.3, except that in this exhibit the budget standard is the flexible budget rather than the simple budget. The flexible budget reflects projected revenues and costs at the actual volume, as opposed to the projected volume, but it incorporates all other assumptions that went into the simple budget. By analyzing these new variances, Carroll Clinic's managers can gain additional insights into why the clinic ended the year with a loss (compared to budget).

Note that the volumes listed in part I of exhibit 6.4 are the same in both the flexible budget and actual results columns. Hence, they show no variances because actual volumes are used to create the flexible budget.

The flexible budget maintains the simple budget assumptions of Revenues = ($100 × Number of payer A visits) + ($90 × Number of payer B visits). However, the flexible budget flexes (adjusts) revenues (and costs) to reflect actual volume levels. Thus, in the part IV flexible budget column, Total revenues = ($100 × 10,000) + ($90 × 11,500) = $1,000,000 + $1,035,000 = $2,035,000, which reflects the initial assumptions regarding reimbursement along with actual volumes.

EXHIBIT 6.4
Carroll Clinic: 2016 Flexible Budget Variance Analysis

	Flexible Budget	Actual Results	Variance: Dollar or Visit	Variance: Percentage
I. Volume (Number of Visits)				
Payer A	10,000	10,000		
Payer B	11,500	11,500		
Total	21,500	21,500		
II. Reimbursement (per Visit)				
Payer A	$ 100	$ 105	$ 5	5.0%
Payer B	$ 90	$ 85	($ 5)	(5.6)
III. Costs				
Variable costs:				
Supplies	$ 322,500	$ 320,000	$ 5,000	0.8%
Fixed Costs:				
Labor	$1,035,000	$1,050,000	($15,000)	(1.4)
Overhead	500,000	550,000	(50,000)	(10.0)
Total	$1,535,000	$1,600,000	($65,000)	(4.2)
IV. Forecasted P&L Statement				
Revenues:				
Payer A	$1,000,000	$1,050,000	$50,000	5.0%
Payer B	1,035,000	977,500	(57,500)	(5.6)
Total revenues	$2,035,000	$2,027,500	($ 7,500)	(0.4)
Variable costs	$ 322,500	$ 320,000	$ 2,500	0.8
Fixed costs	1,535,000	1,600,000	(65,000)	(4.2)
Total costs	$1,857,500	$1,920,000	($62,500)	(3.4)
Profit	$ 177,500	$ 107,500	($70,000)	(39.4)

On the cost side, fixed costs are presumably unaffected by volume changes (in the relevant range), but budgeted variable costs reflect the actual volume of 21,500 visits: 21,500 × $15 = $322,500, where $15 is the assumed variable cost rate in the simple budget.

The flexible budget can be described as follows. The $2,035,000 in total revenues is what the clinic would have expected at the start of the year if the volume estimates had been 10,000 visits for payer A and 11,500 for payer B. In addition, the total variable costs of $322,500 in the flexible budget are the costs that Carroll would have expected for 21,500 total visits. By definition, the fixed costs should be the same, within a reasonable (the relevant) range, regardless of the volume level. On net, the $177,500 shown on the bottom line of the flexible budget represents the profit expected given the initial assumed revenue, cost, and volume relationships, coupled with the actual volume.

Next, we will examine the variances. The profit variance of –$70,000 tells us that, after adjusting for the actual volume, the clinic's profit was $70,000 less than expected. Thus, the situation is actually worse than that indicated by the simple variance analysis. In effect, greater volume should have led to greater profit, but that did not happen.

To understand why, take a look at the revenue variances. Payer A has a $50,000 positive variance, while payer B has a negative $57,500 variance. Because these variances have already been adjusted for actual volume, they reflect reimbursement changes only. In fact, higher reimbursement from payer A and lower reimbursement from payer B (compared to original expectations) created these variances. On net, revenues were $7,500 less than expected, given actual volume. In essence, the lower reimbursement per visit from payer B more than offset the higher reimbursement from payer A.

Next, we will change our focus to the cost side. Exhibit 6.4 tells us that the variable cost variance (which reflects supplies costs only) was $2,500. Because this variance is a positive (good) one, supplies costs were $2,500 less than expected after adjusting for actual volume. Thus, Carroll Clinic's personnel did a good job of managing supplies in spite of the negative variance reported in exhibit 6.3.

On the fixed cost side, the variance analysis remains unchanged between exhibits 6.3 and 6.4. Because fixed costs are not affected by volume, the simple and flexible budget amounts are the same, and hence the variance analysis is the same.

Final Comments on Variance Analysis

The Carroll Clinic example is meant to illustrate variance analysis techniques; it is not a complete analysis. A complete analysis would encompass many more variances. Furthermore, at most organizations, variance analysis is conducted at the department level, as well as at other sublevels such as service lines, and by the organization as a whole. Nevertheless, the Carroll Clinic example is sufficient to give you an idea of the variance analysis process and its benefits to the organization.

Variance analysis helps managers identify the factors that cause actual profits to be different from those expected. If profits are higher than expected, managers can see why and try in the future to exploit those factors even further. If profits are lower than expected, managers can identify the causes and embark on a plan to correct the deficiencies.

Large health services organizations have made significant improvements in their use of variance analysis. The benefit of expanding the level of detail is that it allows managers to isolate and presumably rectify problem areas. The marginal cost of obtaining such detailed information is lower now than ever because information technology initiatives are creating managerial accounting systems that generate large amounts of data that support budgeting and cost-control efforts.

SELF-TEST QUESTIONS

1. What are some key assumptions required to prepare an operating budget?
2. Why is the budgeted P&L statement so important?
3. What is variance analysis, and what is its value to healthcare providers?
4. What is the difference between a simple budget and a flexible budget?
5. How does the use of flexible variance analysis allow managers to isolate problem areas?

THEME WRAP-UP: ACTUAL VERSUS EXPECTED RESULTS

As mentioned in the theme set-up, Mark Mason, SCORN's director, needed to compare the dental clinic's actual first-quarter 2016 expenses against those budgeted. Here is how he conducted the variance analysis:

			Variance	
	First Quarter Budget	Actual Results	Dollar	Percentage
Coordinator's compensation	$13,334	$12,855	$479	3.6%
Hygienists' compensation	7,041	8,614	(1,573)	(22.3)
Assistants' compensation	25,969	27,433	(1,464)	(5.6)
Office staff compensation	9,512	8,470	1,042	11.0
Clinical supplies	10,000	9,344	656	6.6
Office supplies	500	529	(29)	(5.8)
Equipment maintenance	1,250	1,250	0	0
Utilities	1,500	1,355	145	9.7
Telephone	900	793	107	11.9
Total	$70,006	$70,643	($637)	(0.9%)

The dental clinic ended the first quarter with a negative total expense variance of \$637, which means costs were \$637 greater than budgeted. This represents a difference of less than 1 percent. Considering the difficulties in forecasting, Mark believes that overall the dental clinic's staff did a good job of managing expenses.

However, the individual cost item results are not all rosy. The compensation for hygienists and assistants was significantly over budget; in fact, the cost for hygienists was 22.3 percent over budget. Mark needs to look into these line items more closely to make sure they do not get out of control.

Of course, this variance analysis is only for a small portion of the dental clinic's overall budget, which in itself is only one component of SCORN's organizational budget. Still, this illustration gives you an idea of how budgeting and variance analysis are conducted by one health services organization.

Key Concepts

This chapter covers two important managerial activities: planning and budgeting. Here are the key concepts:

- *Planning* encompasses the overall process of preparing for the future, while *budgeting* is the accounting process that ties together planning and control functions.
- The *strategic plan*, which provides broad guidance for the future, is the foundation of any organization's planning process.
- The *operating plan*, often called the *five-year plan*, contains more detailed information than does the strategic plan.
- The *financial plan* is the portion of the operating plan that deals with financial matters.
- Budgeting provides a means for communication and coordination of organizational expectations as well as allocation of financial resources. In addition, budgeting establishes benchmarks for control.
- The *conventional (incremental) approach* to budgeting uses the previous budget as the basis for constructing the new budget. *Zero-based budgeting* begins each budget as a clean slate, and hence all entries have to be justified each budget period.
- *Bottom-up budgeting*, which begins at the subunit level, encourages maximum involvement by department or program managers. Conversely, *top-down budgeting*, which is less participatory, communicates senior management's views.
- Among the numerous types of budgets are the *revenue budget*, *expense budget*, and *operating budget*. The operating budget sets the profit target for the budget period.

- A *variance* is the difference between a budgeted (planned) value, or *standard*, and the actual (realized) value. Variance analysis examines differences between budgeted and actual amounts with the goal of finding out why financial outcomes were either negative or positive.
- The budget created at the beginning of a budget period is called a *simple budget*. When this budget is recast to reflect the actual volume of patients treated, leaving all other assumptions unchanged, the result is a *flexible budget*.
- Simple variance analysis compares actual results with the simple budget, while flexible variance analysis compares actual results with the flexible budget. The advantage of flexible variance analysis is that the calculated variances remove the effect of volume forecast inaccuracies, so the variances focus on factors that are, more or less, controllable by managers.

In chapter 7, we discuss some techniques used to manage operations.

End-of-Chapter Questions

6.1 Why are planning and budgeting so important to an organization's success?

6.2 Briefly describe the planning process. In your description, include summaries of strategic, operating, and financial plans.

6.3 Describe the components of a financial plan.

6.4 How are the revenue, expense, and operating budgets related?

6.5 a. What are the advantages and disadvantages of conventional budgeting and zero-based budgeting?
b. What organizational characteristics create likely candidates for zero-based budgeting?

6.6 If you were the CEO of Bayside Memorial Hospital, would you advocate a top-down or bottom-up approach to budgeting? Explain your rationale.

6.7 What is variance analysis?

6.8 Explain the relationship between a simple budget and a flexible budget.

6.9 What is the advantage of flexible variance analysis compared to simple variance analysis?

END-OF-CHAPTER PROBLEMS

6.1 Consider the following 2016 data for Newark General Hospital (in millions of dollars):

	Simple Budget	Flexible Budget	Actual Results
Revenues	$4.7	$4.8	$4.5
Costs	4.1	4.1	4.2
Profit	0.6	0.7	0.3

a. Calculate and interpret the two profit variances.
b. Calculate and interpret the two revenue variances.
c. Calculate and interpret the two cost variances.
d. How are the variances related?

6.2 Following are the budgets of Brandon Surgery Center for the most recent historical quarter (in thousands of dollars):

	Simple	Flexible	Actual
Number of surgeries	1,200	1,300	1,300
Patient revenue	$2,400	$2,600	$2,535
Salary expense	$1,200	$1,300	$1,365
Nonsalary expense	$ 600	$ 650	$ 585
Profit	$ 600	$ 650	$ 585

The center assumes that all revenues and costs are variable and hence tied directly to patient volume.

a. Explain how each amount in the flexible budget was calculated. (Hint: Examine the simple budget to determine the relationship of each budget line to volume.)
b. Determine the variances for each line of the P&L statement, both in dollar terms and in percentage terms.
c. What do the results in part b tell Brandon's managers about the center's operations for the quarter?

6.3 Refer to Carroll Clinic's 2016 operating budget, contained in exhibit 6.2. Instead of the actual results reported in exhibit 6.3, assume the following results:

I. Volume (Number of Visits)	
Payer A	11,000
Payer B	12,000
Total	23,000
II. Reimbursement (per Visit)	
Payer A	$ 95
Payer B	$ 95
III. Costs	
Variable costs:	
Supplies	$ 350,000
Fixed costs:	
Labor	$1,000,000
Overhead	500,000
Total	$1,500,000
IV. P&L Statement	
Revenues:	
Payer A	$1,045,000
Payer B	1,140,000
Total revenues	$2,185,000
Variable costs	$ 350,000
Fixed costs	1,500,000
Total	$1,850,000
Profit	$ 335,000

a. What are the profit, revenue, and cost variances based on the simple (exhibit 6.2) budget?
b. Construct Carroll's flexible budget for 2016.
c. What are the profit, revenue, and cost variances based on the flexible budget?
d. Interpret your results. In particular, focus on the differences between the variance analysis here and the Carroll Clinic illustration presented in the chapter.

6.4 Again refer to Carroll Clinic's 2016 operating budget, contained in exhibit 6.2. Instead of the actual results reported in exhibit 6.3 or listed in problem 6.3, assume these results:

Carroll Clinic: New 2016 Results	
I. Volume (Number of Visits)	
Payer A	8,500
Payer B	11,000
Total	19,500
II. Reimbursement (per Visit)	
Payer A	$ 90
Payer B	$ 80
III. Costs	
Variable Costs:	
Supplies	$ 320,000
Fixed Costs:	
Labor	$1,050,000
Overhead	550,000
Total	$1,600,000
IV. P&L Statement	
Revenues:	
Payer A	$ 765,000
Payer B	880,000
Total revenues	$1,645,000
Variable costs	$ 320,000
Fixed costs	1,600,000
Total	$1,920,000
Profit	($ 275,000)

a. What are the profit, revenue, and cost variances based on the simple (exhibit 6.2) budget?
b. Construct Carroll's flexible budget for 2016.
c. What are the profit, revenue, and cost variances based on the flexible budget?
d. Interpret your results. In particular, focus on the differences between the variance analysis here and the Carroll Clinic illustration presented in the chapter and in problem 6.3.

CHAPTER 7

MANAGING FINANCIAL OPERATIONS

Theme Set-Up: Revenue Cycle Management

Big City Medical Center is a major not-for-profit healthcare system. It operates five hospitals with roughly 2,000 beds and a physician staff of more than 2,000. Total revenues exceed $1 billion, stemming from almost 100,000 inpatient stays and more than 600,000 outpatient visits.

In 2015, Big City's senior management recognized that the system had a big problem with its revenue cycle: It could not quickly bill and collect the amounts due from its third-party payers. Like all healthcare providers, Big City must pay its employees, buy medical supplies, and run the facilities in which patient services are offered. Thus, it must pay its bills at more or less the same time (or even before) it provides services. After the services are provided, it bills the appropriate payer but does not collect the bulk of its revenues until later. In 2015, Big City waited an average of 60 days to collect from third-party payers.

With annual revenues of $1 billion, Big City bills, on average, about $2.7 million per day ($1,000,000,000 ÷ 365). Because it takes 60 days to collect these bills, the system has a total of $2.7 million × 60 = $162 million in receivables waiting to be collected. Because no money is collected to pay the costs of providing the 60 days of services, Big City must finance (borrow) roughly the amount of revenues that it is owed. The average hospital collects its bills in about 47 days, so Big City does not perform well in this measure of financial condition.

Recognizing the problem, Big City hired a consulting company to help shorten the amount of time it takes to collect from payers. After several meetings with Big City's senior management, the consultants offered a number of suggestions to improve Big City's financial operations, including measures used to monitor the revenue cycle.

As you read this chapter, you will gain an understanding of the revenue cycle and how managers use metrics to monitor and control operations. At the end, you will learn what the consultants recommended to improve Big City's billing and collections procedures.

Learning Objectives

After studying this chapter, you will be able to do the following:

- Describe the revenue cycle and its importance to healthcare managers.
- Explain how receivables are created and managed.
- Discuss in general terms how businesses manage cash and short-term investments.
- Relate the basics of inventory management.
- Understand how managers monitor and control operations.

7.1 INTRODUCTION

In previous chapters, our discussion generally focused on how to estimate costs and profits and how to use this information to plan for the future. This chapter covers a different element of healthcare finance—the management of day-to-day financial operations.

Unlike cost and profit estimation and planning for the future, the management of day-to-day financial operations is highly dependent on the specific type of provider organization (hospital vs. medical practice vs. nursing home). Thus, we treat this topic in somewhat generic terms. Our discussion begins with the revenue cycle and receivables management and continues to the management of two related items: cash and inventories.

It is not enough merely to establish a sound framework for financial operations. Good managers ensure that financial operations continue to run smoothly even when internal and external factors create turbulence in the environment. For the most part, clinical operations are monitored and controlled by the budgeting process, while financial operations are monitored and controlled using a set of metrics (measures) that focus on financial performance. This chapter concludes with a brief discussion of several of these metrics. Our intent here is not to make you an expert, but rather to provide some insights into financial and clinical operations and how they are monitored.

7.2 THE REVENUE CYCLE AND RECEIVABLES MANAGEMENT

One of the hottest topics in healthcare finance today, especially among hospitals, is the revenue cycle, which arises because most healthcare providers do not get paid for providing services at the same time those services are rendered. Providers incur cash costs for facilities, supplies, and labor but do not receive immediate payment to cover those costs. In fact, both hospitals and medical practices, on average, have to wait about 50 days to collect from third-party payers.

The revenue cycle concept is not new, but it is gaining increased emphasis as maintaining profitability in today's healthcare environment becomes harder and harder. One element of the revenue cycle (and perhaps the most important) is the management of receivables—that is, the management of monies owed to a provider (predominantly by third-party payers). Because receivables management is a critical part of the revenue cycle, these topics are discussed together.

THE REVENUE CYCLE

Generally, the *revenue cycle* is the set of recurring business activities and related information processing necessary to bill for and collect the revenues due for services provided (see "Critical Concept: Revenue Cycle"). More pragmatically, the revenue cycle at health services organizations should ensure that patients are properly categorized by payment obligation, that correct and timely billing takes place, and that the correct payment is promptly received.

Revenue cycle activities typically are broken down into four phases, based on their timing: (1) those that occur before the service is provided, (2) those that are simultaneous with the service, (3) those that occur afterward, and (4) those that are continuous.

> **CRITICAL CONCEPT**
> Revenue Cycle
>
> The revenue cycle arises because healthcare businesses must provide (and hence bear the costs of) services up front but are not paid for those services until later. Essentially, the revenue cycle consists of activities associated with gathering patient financial information, billing for services rendered, and then collecting payment on those bills. The process begins when a patient walks in the door (or perhaps even before) and ends when the organization has the cash reimbursement in hand. The shorter the time it takes to complete the revenue cycle, the better the provider's financial situation. At large providers, many people in different functional areas are involved in the revenue cycle. The process is further complicated by the fact that most providers must work with multiple third-party payers, each of which may use different billing formats and pay according to different contractual arrangements. Proper management of the revenue cycle usually requires a significant investment in information technology to support the billing and collections functions.

1. Before-service activities
   - *Preservice insurance verification.* The insurance status of the patient is confirmed immediately after the outpatient visit (or inpatient stay) is scheduled. This practice ensures that the patient actually has the insurance that was indicated when the appointment was made.
   - *Precertification (if necessary).* If the insurance verification indicates that the payer requires **precertification**, it should be sought immediately. Without precertification for services that require it, the provider runs the risk of having the claim (bill) denied even though the services were provided.
   - *Preservice patient financial counseling.* Before the service, the patient should be counseled regarding both the payer's and patient's responsibilities regarding payment. Presenting a large bill to an unsuspecting patient after the service has been rendered is unfair to the patient and can lead to problems in collecting the bill.

Precertification
An insurer's authorization indicating its willingness to pay for a particular service when delivered.

2. At-service activities
   - *Time-of-service insurance verification.* Staff members should check the patient's insurance status at the time of service to ensure that no changes have occurred since the initial verification. They should verify insurance with both the patient and the payer.
   - *Service documentation and claims production.* The services provided should be documented in a way that facilitates correct claims submission. The

documentation process should ensure that (1) the services provided are coded in accordance with the payer's claim system, (2) the code reflects the highest legitimate reimbursement amount, and (3) the claim will be formatted in accordance with payer guidelines and will contain all required information.

3. After-service activities

   - *Claims submission.* The claim should be submitted to the payer as quickly as possible after the service is rendered. However, speed should not take precedence over accuracy, because incomplete and inaccurate billing accounts for a large proportion of late payments.

   - *Third-party follow-up.* If payment is not received within 30 days, a follow-up communication should be sent.

   - *Denials management.* **Claims denial** by third-party payers is a major impediment to prompt reimbursement. Typically, most denials are caused by improper precertification and incomplete or erroneous claims submission. Prompt claims resubmission is essential to good revenue cycle management.

   - *Payment receipt and posting.* When the reimbursement is received, it must be properly deposited and credited. This activity ends the revenue cycle.

Claims denial
The refusal of a third-party payer to honor a submitted bill (claim).

4. Continuous activities

   - *Monitoring.* Once the revenue cycle activities are identified and timing goals are set for each activity, the provider should implement a system of metrics (key indicators) to ensure that these goals are met.

   - *Review and improvement.* The key indicators that monitor the revenue cycle must be continually reviewed with the goals of correcting any deficiencies and constantly striving to improve the process.

The revenue cycle requires constant attention, because the external factors that influence the cycle are constantly changing. Also, problems that occur at any point in the cycle tend to have ripple effects. That is, a problem that occurs early in the cycle can create additional problems at later points in it. For example, failure to obtain required precertification can lead to claims denial, which at best means delayed payment and at worst means no payment at all.

The ability of healthcare providers to convert services rendered into cash is critical to their financial performance (see "For Your Consideration: Revenue Cycle Management in Medical Practices"). Indeed, payment collections for services provided is essential for the survival of all providers. Problems in the revenue cycle lead to lost and late payments, both of which degrade provider revenues and hence financial condition. Think of the provider as giving an interest-free loan to the payer that covers the costs of the services rendered. The faster the loan is repaid, the better for the lender (provider).

FOR YOUR CONSIDERATION
Revenue Cycle Management in Medical Practices

Revenue cycle management is an important contributor to medical practice profitability. Yet, many physicians struggle with the idea that they are business people as well as clinicians.

One problem frequently encountered in medical practices is the lack of physician engagement in revenue cycle management. To create the most efficient revenue cycle process, all physicians, especially the lead physician, must be fully committed to the effort. Without a high level of executive sponsorship, small problems can quickly turn into large ones.

Physicians who are fully engaged in revenue cycle management send a clear signal that the process is of utmost importance to the overall success of the practice and that the entire clinical and administrative team needs to be on board. This commitment is particularly important when new processes or technologies are being introduced into the revenue cycle system.

What do you think about the need for physician involvement in revenue cycle management? Could the office manager and billing and collections staff handle the task? What can be done to encourage physicians and other clinicians to be more supportive of the organization's business practices?

Receivables Management

Because healthcare services are provided before payment is received, healthcare providers extend credit to patients (in reality, the credit typically is extended to third-party payers). The monies owed for each service rendered create an *account receivable* for the provider. (See "Critical Concept: Account Receivable"; the recording of accounts receivable on a provider's financial statements is discussed in chapter 12.) A provider's receivables accumulate over time as more and more services are provided. Eventually, however, the patient or third-party payer pays the account, at which time the provider receives cash and its receivables balance declines. The management of receivables is the most critical part of the revenue cycle, so it warrants a separate discussion.

CRITICAL CONCEPT
Account Receivable

Most patients have health insurance, so when they visit a healthcare provider, the services are rendered but no payment (or only a small copay) is made. The amount owed for the service, typically by a third-party payer (insurer), creates a receivable for the provider. Thus, an account receivable is an amount owed to a provider by a payer for services already rendered. At some future time, perhaps as long as 60 or more days, the payer will remit the amount owed and the receivable will be collected.

CRITICAL CONCEPT
Average Collection Period (ACP)

The average collection period, commonly called days in patient accounts receivable, is the average time that it takes a provider to collect for services rendered. For example, the ACP for hospitals today is about 47 days. That means hospitals, on average, have to wait 47 days from the time they provide a service until payment is received for that service. The best hospitals (top 10 percent) collect in about 35 days, while the worst (bottom 10 percent) receive payment in about 72 days. Of course, some portion of the payment (the copay) often is collected when the service is rendered, and some patients fall into the self-pay category. Still, the bulk of a provider's revenues comes from third-party payers, which creates a delay between the provision of services and the payment for those services.

The Accumulation of Receivables

The total amount of accounts receivable outstanding at any given time is determined by two factors: patient volume and the average length of time between service and collection. For example, suppose Home Infusion provides an average of ten home health visits a day at an average reimbursement of \$100 per visit, for \$1,000 in average daily billings. Assuming 250 workdays a year, the company's annual billings total Average daily billings × Number of days = \$1,000 × 250 = \$250,000.

At Home Infusion, all services are paid for by only two third-party payers: payer A, which pays for half of the billings 25 days after the service is provided, and payer B, which pays for the other half of total billings in 40 days. Home Infusion's average collection period (ACP), also called *days in patient accounts receivable* or *accounts receivable days*, is 32.5 days (see "Critical Concept: Average Collection Period [ACP]"):

$$\text{ACP} = (0.5 \times 25 \text{ days}) + (0.5 \times 40 \text{ days}) = 32.5 \text{ days.}$$

Thus, on average, it takes Home Infusion 32.5 days from the time that a service is provided to receive payment for that service.

Assuming a constant uniform rate of services provided, and hence billings generated, Home Infusion will have, at any given point in time, \$32,500 of receivables outstanding. We know this because the receivables are building up at a rate of \$1,000 per day, and it will take 32.5 days to collect them.

Think of the example this way: Assume Home Infusion just started operations, so it will provide and bill for \$1,000 of services on day 1, day 2, day 3, and so on. These billings will accumulate for 32.5 days, at which point \$32,500 of billings will have accumulated as receivables. On day 33 (approximately), the \$1,000 owed for day 1 services is collected. After day 33, the company will collect \$1,000 per day but, at the same time, provide another \$1,000 of services that will add to billings. The amount of billings outstanding (the receivables) thus will stabilize at \$32,500.

What is the financial implication of carrying \$32,500 in receivables? The \$32,500 in billings, except for a profit component, represents the cost of the home health services rendered—salaries, supplies, and so on—which have to be paid either before or as the services are provided. Thus, the funds required to pay the bills associated with the services must be obtained elsewhere until the receivables are collected. Home Infusion uses a bank loan to pay the bills (finance the receivables), which has an interest rate of 8 percent. Over a year, the firm must pay the bank roughly 0.08 × $32,500 = $2,600 in interest to finance (carry) its $32,500 receivables balance. (We use the term *roughly* here because Home Infusion's cost of providing $32,500 worth of services is somewhat less than $32,500, as it earns a profit on each visit.)

Monitoring the Receivables Position

If a receivable is never collected, the revenue is never received. Thus, healthcare managers must closely monitor receivables to ensure that they are being collected in a timely manner and to uncover any deterioration in **receivables quality**. Early detection can help managers take corrective action before the situation has a significant negative impact on the organization's financial condition.

Receivables quality A subjective measure of the speed and likelihood that a business's receivables will be collected.

One way to monitor receivables is to compare the organization's ACP to the national average ACP in the sector. For example, if the home health sector ACP is 37 days and Home Infusion's ACP is 32.5 days, then Home Infusion's collections department is doing a better-than-average job.

Note, however, that even though Home Infusion's payers are, on average, paying faster than the 37-day national average, payer A pays in 25 days while payer B takes 40 days. Thus, the firm's collections department should take a hard look to see if the ACP of the 40-day payer can be reduced to the national average, or even to the 25 days of the faster payer.

Why is minimizing a business's ACP important? To illustrate, consider the situation if Home Infusion's ACP were 37 days, and hence its receivables balance were $37,000. Assuming an 8 percent cost of financing (carrying) its receivables, the annual carrying cost to Home Infusion is about 0.08 × $37,000 = $2,960. However, at its actual ACP of 32.5 days, its carrying costs are roughly only 0.08 × $32,500 = $2,600. By reducing its ACP by 4.5 days, Home Infusion reduced its receivables carrying costs by about $360 annually.

No big deal, you may say. True, but now consider a large hospital with $100 million in receivables and a 60-day ACP, which implies average daily billings of $100 million ÷ 60 days = $1.67 million. A reduction of ACP by five days would reduce the receivables balance to $1.67 million × 55 days = $91.85 million, or by about $8 million. Assuming the same 8 percent cost of carrying receivables, the savings would roughly amount to a substantial 0.08 × $8,000,000 = $640,000. In addition, the hospital would receive a one-time cash flow of $8 million as the receivables balance is reduced. It should be apparent that immediate cash flow as well as annual savings can be obtained by reducing a business's

ACP, and hence its receivables balance. This idea is the driving force behind revenue cycle management—the faster the bills for services rendered are produced and collected, the better for the organization.

Aging schedule
A table that expresses a business's accounts receivable in increments according to how long it takes to collect each account.

A second tool for monitoring receivables is the **aging schedule**, which breaks down a business's receivables by age of account. Aging schedules are important to good receivables management for two reasons. First, as just described, the longer it takes to collect receivables, the greater the cost of carrying (financing) those receivables. Thus, aging schedules that show a large percentage of "old" accounts imply high carrying costs. Second, accounts that are long past due often become problematic, meaning that they end up not being collected and hence are written off as bad debts.

To illustrate, exhibit 7.1 contains the December 31, 2016, aging schedules of two home health companies: Home Infusion and Home Care. Both firms offer the same services and show the same total receivables balance. However, Home Infusion's aging schedule indicates that it is collecting its receivables faster than Home Care is. Only 50 percent of Home Infusion's receivables are more than 30 days old, while 60 percent of Home Care's receivables fall in the over-30-days category. More important, Home Care has receivables that are more than 90 days old. Knowing that the ACP standard for the sector is 37 days, Home Care's managers should be concerned about both the efficiency of the firm's collections effort and the ability of the late payers to make the payments due.

We have just scratched the surface of this topic. Furthermore, we have focused only on third-party payment. In general, providers also have to worry about collecting directly from patients, either the entire amount for uninsured patients or the copayment (or coinsurance) amount for insured patients. The bottom line, however, is that management of a provider's receivables is important (see "For Your Consideration: Managing Hospital Receivables"). Providers need to collect payment as fast as they can for services they render.

EXHIBIT 7.1
Aging Schedules for Two Home Health Companies

	Home Infusion		Home Care	
Age of Account (Days)	**Value of Account**	**Percentage of Total Value**	**Value of Account**	**Percentage of Total Value**
0–30	$16,250	50	$13,000	40
31–60	9,750	30	8,125	25
61–90	6,500	20	6,500	20
Over 90	0	0	4,875	15
Total	$32,500	100%	$32,500	100%

FOR YOUR CONSIDERATION
Managing Hospital Receivables

Although the general principles of receivables management discussed in this chapter are applicable to all providers, hospitals (especially large ones) face unique problems. The most obvious problem is the complexities in billing that result from having to deal with a large number of governmental and private insurers that use different payment methodologies. Hospitals have to maintain large staffs of specialists just to manage the billing and collections function.

To illustrate the problem, consider the following data on the receivables mix for the hospital field:

Payer	Percentage of Total Accounts Receivable
Medicare	26.5
Managed care	29.8
Self-pay	13.4
Commercial insurers	9.9
Medicaid	9.8
Other	10.6
Total	100.0

Multiple payers reimburse for services provided in many of the categories listed here, so the number of individual insurers can easily run into the hundreds. It is easy to imagine the problems that arise when dealing with a large and diverse collection of payers.

The following data provide information on how long it takes hospitals to collect receivables:

Average Collection Period (Days in Patient Accounts Receivable)

Percentile	Average Collection Period (Days)
10th	34.7
25th	40.0
Median	47.3
75th	58.0
90th	71.6

(continued)

FOR YOUR CONSIDERATION
Managing Hospital Receivables *(continued)*

Aggregate Aging Schedule

Age of Account (Days)	Percentage of Total Accounts Receivable
0–30	51.1
31–60	16.6
61–90	9.0
91–120	5.4
Over 120	17.9
Total	100.0

Hospitals clearly have some difficulty collecting bills in a timely manner. On average, collecting a receivable takes a little less than 50 days. However, this number has decreased in recent years as hospital managers have become increasingly aware of the costs associated with carrying receivables and as electronic billing and collections have become more prevalent. In spite of the positive trend, more than 20 percent of receivables still are more than 90 days old. In addition, about 5 percent of patient bills are never paid at all, with the percentage roughly evenly split between bad debt losses (patients and insurers that have the ability to pay but do not) and charity (indigent) care.

To help providers collect from managed care plans in a timely fashion, many states have enacted prompt-payment laws, which require payers to pay within a mandated period or face penalties. For example, New York requires that all undisputed claims by providers be paid by managed care plans within 45 days of receipt. If prompt payment is not made, fines are assessed.

Note: This Healthcare in Practice is based on data published in *Hospital Accounts Receivable Analysis,* first quarter 2016, Frederick, MD: Aspen.

SELF-TEST QUESTIONS

1. What is the revenue cycle?
2. What are the four phases of activities that make up the revenue cycle?
3. Why is proper management of the revenue cycle critical to the financial performance of healthcare providers?

? SELF-TEST QUESTIONS (CONTINUED)

4. Explain how a firm's receivables balance is built up over time and why costs are associated with carrying receivables.
5. Briefly discuss two means by which a firm can monitor its receivables position.

7.3 CASH MANAGEMENT

Although the management of a provider's revenue cycle focuses on receivables, it could not be optimized without good management of the business's cash and short-term investments.

All health services organizations need cash—both actual cash on hand and cash held in commercial checking accounts—to pay for labor and supplies, to buy facilities and equipment, to pay taxes (if applicable), to service (pay interest on) debt, and so on. In essence, maintaining sufficient cash ensures a business's **liquidity**, which is its ability to meet its cash obligations as they become due. A business that is illiquid cannot meet its payment obligations, and hence its operations suffer. If it remains illiquid for some time, it will ultimately fail.

Liquidity
The ability of a business to meet its cash obligations as they become due.

However, cash itself is a nonearning asset; that is, it earns no interest. Furthermore, commercial checking accounts, except for those of the very smallest businesses, do not pay interest, although banks are permitted to grant "earnings credits," which can be used to offset fees charged for other cash management services. Because cash earns no (or very little) interest, the goal of cash management is to minimize the amount of cash on hand but, at the same time, have enough to meet the business's immediate cash obligations.

The value of careful cash management depends on the current level of interest rates. For example, in the early 1980s, with short-term interest rates higher than 15 percent, businesses were devoting a great deal of care to cash management. During the economic downturn of the early 21st century, with short-term interest rates near zero, the value of cash management was greatly reduced. Clearly, only businesses with very large cash balances had incentives to maintain tight control over their cash positions.

Because cash management is an element of business operations in which economies of scale are a factor, banks have placed considerable emphasis on developing and marketing these services. Thus, banks can generally provide cash management services to smaller businesses at lower costs than such businesses would incur if operating in-house cash management systems.

FLOAT MANAGEMENT

A well-run business has more money in its checking account than the balance shown on its checkbook. *Float* is defined as the difference between the balance shown on the bank's records and the balance on the business's checkbook (see "Critical Concept: Float"). Because

CRITICAL CONCEPT
Float

Float is the difference between the checking account balance at the bank and the balance shown on the business's checkbook. For example, if a business has a bank balance of $75,000 and its checkbook shows a balance of $50,000, the business has $25,000 of float. Float is created when checks received by a business are processed by the banking system faster than checks that are written by the business. Float can be thought of as an interest-free loan from the bank. Thus, the larger the float, the better for the business. The use of technology such as electronic imaging and electronic funds transfer is decreasing the time it takes for checks to clear the banking process; thus the opportunities to create float are more dependent on internal processes.

float can be thought of as an interest-free loan from the bank, the larger the float, the better. (Personal float is also a good idea. Perhaps the best way to obtain personal float is to use a credit card to make purchases and then to pay the full amount of the credit card bill each month on or before the due date. In effect, the credit card company is providing you with an interest-free loan for the amount of purchases made that month, and hence extending float.)

To illustrate float, assume that Gainesville Clinic writes, on average, checks in the amount of $5,000 each day. (As the checks are written, the amounts are deducted from the checkbook balance at the clinic.) It takes six days for these checks to be mailed, delivered, deposited, and cleared, and hence for the amounts to be reflected on the bank's records. This lag causes the clinic's own checkbook to show a balance that is 6 × $5,000 = $30,000 less than the balance at the bank.

Now assume that the clinic receives checks in the amount of $5,000 daily, and it takes four days for the checks to be processed by the business office, deposited in the clinic's bank account, and cleared by the banking system. Because of the delay in depositing and clearing the checks, the clinic's balance at the bank is 4 × $5,000 = $20,000 less than that on its checkbook.

The clinic's overall float, then, is a combination of the incoming and outgoing check float components. The bank balance is $30,000 more than the checkbook because of checks written, but $20,000 less because of checks deposited. On net, its balance at the bank is $10,000 larger than the balance on its checkbook, so Gainesville Clinic's float is a positive $10,000.

The extent of an organization's float depends on its ability to speed up collections on checks received and to slow down collections on checks written. Efficient businesses go to great lengths to (1) speed up the processing of incoming checks, thus putting the funds to work faster, and (2) stretch out their own payments as long as possible (without engaging in unethical or illegal practices).

Short-Term Investments (Marketable Securities) Management

Many businesses hold temporary portfolios of securities called *marketable securities*, also called *short-term investments* or *near cash* (see "Critical Concept: Marketable Securities

[Short-Term Investments]"). In practice, cash and marketable securities management cannot be separated because management of one implies management of the other. Businesses have two primary reasons for holding marketable securities:

1. They serve as an interest-earning substitute for cash balances.
2. They hold funds that are accumulated to meet a specific large, near-term obligation, such as a tax payment, a construction project, or a new equipment purchase.

CRITICAL CONCEPT
Marketable Securities (Short-Term Investments)

Marketable securities are short-term investments held by businesses in lieu of cash. Because cash (including commercial checking accounts) earns no interest, as little cash as possible should be held—only enough necessary to meet immediate needs. Businesses should invest any excess cash in safe, short-term securities, such as money market funds or Treasury securities. By doing so, businesses convert a nonearning asset (cash) into an earning asset (securities). Of course, the amount earned on marketable securities depends on the prevailing level of interest rates. Still, some return is better than no return.

In general, the key characteristic sought in marketable securities investments is safety. Thus, most healthcare managers are willing to give up some return to ensure that funds are available, in the amounts expected, when needed. Large businesses, with large amounts of surplus cash, often directly own securities such as Treasury bills or negotiable certificates of deposit.

Smaller businesses are more likely to invest excess cash with a bank or a money market mutual fund because a small firm's volume of investment simply does not warrant hiring specialists to manage a marketable securities portfolio. Interest rates on mutual funds are somewhat lower than rates on direct investments of equivalent risk because of management fees. However, for smaller companies, overall returns may well be higher on mutual funds because no in-house management expense is required.

SELF-TEST QUESTIONS

1. What is *float*?
2. How do firms use float to increase cash management efficiency?
3. Why do firms hold marketable securities portfolios?
4. How do the cash management practices of large and small businesses differ?

7.4 SUPPLY CHAIN MANAGEMENT

Supply chain management involves the requisitioning, ordering, receipt, storage, and payment of supplies, including clinical supplies (e.g., tongue depressors) and office supplies (e.g., consent forms). Inventories are an essential part of virtually all healthcare operations (see "Critical Concept: Supply Chain Management"). Inventory levels depend heavily on volume—the greater the amount of services provided, the greater the need for supplies, both clinical and administrative. At many organizations, supply chain management is called inventory management or materials management. (To those who work in this field, each term has a slightly different meaning. For most of us, they connote the same thing—managing a business's inventories.)

CRITICAL CONCEPT
Supply Chain Management

Supply chain management (also known as inventory management or materials management) involves the requisitioning, ordering, receipt, storage, and payment of supplies. The process starts with the decision about how many items to keep on hand and ends when the supplies used to provide services are ultimately paid for by patients or third-party payers. Inventories are expensive to buy and to carry (keep on hand). Furthermore, some inventory items, such as drugs and reagents, have limited shelf lives (become unusable if not used by a certain date); for example, according to the manufacturer, Bayer aspirin has a shelf life of two years. Thus, the goal of inventory management, like cash management, is to have enough usable items on hand, but not too many because higher inventory levels mean higher costs.

Perhaps the greatest problem in inventory management is the fact that inventories must be acquired ahead of time. The necessity of forecasting volume before establishing inventory levels makes inventory management a difficult task. Also, because errors in inventory levels can lead either to catastrophic consequences for patients or to excessive inventory costs, inventory management in health services organizations is as important as it is difficult.

Base stock
The amount of inventory held to meet expected usage.

Safety stock
The amount of inventory, above the base stock, held to meet unexpected usage increases or delays in receipt of reorders.

Stockout
The situation in which a needed inventory item is not available at the provider.

Each item of inventory can be thought of as having two components. The first is a **base stock**, which is designed to meet forecasted volume. For example, a clinic might stock 100 test strips for prothrombin time testing, which is used to assess how long it takes for blood to clot. Regarding resupply, it takes one week to order and receive the strips, and the clinic expects to use 25 strips each week. Thus, the clinic orders the strips when 25 (one week's supply) remain and receives the resupply order as the last strips on hand are being used.

On top of the base stock, the clinic holds ten additional test strips to meet any unexpected usage increases or delays in receiving base stock reorders. These additional inventory items are called the **safety stock**. (Note that the same concept could be applied to cash management.) The reasoning behind maintaining a safety stock is that a **stockout**, whereby an item is not available, can be a matter of life or death for a provider's patients. Thus, the clinic actually orders prothrombin strips when the inventory level reaches 35 (25 base stock plus 10 safety stock).

In large organizations, inventory management requires close coordination among the patient services, purchasing, and finance departments. The patient services department is generally the first to spot changes in demand. These changes must be worked into the purchasing and operating schedules, and the financial manager must arrange any financing needed to support inventory buildups. Improper communication among departments, poor volume forecasts, or both can lead to disaster.

The key to good inventory management is information technology. Without information systems that support inventory management, the control system will become bogged down with slow-moving hard-copy data. To illustrate, most healthcare businesses now employ computerized inventory control systems. The computer starts with an inventory count in memory. As withdrawals are made, they are recorded in the computer, and the inventory balance is revised. When the point is reached that items must be reordered, the computer automatically places the order, and when the new items are received, the recorded balance is increased. (For more information on broad efforts to improve supply chain management with technology, see "For Your Consideration: The GS1 System of Standards.")

A good inventory management system must be dynamic. A large provider stocks thousands of different items of inventory. The usage of these various items can increase or decrease separately from rising or falling aggregate utilization of services. As the usage rate for an individual item begins to rise or fall, the inventory management system must adjust to avoid running short or having excess, and potentially unusable, items. If the change in

FOR YOUR CONSIDERATION
The GS1 System of Standards

Founded in 1977, GS1 is an international not-for-profit organization dedicated to the improvement of supply chain efficiency. GS1's primary activity is the development of the GS1 System, a series of standards composed of four key elements: bar codes, which are used to automatically identify items; eCom, which creates standardized business inventory messaging data; global data synchronization, which allows multiple businesses to have consistent inventory data; and EPCglobal, which establishes a system that uses radio frequency chips to track items across the entire supply chain from supplier to end user.

In the US healthcare sector, many companies—from manufacturers to distributors to end users such as hospitals—are actively supporting the adoption of GS1 standards. The goals of the companies involved include enhanced patient safety, improved supply chain management, enhanced drug control, and better connectivity to electronic medical records.

What do you think of the GS1 standards concept? How can bar codes and radio frequency chips enhance patient safety? Do you think that the adoption of GS1 standards will increase or decrease supply chain costs?

Just-in-time system
An inventory management approach in which items arrive just a short time before they are used, as opposed to sitting on the shelf for long periods.

Stockless inventory system
A system in which suppliers deliver small quantities of inventory directly to the using departments; a refinement of the just-in-time system.

Consigned inventory system
A system in which the supplier owns and manages the inventory until it is consumed (used).

the usage rate appears to be permanent, then the provider organization should recompute base inventory levels, reconsider the appropriate safety stock levels, and reprogram the computer model used in the inventory control process.

Many health services organizations are now using the **just-in-time system**, which is gaining popularity in all industries. To illustrate, consider Bayside Memorial Hospital, which consumes large quantities of medical supplies each year. A few years ago, the hospital maintained a 25,000-square-foot warehouse to hold its medical supplies. However, as cost pressures mounted, the hospital closed its warehouse and converted to a just-in-time system.

The process began with daily deliveries to the hospital's loading dock, where the supplies were sorted and taken to smaller storerooms in the hospital. After a few years, the system was recalibrated to a similar **stockless inventory system**. Now, the supplier fills orders in exact, sometimes small, quantities and delivers them directly to departmental storage cabinets inside the hospital, including those in the operating rooms and on nursing floors.

Bayside's managers estimate that the stockless system has saved the hospital about $1.5 million a year since it was instituted, including $350,000 from staff reductions and $650,000 from inventory reductions. In addition, the hospital has converted space previously used as storerooms to patient care and other cash-generating uses. The distributors that offer stockless inventory systems typically add 3 percent to 5 percent service fees, but many hospitals still can realize savings on total inventory costs.

As stockless inventory systems become more prevalent in hospitals, more and more hospitals are relying on outside contractors who assume both inventory management and supplier roles. In effect, hospitals are beginning to outsource inventory management. For example, some hospitals are experimenting with an inventory management program in which the supplier delivers supplies just as in a stockless system. The difference is that the supplier owns the products until they are used by the hospital, at which time the hospital pays for the items. Such an approach is called a **consigned inventory system**.

In addition to reducing inventories, outside inventory managers often are better at ferreting out waste than are their in-house counterparts. For example, an inventory management company found that one hospital was spending $600 for products used in open-heart surgery, while a competitor hospital was spending only $420. Because no meaningful difference resulted in the procedure or outcomes, the higher-cost hospital was able to convince the surgeons to change the medical devices used in the surgery and the hospital was able to pocket the difference.

? Self-Test Questions

1. Why is good supply chain management important to a firm's success?
2. What is the difference between a base stock and a safety stock?
3. Describe some recent trends in inventory management by healthcare providers.

7.5 MONITORING OPERATIONS

Thus far in this chapter, we have discussed many concepts related to managing financial operations. An important part of any healthcare manager's job is to ensure that the day-to-day operations of the business run smoothly and meet performance expectations. For the most part, this responsibility is fulfilled by monitoring a set of **metrics** that measure various aspects of operational performance. When the metric fails to meet organizational standards, a manager must act to correct the deficiency.

Metric
A value used to assess one element of performance.

Providers typically use a large number of metrics to monitor operations. Furthermore, many of the specific metrics used depend on the nature of the healthcare business. For example, a hospital metric to measure volume is number of inpatient days, whereas a medical practice volume metric is number of visits.

To give you a better appreciation of how managers monitor clinical operations, we define and illustrate several commonly used operational metrics. Because separating operational from financial performance is often impossible, some of the metrics discussed have a financial component. We are just scratching the surface in this discussion. For a more comprehensive list of operational metrics, visit the Health Administration Press Book Companion website at ache.org/books/FinanceFundamentals3.

Volume Metrics

One major concern of health services managers is patient volume. After all, providers typically have a large investment in land, buildings, and equipment and hence have to generate the number of patients necessary to cover the fixed costs of treatment.

In a fee-for-service payment system, a declining patient volume means falling revenue, which ultimately must be offset by decreasing costs. At first, labor and inventory costs can be cut, but if the volume decline is large, managers must consider shedding facilities. An increasing volume results in just the opposite situation. Inventories and labor must be added, and perhaps plans for new facilities developed, to handle the expected additional volume to accommodate the growth. Thus, the measurement of volume is critical to good management.

Inpatient Volume

For hospitals, **occupancy rate** measures the utilization of inpatient facilities. Because facilities costs are incurred on all assets, whether used or not, higher occupancy spreads these costs over more patients and hence increases per-patient profitability. To illustrate this metric, consider Riverside Memorial Hospital, which on one day in 2016 had 261 inpatients in its 450 beds. Thus, its occupancy rate was 58 percent:

Occupancy rate
The proportion (percentage) of hospital beds occupied.

$$\text{Occupancy rate} = \text{Number of inpatients} \div \text{Number of beds}$$
$$= 261 \div 450 = 0.58 = 58\%.$$

To interpret operating and financial metrics, managers compare the value against some standard and track the metric over time. The average occupancy rate for all hospitals is 49.5 percent. Thus, Riverside has a higher occupancy rate and hence is using its inpatient assets more productively than the average hospital. Furthermore, Riverside's occupancy rate has been climbing slowly over time, which is a good sign for the hospital. (The top 10 percent of hospitals have an occupancy rate of more than 75 percent, so Riverside has a way to go to be among the best.)

Note, however, that we have measured occupancy rate for only one day. Day-to-day fluctuations in volume are important indicators of seasonal volume changes. Once Riverside's managers identify seasonal utilization patterns, they can plan for and manage their inpatient operations.

In addition to monitoring daily inpatient volume, Riverside's managers will track occupancy on a weekly, monthly, quarterly, and annual basis. Such utilization (volume) metrics are important to the efficient management of any healthcare provider.

Outpatient Volume

To understand outpatient volume, one could just record the number of outpatient visits, which would be the measure for hospital outpatient departments, clinics, and medical practices. For outpatients, especially at medical practices, one common measure of volume is the **number of visits per physician**. This measure can be compared to other organizations (which typically are different sizes) or over time as the physician staffing level changes.

Number of visits per physician
The patient volume of an outpatient facility on a per-physician basis.

Assume that Medford Family Practice has five full-time equivalent (FTE) physicians and a total of 26,987 patient visits in 2016. The annual number of visits per physician is 5,397:

$$\text{Number of visits per FTE physician} = \text{Number of visits} \div \text{Number of physician FTEs}$$
$$= 26{,}987 \div 5 = 5{,}397.$$

The average volume for primary care physician practices is 5,090 visits per physician, so Medford is performing better than the average practice in using its physician resources. However, practices considered by the Medical Group Management Association to be top performers have more than 7,000 visits per physician, so Medford should consider actions to increase volume.

If the practice has unmet demand (e.g., long appointment wait times), perhaps it should add support personnel to enable the physicians to be more productive. Or, if the practice has an insufficient number of patients, it may consider instituting an aggressive marketing program or cutting the number of personnel.

Patient Characteristic Metrics

In addition to raw volume, health services managers must have other information about the organization's patients. For example, in a hospital setting, what proportion of patients uses outpatient services as opposed to being admitted as inpatients? What proportion of patients is insured by Medicare, Medicaid, commercial insurers, or other payers?

A host of measures defines the characteristics of a provider's patients. Clearly, this information is important, because patient characteristics define the nature of the services required and the reimbursement methods used.

Patient (Outpatient or Inpatient) Mix

Hospitals typically offer both inpatient and outpatient services. Historically, outpatient services were regarded to be more profitable than inpatient services. However, comparative profitability between inpatient and outpatient services is highly dependent on overhead allocation amounts and the type of organization, so making universal judgments is difficult.

The **outpatient revenue percentage** measures the percentage of a hospital's total patient services revenues that stem from outpatient services. Riverside has $163,832,000 in total patient service revenues composed of $40,092,000 in outpatient revenues and $123,740,000 in inpatient revenues, for an outpatient revenue percentage of 24.5 percent:

Outpatient revenue percentage
Outpatient revenues as a percentage of total revenues.

Outpatient revenue percentage = Outpatient revenues ÷ Total patient services revenues
= $40,092,000 ÷ $163,832,000 = 24.5%.

The national average outpatient revenue percentage is 58.4 percent, so Riverside has a much smaller outpatient program, relative to its size, than the average hospital does. Regardless of relative profitability, a larger percentage of revenue from outpatient services would render Riverside's revenue stream less dependent on a single source of revenue—inpatient services. Thus, it might be prudent for Riverside's managers to take steps to increase the volume of outpatient services. Such steps might include increasing capacity, offering more outpatient services (perhaps hiring more hospital-based physicians), or expanding the marketing effort to ensure that prospective patients think about Riverside as more than just a hospital.

Finally, note that because all of Riverside's patients are either outpatients or inpatients, an outpatient revenue percentage of 24.5 percent implies an inpatient revenue percentage of 100.0 – 24.5 = 75.5%.

Payer Mix

Medicare payment percentage measures the exposure of a hospital to Medicare patients and hence to payments set by political, rather than economic, processes. For inpatient services, Riverside Memorial Hospital had 7,642 Medicare discharges in 2016 out of a total of 18,281 discharges. Thus, its Medicare payment percentage is 41.8 percent:

Medicare payment percentage
Medicare discharges (or revenues) as a percentage of total discharges (or revenues).

Medicare payment percentage = Medicare discharges ÷ Total discharges
= 7,642 ÷ 18,281 = 41.8%.

Compared to a national average of 40.3 percent, Riverside has a somewhat higher percentage of Medicare patients than the average hospital does. To the extent that Medicare payments are lower than payments from other third-party payers, a higher Medicare payment percentage puts pressure on operating revenues. Conversely, if Medicare payments are higher than reimbursements by Medicaid or by managed care plans, then in some situations, a higher Medicare payment percentage could be positive.

Similar metrics can be constructed for Medicaid, managed care plan, and bad debt and charity care patients. Also, note that many payer mix metrics can be either volume based (such as visit or inpatient day) or revenue based.

Average Length of Stay

Average length of stay (ALOS)
The average time an inpatient spends in the hospital (per stay).

Average length of stay (ALOS), or just length of stay, is the number of days that an average inpatient is hospitalized with each admission. Riverside had a total of 95,061 inpatient days in 2016 from 18,281 discharges. Thus, the ALOS is 5.2 days:

$$\begin{aligned}\text{ALOS} &= \text{Inpatient days} \div \text{Total discharges}\\ &= 95{,}061 \div 18{,}281 = 5.2 \text{ days.}\end{aligned}$$

On average, Riverside keeps its patients in the hospital longer than does the average hospital, with an ALOS of 4.5 days. Still, Riverside has a lower cost structure, and hence lower costs per discharge, than does the average hospital. Riverside's managers would benefit from ensuring that its ALOS is consistent with the intensity of services provided. They may be able to lower the hospital's ALOS, which would mean even lower costs and greater profitability of inpatient services.

Price and Cost Metrics

Although volume is important to a provider's financial success, a high volume coupled with losses on each patient encounter will lead to disaster. To achieve financial soundness, the individual services provided must be profitable. Following are some metrics that focus on prices and costs.

Inpatient Prices

Price per discharge
The average revenue on each inpatient stay.

Price per discharge measures the average revenue collected on each inpatient discharge. In 2016, Riverside Memorial Hospital reported $123,740,000 in inpatient service revenue and discharged 18,281 patients, so the net price per discharge is $6,769:

$$\begin{aligned}\text{Net price per discharge} &= \text{Net inpatient revenue} \div \text{Total discharges}\\ &= \$123{,}740{,}000 \div 18{,}281 = \$6{,}769.\end{aligned}$$

Considering the national average of $10,154, Riverside collects much less per discharge than the average hospital does. However, if Riverside's cost per discharge is lower than average, perhaps its net price per discharge is appropriate. The net price per discharge cannot be completely interpreted without knowing Riverside's cost per discharge.

Inpatient Costs

Cost per discharge measures the dollar amount of resources, on average, expended on each discharge. Because Riverside's inpatient operating expenses for 2016 were $114,865,000, its cost per discharge was $6,283:

Cost per discharge
The average cost of each inpatient stay.

Cost per discharge = Inpatient operating expenses ÷ Total discharges
= $114,865,000 ÷ 18,281 = $6,283.

Riverside's cost per discharge is far below the national average of $10,162. Thus, though Riverside's price per discharge is below average, its cost per discharge is even more so. The hospital's average profitability on each discharge is more than that for the hospital sector.

Inpatient Profits

We can easily calculate **profit per discharge**, given net price per discharge and cost per discharge, as follows:

Profit per discharge
The average profit made on each inpatient stay.

Profit per discharge = Net price per discharge – Cost per discharge
= $6,769 – $6,283 = $486.

The average hospital loses money on each discharge at around –$27, so Riverside is performing comparatively well on its revenue from inpatient services.

Key Performance Indicators and Dashboards

As mentioned earlier, our discussion of metrics is introductory: Many additional metrics are available to help managers control operations, and they are usually created on annual, quarterly, monthly, or even weekly or daily bases. However, tracking a large number of metrics on a daily or weekly basis would overload managers and, as a result, important findings could be missed.

To help solve the data overload and timeliness problems, many healthcare organizations use key performance indicators (KPIs) and dashboards. KPIs are a limited number of metrics that measure performance critical to the success of an organization. In essence, KPIs assess the current state of the business, measure progress toward organizational goals, and

> **CRITICAL CONCEPT**
> Key Performance Indicators (KPIs) and Dashboards
>
> A key performance indicator is a metric chosen by a business to monitor one aspect of operational or financial performance routinely. For example, number of visits for a clinic (or net admissions for a hospital) might be the KPI that monitors volume. A dashboard is a way to present KPIs in an easily readable format. The dashboard presents metrics as dials or with color codes to signify whether benchmarks are being met. Some KPIs (e.g., volume) are reviewed daily, while others are reviewed less often.

prompt managerial action to correct deficiencies (see "Critical Concept: Key Performance Indications [KPIs] and Dashboards").

The KPIs chosen by any business depend on the line of business and its mission, objectives, and goals. In addition, KPIs usually differ by timing. For example, a hospital might have a daily KPI of number of net admissions (admissions minus discharges), while the corresponding quarterly and annual KPI might be occupancy rate.

Clearly, the number of KPIs used must be kept to a minimum to allow managers to focus on the most important aspects of operational performance. Yet, managers need a sufficient number to ensure that they can monitor all critical areas of clinical and financial operations. Determining the optimum number of KPIs requires a tough balancing act.

> ***Dashboards***
> Gauges or visuals that present key information in a form that is easy to read and interpret.

Dashboards—gauges or visuals that present key information in a form that is easy to read and interpret—are a common way to present an organization's KPIs. The term stems from an automobile's dashboard, which presents key information (e.g., speed, engine temperature, oil pressure) about the car's performance. Often, KPIs are shown as gauges, which allow managers to interpret the indicators quickly. Dashboards allow managers easily to monitor the business's most important metrics on a regular basis (daily for some metrics) in a form that is easy to read and interpret.

Self-Test Questions

1. Why are operational and financial metrics important to good management?
2. Describe three metrics commonly used to track operations.
3. What is a key performance indicator (KPI)? A dashboard?
4. How are KPIs and dashboards used to monitor operations?

Theme Wrap-Up: Revenue Cycle Management

In 2015, the managers at Big City Medical Center were concerned that collecting receivables from third-party payers took about 60 days, while the average hospital was collecting in roughly 47 days. To help address the problem, Big City hired a consulting firm. How did Big City improve its revenue cycle performance?

For starters, Big City created an executive-level position—chief revenue officer (CRO)—to focus organizational attention on the revenue cycle and on achieving best-practice results. Big City recognized that the revenue cycle is not simply a function of the finance department; it requires cooperation from a large number of Big City's clinical employees and physicians (who start the entire billing process with their diagnoses). In addition, revenue cycle improvement requires close and continuous dialogue with Big City's payer partners, primarily City Health Plan, Metropolis Blue Cross and Blue Shield, Medicare, and Medicaid.

To help meet Big City's revenue cycle goals, the CRO assembled a system-level revenue cycle management team that has full responsibility for revenue cycle management, including information technology, at all five of Big City's hospitals. Of course, implementation of all directives was accomplished through each hospital's chief financial officer and receivables management staff.

To monitor progress, the CRO established a set of revenue cycle performance metrics. The choice of metrics was driven by a focus on performance reporting and employee accountability. Without the ability to measure progress, to identify areas suitable for improvement, and to hold employees responsible for meeting goals, it would be difficult to make much progress. In total, almost 50 metrics were selected. Such a large number was required because it was essential to monitor hospital-specific and payer-specific performance in addition to aggregate (system) performance.

However, much of the attention was paid to six KPIs, which were called the *Big City Six*: (1) days in accounts receivable (ACP), (2) proportion of receivables more than 90 days old, (3) percentage of claim rejections (based on revenues), (4) percentage of final denials (based on revenues), (5) cash as a percentage of revenue, and (6) billed revenues per FTE revenue cycle management employee.

To give Big City's management a quick view of revenue cycle performance, the team compared each KPI against a management-established goal (standard) and best-practices benchmark. Then, variances were calculated in both numerical and percentage formats. (For example, if the initial standard was an ACP of 55 days and the first quarter's value was 60 days, then the variance was −5 days, or −5 ÷ 55 = −9%.)

After two years of effort, Big City saw a decrease in its ACP to 48.3 days, which puts the system just above the national average of 47 days and indicates that Big City is performing close to average. The money saved by reducing receivables provided a one-time cash flow of more than $30 million and now saves more than $1.5 million a year in receivables financing costs.

Key Concepts

This chapter examines some day-to-day financial issues related to revenue cycle and cash, inventory, and receivables management, including operational monitoring. Here are the key concepts:

- The *revenue cycle* includes all activities associated with billing and collections for services provided.

- The revenue cycle can be broken down into these activity categories, depending on when they occur: (1) *before-service activities*, (2) *at-service activities*, (3) *after-service activities*, and (4) *continuous activities*.
- When a health services organization does not receive immediate payment for services rendered, an *account receivable* is created. Receivables accumulate until staff members collect the amounts due.
- Businesses can use an *aging schedule* and a*verage collection period (ACP)* to help keep track of their receivables position and to help avoid the buildup of possible bad debts.
- The primary goal of *cash management* is to reduce the amount of cash held to the minimum necessary to conduct business.
- *Float* is the difference between the amount of cash in a checking account and the amount shown on the business's checkbook. The larger the float, the better.
- Float is increased by speeding up the collection of checks received and slowing down the processing of checks written.
- *Marketable securities (short-term investments)* serve as both a substitute for cash and a temporary investment for funds that are not needed now but will be needed in the near future. Safety is the primary consideration when selecting marketable securities.
- Proper *supply chain (inventory) management* requires close coordination among several departments. Because the cost of holding inventories is high but stockouts can be disastrous, inventory management is very important.
- Inventories consist of a *base stock* to meet expected usage and a *safety stock* to account for unexpected increases in usage or delays in receiving reorders.
- *Just-in-time*, *stockless inventory*, and *consigned inventory* systems are used to minimize inventory costs and, simultaneously, to improve operations.
- Healthcare managers use *metrics* to monitor performance. Some metrics focus on operational performance, while others (discussed in more detail in chapter 13) focus on financial performance.
- *Key performance indicators (KPIs)* are a limited number of metrics that focus on measures that are most important to an organization's mission success. Often, KPIs are presented in a format that resembles a dashboard.

In part III (beginning with chapter 8), we begin a new topic: financing and capital investment decisions.

End-of-Chapter Questions

7.1 What is the revenue cycle? Why is it important to healthcare organizations?

7.2 What is a receivable? Explain how receivables are built up over time.

7.3 Define *average collection period*. How is it used to monitor a firm's accounts receivable?

7.4 What is an aging schedule? How is it used to monitor a firm's accounts receivable?

7.5 What is the goal of cash management?

7.6 Briefly describe float and why it is a useful cash management concept.

7.7 a. Give two reasons that businesses hold marketable securities (short-term investments).

b. Which types of securities are most suitable to hold as marketable securities?

c. Suppose Southwest Regional Medical Center has just raised $6 million in new capital that it plans to use to build three freestanding clinics, one each year over the next three years. (For the sake of simplicity, assume that equal payments have to be made at the end of each of the next three years.) What securities should the firm buy for its firm's marketable securities portfolio, assuming that the firm has no other excess cash? (Hint: Consider both the type and maturity of the securities.)

d. Now, consider the situation faced by the Huntsville Physical Therapy Group. It has accumulated $20,000 in cash above its target cash balance, and it has no immediate needs for this excess cash. However, the firm may at any time need some or all of the $20,000 to meet unforeseen cash needs. What securities should be bought for the firm's marketable securities portfolio?

7.8 a. What is a just-in-time inventory system?

b. What are the advantages and disadvantages of just-in-time systems?

c. Can just-in-time inventory systems be used by healthcare providers? Explain your answer.

7.9 What are key performance indicators (KPIs)? What is a dashboard, and how is it used?

End-of-Chapter Problems

7.1 On a typical day, Park Place Clinic writes $1,000 in checks. Generally, those checks take four days to clear. Each day the clinic typically receives $1,000 in checks, which take three days to clear. What is the clinic's float?

7.2 Drugs R Us operates a mail-order pharmaceutical business in San Francisco. The firm receives an average of $325,000 in payments per day. On average, it takes four days from the time customers mail their checks until the firm receives them. The company is considering establishing a lockbox system, in which customers' payments would be sent to nearby banks (local in terms of the purchasers) instead of directly to San Francisco. Banks in the lockbox locations would then wire the daily receipts to a single (concentration) bank.

The lockbox system, which would consist of ten local depository banks and a concentration bank, would cost Drugs R Us a total of $6,500 per month. Under this system, customers' checks would be received at the ten lockbox locations one day after they are mailed, and the daily total from each of the ten lockbox locations would be wired to the concentration bank at a cost of $9.75 per transfer.

Assume that the firm could earn 10 percent on short-term investments; further assume 260 working days, and hence 260 transfers from each lockbox location, per year.

a. What is the total annual cost of operating the lockbox system?
b. What is the dollar benefit of the system to Drugs R Us?
c. Should the firm initiate the lockbox system?

7.3 Fargo Memorial Hospital has annual patient service revenues of $14,400,000. It has two major third-party payers, and some of its patients are self-payers. The hospital's patient accounts manager estimates that 10 percent of the hospital's billings are paid (received by the hospital) on day 30, 60 percent are paid on day 60, and 30 percent are paid on day 90.

a. What is Fargo's average collection period? (Assume 360 days per year throughout this problem.)
b. What is the hospital's current receivables balance?
c. What would be the hospital's new receivables balance if a newly proposed electronic claims system resulted in collecting from third-party payers in 45 and 75 days, instead of in 60 and 90 days?
d. Suppose the hospital's annual cost of carrying receivables is 10 percent. If the electronic claims system costs $30,000 a year to lease and operate, should it be adopted? (Assume that the entire receivables balance has to be financed.)

7.4 Milwaukee Surgical Supplies Inc. has gross sales for the year of $1,200,000. The collections department estimates that 30 percent of the customers pay on the tenth day, 40 percent pay on the thirtieth day, and the remaining 30 percent pay, on average, on the fortieth day after the purchase. (Assume 360 days per year.)

a. What is the firm's average collection period?
b. What is the firm's current receivables balance?

c. What would the firm's new receivables balance be if Milwaukee Surgical toughened up on its collection policy, with the result that the 70 percent of customers that did not pay by the tenth day paid on day 30?
d. Suppose that the firm's cost of carrying receivables was 8 percent annually. How much would the toughened credit policy save the firm in annual receivables carrying expense? (Assume that the entire amount of receivables has to be financed.)

7.5 Sacred Heart Hospital has the following receivables amounts, listed by age:

Age of Account (Days)	Value of Account	Percentage of Total Value
0–30	$ 5,450,000	
31–60	3,666,000	
61–90	1,278,000	
91–120	867,000	
Over 120	49,000	
	$11,310,000	

a. Complete the aging schedule by filling in the percentage of total value column.
b. Interpret your results.
c. Using these data, estimate the hospital's ACP (days in patient accounts receivable). (Hint: Assume that the average age in the first category is 15 days [the midpoint of the range], the average age in the second category is 45 days, and so on. Ignore the receivables older than 120 days.)

7.6 Sacramento Memorial Hospital has the following annual financial data and operational metrics:

Number of beds	250
Total inpatient admissions	12,250
Total outpatient visits	90,754
Total patient revenues	$111,900,050
Outpatient mix	16.2%
Medicare payment percentage (revenues)	28.0%
Average length of stay	5.8 days
Net price per discharge	$7,653
Cost per discharge	$6,292

a. What is the hospital's profit per discharge?
b. What is the hospital's total inpatient and total outpatient revenue? (Hint: Apply patient mix metrics to total revenues.)
c. Verify your part b answer for total inpatient revenue using volume and profitability metrics.
d. What are the hospital's total revenues from Medicare patients?
e. What is the total number of inpatient days?
f. What is the hospital's occupancy rate? (Hint: Start by calculating available bed days.)

7.7 Northeast Medical Group, a family practice, has the following financial data and operational metrics:

Number of physicians	5
Total revenue	$2,748,360
Total operating costs	$ 1,557,615
Total procedures per physician	12,353
Patients per physician	1,941
Visits per physician	5,333

a. What is the group's revenue per physician?
b. What is the group's operating cost per physician?
c. What is the group's total operating profit?
d. What is the group's profit per physician? Per patient? Per visit? Per procedure?
e. Assume that the group plans to reinvest $50,000 of its profits in the practice by buying a new EKG (electrocardiogram) machine. Also, assume that the remainder of profits will be distributed equally to the group's physicians as salary. What compensation will each physician receive?

PART III

FINANCING AND CAPITAL INVESTMENT DECISIONS

Hospitals need land, buildings, and equipment (assets) to provide inpatient and outpatient services, while clinics and physician practices require similar assets to provide outpatient services. To obtain these assets, healthcare organizations need capital (money). A large hospital requires a large amount of capital (some hospitals have more than $1 billion of capital), while a small home health care business requires a small amount of capital. In this section, we describe how businesses raise capital and how they decide what assets to acquire with those funds.

Chapter 8 discusses how healthcare organizations are financed. Two primary types of capital are available to healthcare businesses: *Debt capital* is borrowed money supplied by lenders; *ownership (equity) capital* is obtained from owners (for a for-profit business) or from the community at large (for a not-for-profit business). Because debt and ownership capital have different characteristics, managers must learn the impact of these differences on the financial condition of the business.

Chapters 9 and 10 cover capital investment decisions: Once capital is in the healthcare provider's hand, how should it be best spent? In other words, what capital investments (investments in land, buildings, and equipment) should be made? To make the best possible decisions, managers must assess the financial impact of proposed capital investments. Completing such an assessment requires an understanding of discounted cash flow analysis, financial risk, and other issues related to capital investment decisions.

CHAPTER 8

BUSINESS FINANCING AND THE COST OF CAPITAL

THEME SET-UP: STARTING A NEW MEDICAL PRACTICE

A few months ago, six primary care physicians in Seattle met to discuss the feasibility of creating a new medical group practice. Of the six, four were operating solo practices, while the other two were just completing family practice residencies. Although a solo practice offers some advantages, such as complete control, it presents numerous disadvantages.

Perhaps the largest disadvantage is that the business's administrative and clinical overhead costs must be borne by a single physician, while larger group practices can benefit from economies of scale (the spreading of fixed administrative and clinical costs over more patients). In addition, solo practitioners are, in effect, always on call for handling medical emergencies outside of regular working hours. Finally, a solo practice lacks the bargaining power with third-party payers that is enjoyed by physician group practices.

The bottom line is that more and more individual physicians are forming groups. The six physicians recognized the trend toward multiphysician practices, and they agreed to form a new business, Puget Sound Family Practice.

Starting a new group practice is not easy. First, the members must settle legal issues, such as what type of business organization to establish (the physicians decided on a professional corporation) and who will have the greatest say in running the practice. Next, they must obtain a space (purchased or rented) and equip it. Then, clinical and administrative staffs have to be hired and trained to ensure that the practice runs smoothly and that patients receive quality care in a timely, patient-friendly setting.

All of these start-up tasks require capital. In fact, the initial analysis of capital needs for Puget Sound Family Practice indicated that about $1.8 million was required to get the business up and running. The next steps in the start-up process are to (1) decide how to raise the required capital and (2) estimate how much the financing will cost.

By the end of the chapter, you will see how the physicians at Puget Sound Family Practice decided to fund the new business. Furthermore, you will get a feel for the cost of the capital raised and how that cost will influence the practice's decisions regarding equipment purchases and other capital expenditures.

Learning Objectives

After studying this chapter, you will be able to do the following:

- Describe how interest rates are set on debt financing.
- Discuss the various types of long-term and short-term debt instruments and their features.
- Define the two types of equity and their features.
- Briefly describe the capital structure decision.
- Explain the corporate cost of capital and its use.

8.1 INTRODUCTION

If a business is to operate, it must have assets (land, buildings, equipment). To acquire these assets, it must raise capital. **Capital** comes in two basic forms: debt and equity. Most healthcare organizations use some debt capital that lenders such as banks provide. Alternatively, equity capital is furnished by the owners for investor-owned businesses or by the community at large for not-for-profit businesses. This chapter discusses many facets of business financing, starting with how interest rates are set on borrowed capital.

Capital
For finance purposes, the funds used to acquire a business's assets, including land, buildings, equipment, and inventories. Note that in economics, capital generally refers to the assets owned by a business.

8.2 SETTING INTEREST RATES

The *interest rate* is the price paid to obtain debt capital. Many factors influence the interest rates set on business loans, but the two most important are risk and inflation (see "Critical Concept: Interest Rate"). The Puget Sound Family Practice example demonstrates how these factors operate, as the owners of the practice do not have sufficient personal funds to start the business and must supplement their funds with a loan.

Risk

The risk inherent in the prospective group practice, and thus in the ability to repay the loan, affects the return lenders will require. In effect, lenders assess the likelihood of the practice earning enough to make the required payments in full and on time. If they determine that the practice is highly likely to achieve this level of earnings, the loan carries minimal risk for the lender. On the other hand, if the practice will likely have difficulty making the payments, the lender faces a higher risk on making the loan.

Lenders are unwilling to lend to high-risk businesses unless the interest rate on such loans is higher than on loans to low-risk businesses. In this instance, the lender typically requires personal guarantees from the owner-physicians so that if the practice fails, the owners are personally liable for repaying the loan.

> **CRITICAL CONCEPT**
> Interest Rate
>
> The interest rate is the price paid by borrowers to obtain debt capital. Put another way, it is the price charged by lenders to provide debt financing. For example, First National Bank might provide a loan to Puget Sound Family Practice with an 8 percent interest rate, which means that the practice must pay the bank $0.08 \times \$1{,}000 = \$80$ per year for each $1,000 borrowed. The interest rate set on a loan is primarily dependent on two factors: the riskiness of the loan and the expected inflation during the term of the loan.

Inflation

Inflation has a major impact on interest rates because it erodes the purchasing power of the dollar and lowers the value of investment returns. Suppose a loaf of bread at the local supermarket cost $1.29 five years ago. Today, that same loaf costs $1.69. Furthermore, assume a lender made a business loan five years ago that pays $1,000 in annual interest. When the loan was made, the interest received would buy $1,000 ÷ $1.29 = 775 loaves of bread. Today, the same interest payment would buy only $1,000 ÷ $1.69 = 592 loaves. Thus, the interest payments received by a lender who made a loan five years ago will buy less bread today than when the loan was made. In effect, price inflation has reduced the purchasing power of the interest payments received on the loan.

Lenders are well aware of the impact of inflation, and hence the greater the expected rate of inflation, the greater the interest rate required to offset the loss of purchasing power. In the bread example, the price increased 40 cents over five years, which represents an inflation rate of 5.5 percent. The interest rate on loans over this time has to be at least 5.5 percent just to cover the effects of inflation.

Of course, we just looked at bread. A more meaningful measure of inflation is the increase in overall prices in the economy, often measured by the Consumer Price Index. In addition, the relevant rate of inflation to a lender is the rate expected in the future, not the rate experienced in the past. Thus, rather than the past rate of 5.5 percent, the lender looks to the anticipated rate. If it expects a 4 percent inflation rate in the future, then 4 percent is the relevant amount used to set current interest rates.

Finally, the inflation rate built into the interest rate on a loan is the average rate expected over the life of the loan. Thus, the inflation rate relevant to a one-year loan is the rate expected for the next year, whereas the inflation rate relevant to a ten-year loan is the average rate of inflation expected over the next ten years.

? SELF-TEST QUESTIONS

1. What is the "price" of debt capital?
2. What are the two primary factors that affect a loan's interest rate?

8.3 DEBT FINANCING

Many types of debt financing are available. Some types, such as home mortgages and personal auto loans, are used by individuals, while other types are used primarily by businesses. Some debt is used to meet short-term needs, while other debt is for longer terms.

When money is borrowed, the borrower (whether a business or an individual) has a contractual obligation to repay the loan, so debt obligations are "fixed by contract." The repayment consists of two parts: the amount borrowed, or **principal**, and the amount of interest stated on the loan.

Principal
The amount of money borrowed in a loan transaction.

In section 8.3, we discuss the types of debt most commonly used by health services organizations. In subsequent sections, we explore the most important features of debt financing.

Long-Term Debt

Long-term debt is defined as debt that has a **maturity** greater than one year. The amount borrowed (principal amount) on a long-term loan must be paid back to the lender at some time in the future longer than one year from the date of the loan. Long-term debt typically is used to finance assets that have a long life, such as buildings and equipment. The two major types of long-term debt used by health services organizations are term loans and bonds.

Maturity
The amount of time until a loan matures (must be repaid). Short-term debt has a maturity of one year or less, while long-term debt has a maturity greater than one year.

Term Loans

A *term loan* is long-term debt financing that is arranged directly between the borrowing business and the lender (see "Critical Concept: Term Loan"). In essence, the lender provides the capital, and the borrower agrees to pay the stated interest rate over the life of the loan and return the amount borrowed.

Typically, the lender is a financial institution such as a commercial bank, a mutual fund, or an insurance company, but it can also be a wealthy private investor. Most term loans have maturities of three to ten years. Like personal auto loans, term loans usually are paid off in equal installments over the life of the loan, so part of the principal amount is repaid with each loan payment.

CRITICAL CONCEPT
Term Loan

A term loan is a type of long-term debt financing used by businesses. It typically has a maturity of three to ten years and is obtained directly from financial institutions, such as commercial banks. The interest rate on a term loan may be fixed for the life of the loan or may be variable, which means that the rate changes (floats) as the general level of interest rates in the economy changes. Term loans typically are amortized, which means that the borrower pays back some of the principal amount along with each interest payment.

The interest rate on a term loan either is fixed for the life of the loan or is variable, known as a **floating rate**. If fixed, the interest rate stays the same over the life of the loan. If variable, the interest rate is usually set at a certain number of percentage points above some index rate. When the index rate goes up or down, so does the interest rate that must be paid on the outstanding balance of the loan.

Floating rate
A type of interest specified on a loan whereby the rate changes over time as interest rates in the economy rise and fall.

To illustrate a term loan, Apria Healthcare Group, a company whose website states that it runs about 325 home respiratory and infusion locations across the United States, recently obtained a $125 million five-year term loan from Bank of America. The loan's floating (variable) interest rate was set at 175 **basis points** (1.75 percentage points) above the index rate. (The index used on the loan was the London Interbank Offered Rate, which is the interest rate that London banks charge to one another on short-term, dollar-denominated loans.)

Basis point
One-hundredth of a percentage point (e.g., 50 basis points equal 0.5 percent, or one-half a percentage point).

Bonds

A *bond* is a long-term loan under which a borrower agrees to make payments of interest and principal, on specific dates, to the holder of the bond (see "Critical Concept: Bond"). Although bonds are similar in many ways to term loans, a bond issue generally is offered

> **CRITICAL CONCEPT**
> Bond
>
> A bond is a type of long-term debt used to raise large amounts of capital. Investor-owned corporations issue corporate bonds; the US government issues Treasury bonds; and states, counties, cities, and not-for-profit healthcare providers issue municipal bonds. Bonds typically have maturities in the range of 10 to 30 years. Because of the high administrative costs involved in selling bonds (compared to term loans), bonds are not typically used unless the amount required is greater than $10 million, although smaller issues do occasionally occur. To ensure that the entire issue is sold (the full amount of money is raised), bonds typically are issued in small denominations ($1,000 or $5,000) and sold through brokers to institutions and the public.

to the public by the borrowing entity and sold to many different investors. Indeed, thousands of individual and institutional investors may participate when a business sells a bond issue, while a term loan generally has only one lender.

In addition, bonds have a terminology of their own. The issuer of a bond is equivalent to the borrower on a term loan, the bondholder is the lender, and the interest rate often is called the coupon rate.

Because bonds are sold to many investors, large amounts of capital can be raised in a bond issue. To illustrate, HCA (Hospital Corporation of America) raised more than $1.5 billion of debt capital in a single bond issue in 2017. Each bond had a principal amount of $1,000, so more than a million individual bonds were sold to thousands of investors to complete the issue. To reach so many investors, bonds generally are sold through brokers rather than directly by the borrowing company.

Bonds are categorized as either government (Treasury), corporate, or municipal. Treasury bonds are used to raise money for the federal government. Investor-owned businesses issue corporate bonds, while states, counties, cities, and not-for-profit healthcare organizations issue municipal bonds.

Although bonds generally have maturities in the range of 10 to 30 years, organizations use both longer and shorter maturities. In fact, in 1995, HCA (then Columbia/HCA) issued corporate bonds with a 100-year maturity. Unlike term loans, bonds usually pay only interest over the life of the bond, and the entire amount borrowed is returned to lenders at maturity. Most bonds have a fixed interest rate, which locks in the current rate for the entire maturity of the bond and hence minimizes interest payment uncertainty. However, some bonds have floating, or variable, rates, so the interest payments move up and down with the general level of interest rates in the economy.

Although municipal, or *muni*, bonds typically are issued by states, counties, and cities, not-for-profit healthcare providers are entitled to issue such securities through government-sponsored healthcare financing authorities. Whereas the vast majority of Treasury and corporate bonds are held by institutions—primarily mutual funds—nearly half of all outstanding municipal bonds are held by individual investors. However, the Republican tax reforms passed by Congress in 2017 may change the ways in which not-for-profit hospitals manage their finances.

The primary attraction of most municipal bonds is the fact that bond owners (lenders) do not have to pay income taxes on the interest earned. Because such bonds are tax-exempt, the interest rate set on municipal bonds is less than the rate set on similar corporate bonds. The idea is that municipal bond buyers are willing to accept a lower interest rate because they do not have to pay income taxes on the interest payments received. However, since the 2017 tax reforms set lower corporate and individual tax rates, the benefit of the interest tax exemption will be less. This may lead to smaller differences between the interest rates set on corporate and municipal bonds.

Short-Term Debt

Short-term debt, with a maturity of one year or less, generally is used to finance temporary needs, such as increasing the level of inventories to meet busy-season demand. Short-term debt has several advantages over long-term debt. For example, administrative (e.g., accounting, legal, selling) costs generally are lower for short-term debt than for long-term debt. Also, long-term loan agreements usually contain more restrictions on the firm's future actions, whereas short-term debt agreements typically are less onerous in this regard. Finally, the interest rate on short-term debt generally is lower than the rate on long-term debt because longer maturities pose more risk to lenders.

In spite of these advantages, short-term debt has one serious disadvantage: It subjects the borrower to more risk than does long-term financing. The increased risk occurs for two reasons. First, if a business borrows on a long-term basis, its interest costs will be relatively stable over time, but if it uses short-term debt, its interest expense can fluctuate widely, at times possibly going quite high. For example, the short-term rate that banks charge their best business customers (the prime rate) more than tripled over a two-year period in the early 1980s, rising to 21 percent from about 6 percent. Thus, businesses that used large amounts of short-term debt financing during those years saw their interest costs rise to unimaginable levels, forcing many into bankruptcy. (If the long-term debt has a floating rate, the problem of fluctuating interest rates also applies.)

Second, the principal amount on short-term debt comes due on a regular basis (one year or less). If the financial condition of a business temporarily deteriorates, it may find itself unable to repay this debt when it matures. Furthermore, the business may be in such a weak financial position that the lender will not extend the loan. Such a scenario can result in severe problems for the borrower, which, like unexpectedly high interest rates, could force the business into bankruptcy.

Commercial banks are the primary provider of short-term debt financing. Although banks make longer-maturity (term) loans, the bulk of their lending is on a short-term basis (about two-thirds of all bank loans mature in a year or less). Bank loans to businesses are frequently written as 90-day notes, so the loan must be repaid or renewed at the end of the 90 days.

Alternatively, a business may obtain short-term financing by establishing a line of credit with a bank (see "Critical Concept: Line of Credit"). A credit line is an agreement that specifies the maximum credit the

CRITICAL CONCEPT
Line of Credit

A line of credit is a common type of short-term debt financing used by healthcare businesses. Typically, lines of credit, which are offered by commercial banks, specify a maximum loan size over a specified period—often a year. The borrowing business can borrow up to the maximum amount (and pay it back) at any time while the line is in effect. However, any funds borrowed on the line must be repaid to the bank when the line expires. Lines of credit typically are used to meet a business's short-term capital needs, such as to build up inventories in advance of the busy season.

bank will extend to the borrower over a designated period, often a year. Say that in December a bank notifies managers of Pine Garden Nursing Care that it will extend up to $100,000 of credit during the forthcoming year. At any time during the year, Pine Garden can borrow up to $100,000, the full amount of the line. Borrowers typically pay an up-front fee to obtain the line, and interest must be paid on any amounts borrowed. Furthermore, the line must be fully repaid by the end of the year.

SELF-TEST QUESTIONS

1. What are the primary features of a term loan? Of a bond?
2. What is a corporate bond? A Treasury bond? A municipal bond?
3. What are the advantages and disadvantages of using short-term debt financing? Of using long-term debt financing?
4. Describe the features of a line of credit.

8.4 DEBT CONTRACTS

Restrictive covenant
A provision in a loan agreement that protects the interests of the lender by restricting the actions of the borrower.

Trustee
An individual or institution, often a bank, that represents the interests of bondholders.

Default
Failure by a borrower to make a promised interest or principal repayment.

Call provision
A provision in a bond contract that gives the issuing company the right to redeem (call) the bonds prior to maturity.

Debt contracts, which are known by various names, such as *loan agreement* or *bond indenture*, spell out the rights and obligations of borrowers and lenders. These contracts vary substantially in length depending on the type of debt. Some contracts, particularly bond indentures, can be several hundred pages long.

Many debt contracts include provisions, called **restrictive covenants**, which are designed to protect lenders from managerial actions that would be detrimental to lenders' interests. For example, a typical bond indenture may contain several restrictive covenants, such as specifying that the borrower maintain a certain amount of cash on hand. By specifying this minimum cash level, lenders have some assurance that the debt payments coming due in the near future can be met.

When debt is supplied by a single creditor, a one-to-one relationship exists between the lender and borrower. Bond issues, on the other hand, can have thousands of buyers (lenders), so a single voice is needed to represent bondholders. This function is performed by a **trustee**, usually an institution such as a bank, which represents the bondholders and ensures that the terms of the contract (indenture) are carried out.

What happens if a borrower fails to make a payment required by a debt contract—that is, if the borrower **defaults**? Usually, the debt contract spells out the actions that can be taken by lenders when this occurs. Regardless of the contract terms, on default, lenders have the legal right to force borrowers into bankruptcy, which could result in closure and liquidation. Note, however, that although lenders have this right, they may not be wise to act on it. In some default situations, lenders may determine they are better off helping the borrowing business get through the bad times rather than force the business to close.

Finally, many bond contracts have **call provisions**, which give the borrower the right to redeem (call) the bonds prior to maturity. In these situations, the issuer can pay

Call provison reduces borrowers risk

off the principal amount and any interest due and retire the issue. The call privilege is valuable to the borrower but potentially detrimental to bondholders, because bonds typically are called when interest rates have fallen. This action enables the borrower to replace an old, higher-interest issue with a new, lower-interest issue and hence reduce interest expense. However, the old bondholders are now compelled to reinvest the principal returned in new bonds that have a lower interest rate.

Investment-grade debt
Debt with a BBB– or higher rating. Generally considered suitable (relatively low-risk) investments for conservative individuals and institutions.

Self-Test Questions

1. What is a restrictive covenant?
2. What is the purpose of a trustee?
3. What happens when a borrower defaults?
4. What is a call provision, and when are bonds typically called?

8.5 DEBT RATINGS

Junk debt
Debt with a BB+ or lower rating. Generally considered to be more speculative than is investment-grade debt and hence inappropriate for conservative investors.

Major debt issuers, as well as their specific debt issues, are assigned creditworthiness (quality) ratings that reflect the probability of default. The three primary rating agencies are Fitch Ratings, Moody's Investors Service, and Standard & Poor's (S&P). All three agencies rate both corporate and municipal debt.

The three rating agencies have similar rating designations; S&P's are shown in exhibit 8.1. **Investment-grade debt** has a rating of BBB– or higher, while BB (double B) or lower-rated debt is called **junk debt** (or, sometimes, speculative debt) because it has a much higher probability of going into default than do higher-rated issues. Although the rating assignments are subjective, they are based on both qualitative characteristics, such as the quality of a business's management, and quantitative factors, such as a business's financial strength.

Debt ratings are important both to borrowers and to lenders for several reasons (see "Critical Concept: Debt Ratings"). First, the rating is an indicator of the issue's default risk, so the rating has a direct influence on the interest rate required by lenders: The lower the rating, the greater the risk and hence the higher the interest rate.

Second, most corporate bonds are purchased by institutional investors rather than by individuals. Many of these institutions are restricted to investment-grade securities. In

CRITICAL CONCEPT
Debt Ratings

Major debt issues are rated by several different rating agencies, such as S&P's, on their probability of default (creditworthiness). In general, ratings range from AAA, which indicates the safest issues (most creditworthy), through AA, A, BBB, BB, and so on to D (in default). Because debt ratings indicate risk, the lower the rating, the higher the interest rate that must be set on the issue to make it attractive to buyers. To assess creditworthiness, rating agencies consider both quantitative factors, such as financial condition, and qualitative factors, such as quality of management and competitive position of the borrower.

Exhibit 8.1
Standard & Poor's Debt Ratings

Capacity to Repay	Rating Category
Extremely strong	AAA
Very strong	AA
Strong	A
Adequate	BBB
Major future uncertainties	BB
Major uncertainties	B
Currently vulnerable	CCC
Currently highly vulnerable	CC
Filed bankruptcy petition	C
In default	D

Note: For ratings ranging between AA and BB, plus or minus modifiers may also be applied. For example, in the AA grade, the strongest bonds may receive a grade of AA+ while the weakest may receive a grade of AA–.

addition, most individual investors who buy municipal bonds are unwilling to take much risk in their bond purchases. Thus, if a new issue is rated below BBB–, it is more difficult to sell because the number of potential purchasers is reduced.

As a result of their higher risk and more restricted market, low-grade bonds typically carry much higher interest rates than do high-grade bonds. To illustrate, in mid-2016 the interest rate on ten-year CCC-rated corporate bonds was about 4.9 percentage points higher than the rate on AAA-rated bonds.

Credit enhancement (bond insurance) Insurance that guarantees the payment of interest and repayment of principal on a bond if the borrower (issuer) defaults. Insured bonds carry the rating of the insurer rather than the issuer.

Because debt ratings affect the cost of financing significantly, healthcare borrowers (particularly not-for-profits) historically have used **credit enhancement (bond insurance)** to raise the rating on a bond issue. Regardless of the inherent creditworthiness of the issuer, bond insurance guarantees that bondholders will receive the promised interest and principal payments. Thus, bond insurance protects lenders against default by the issuer. Because the insurer gives its guarantee that payments will be made, an insured bond carries the credit rating of the insurance company rather than that of the issuer.

Credit enhancement gives the issuer access to a lower interest rate, but not without a cost. Insurers charge an up-front fee related to the underlying rating of the issue: The lower the borrower's inherent credit rating, the higher the cost of insurance. Before the credit collapse of 2008, most municipal bond issues were sold with credit enhancement. However, the banking crisis caused the bond issuers to lose their AAA ratings, so bond insurance lost its luster (see "For Your Consideration: Rating Agency Criticisms"). Today, only about 5 percent of municipal bonds are insured.

FOR YOUR CONSIDERATION
Rating Agency Criticisms

Large credit rating agencies (RAs), such as S&P, have come under increasing criticism in recent years for a number of reasons. First, the RAs maintain close relationships with the management of the companies they rate. These connections are characterized by frequent meetings, during which the RAs provide advice on actions companies should take to maintain current ratings. This practice fosters a familial atmosphere that interferes with independent, unbiased rating judgments. Furthermore, because the RAs are paid by the companies they rate, rather than the investors they are meant to protect, a clear conflict of interest exists.

Second, because the rating business is reputation based (why pay attention to a rating that is not recognized by others?), barriers to market entry are high and the RAs are oligopolists (an oligopoly is a market dominated by just a few sellers). Thus, the RAs are somewhat immune to forces that apply to competitive markets and, to an extent, can set their own rules.

Finally, in many instances, the debt markets (through lower bond prices) have recognized a company's deteriorating credit quality many months before a rating downgrade occurred. This fact has led many observers to suggest that, rather than rely on ratings, investors and regulators should use credit spreads to make judgments about credit risk. (Credit spreads reflect the difference in yields between interest rates on "safe" debt, such as Treasury securities, and rates on risky debt, such as B-rated bonds.)

What do you think? To what extent are credit ratings valid? Do the criticisms of RAs have merit? Can the current credit rating system be improved? If so, how?

SELF-TEST QUESTIONS

1. What are debt ratings?
2. What are some criteria that the rating agencies use when assigning ratings?
3. What impact do ratings have on a borrower's cost of debt?
4. Why would healthcare borrowers seek bond insurance?

8.6 EQUITY FINANCING

The second primary source of capital to healthcare businesses is equity financing. Equity financing is provided by owners in for-profit businesses, and by religious or governmental entities or the community at large in not-for-profit businesses. Although many similarities can be seen between the equity in for-profit and in not-for-profit businesses, some key differences exist as well. In this section, we describe the most important features of equity financing.

Equity in For-Profit Businesses

In for-profit businesses, equity financing is supplied by the owners of the business, either directly through the purchase of an equity (ownership) interest in the business or indirectly through earnings retention.

Most large for-profit healthcare businesses are organized as corporations, in which case the owners are shareholders who contribute equity to the company by buying shares of newly issued stock. (The sale of outstanding [previously issued] stock from one individual to another does not create equity financing for the business.) Smaller businesses are organized as proprietorships or partnerships, or as some other hybrid form of business such as a professional corporation. Regardless of type, equity capital is raised when owners provide start-up or additional capital to the business.

Owners of for-profit businesses have certain rights and privileges. Perhaps the most important is a claim on the residual earnings of the business. A business's residual earnings, which are the profits that remain after all expenses have been paid, belong to the owners. Some portion of these earnings may be paid out to owners as dividends (in the case of corporations) or bonuses (in the case of proprietorships or partnerships), while the remainder is retained (reinvested) in the business. Such retentions are a major source of equity capital in for-profit businesses.

In addition to the claim on residual earnings, owners of for-profit businesses have the right of control. In small businesses, the owners typically are the managers of the business and hence directly control its operations. In large businesses (corporations), the owners (shareholders) elect the firm's directors, who in turn elect the officers who manage the business.

Businesses need equity capital because it provides a financing base with no maturity date. Thus, businesses can use equity financing for long periods without concern that the capital must be repaid. Furthermore, dividends (or bonuses) to equity holders are not guaranteed; they are paid only when the business's managers believe it is prudent to do so. Thus, equity financing does not entail the same mandatory periodic payment to capital suppliers as does debt financing. For more information about payments to equity capital suppliers, see online chapter 16, "Distributions to Owners: Bonuses, Dividends, and Repurchases" (available at http://ache.org/books/FinanceFundamentals3).

Finally, lenders do not make business loans if the business has no equity to share the risk, so equity financing is an important precondition to obtain debt financing.

Equity in Not-for-Profit Businesses

Historically, most not-for-profit health services organizations, particularly hospitals, received their initial, start-up equity capital from religious, educational, or governmental entities.

Today, some organizations continue to receive funding from these sources, but since the 1970s, they have provided a much smaller proportion of equity funding, forcing not-for-profit healthcare entities to rely more on profits and outside contributions.

Not-for-profit businesses obtain much of their equity capital from retained earnings. In fact, all profits earned by a not-for-profit organization must be retained in the organization, as it has no owners to receive dividends (see "For Your Consideration: The Green Bay Packers"). In theory, not-for-profit organizations provide dividends to the community at large by offering healthcare services to the poor, educational programs, and other charitable endeavors.

In addition to retained earnings, not-for-profit businesses raise equity capital through charitable contributions. Individuals, as well as businesses, are motivated to contribute to not-for-profit healthcare organizations for a variety of reasons, including concern for the well-being of others, the recognition that often accompanies large contributions, and tax deductibility.

Because only contributions to not-for-profit organizations are tax deductible, this source of funding is, for all practical purposes, not available to investor-owned businesses.

FOR YOUR CONSIDERATION
The Green Bay Packers

What do the National Football League's Green Bay Packers have in common with the Mayo Clinic? It turns out that they are both not-for-profit organizations, but there is a surprising difference: The Packers have shareholders.

The Green Bay Packers Inc. became a publicly owned, not-for-profit corporation in 1923, when the original articles of incorporation were filed with Wisconsin's secretary of state. The corporation is governed by a board of directors and a seven-member executive committee. Today, 5,011,558 shares are owned by 360,760 shareholders, but these shares are not like most stock. They pay no dividends and cannot be sold on the open market; they can only be sold back to the corporation at the same price at which they were purchased. Furthermore, any profits earned by the corporation must be donated to charity.

One of the more remarkable business stories in American history, over the years the team has been kept financially viable by its shareholders. Fans have come to the team's financial rescue on several occasions, including the sale of $67 million in stock in 2012 for a stadium expansion. To protect against someone taking control of the team, the articles of incorporation prohibit any person from owning more than 200,000 shares.

Did you know that, although rarely done, some types of not-for-profit corporations can issue stock? In what situations might such a model be used in healthcare? What restrictions would be placed on the stock and the stockholders?

Although charitable contributions are not a substitute for profit retentions, charitable contributions can be a significant source of equity capital for not-for-profit businesses.

Equity in not-for-profit healthcare organizations serves the same function as in for-profit businesses. It provides a permanent financing base and supports the business's ability to use debt financing. Note that, in not-for-profit businesses, equity financing may be called fund capital or net assets, but for all practical purposes it is equivalent to a for-profit business's equity financing.

? Self-Test Questions

1. What are the sources of equity financing for for-profit businesses? For not-for-profit businesses?
2. What is the purpose of equity financing?
3. Do both for-profit and not-for-profit healthcare organizations have access to contribution capital?

8.7 THE CHOICE BETWEEN DEBT AND EQUITY FINANCING

Capital structure
The business's mix of debt and equity financing, often expressed as the percentage of debt financing.

The mix of debt and equity financing used by a business is called its **capital structure**. One of the most perplexing issues for healthcare organizations is how much debt financing, as opposed to equity financing, to use. In section 8.7, we discuss some issues related to the choice between debt and equity financing.

Impact of Debt Financing on Risk and Return

To understand the consequences of capital structure decisions fully, it is essential to understand the effects of debt financing on a business's risk and return as reflected in a profit and loss (P&L) statement. Consider the situation that confronts Super Health Inc., a for-profit (investor-owned) retail clinic that is currently being formed. Its founders have identified two financing alternatives for the business: all-equity or 50 percent debt financing.

Note that the asset requirements for any business depend on the nature and size of the business rather than on how the business will be financed. Assume that Super Health requires \$200,000 in assets (e.g., equipment, inventories) to begin operations. If the \$200,000 is financed with 100 percent equity, Super Health's owners will put up the entire \$200,000 needed to purchase the assets. However, if 50 percent debt financing is used, the owners will contribute only \$100,000, with the remaining \$100,000 obtained from a lender—say, a bank loan with a 10 percent interest rate. (We have purposely kept the dollar values unrealistically small for ease of illustration.)

Exhibit 8.2 contains the business's projected P&L statements under the two financing alternatives. What is the impact of the two financing alternatives on Super Health's projected first-year profitability?

Assume revenues are projected to be $150,000 and operating costs are forecasted at $100,000, so the firm's operating income is expected to be $50,000. Because a business's mix of debt and equity financing does not affect revenues and operating costs, the operating income projection is the same under both financing alternatives.

However, interest expense must be paid if debt financing is used. Thus, the 50 percent debt alternative results in a 0.10 × $100,000 = $10,000 annual interest charge, while no interest expense is incurred if the firm is all-equity financed. The result is taxable income of $50,000 under all-equity financing and a lower taxable income of $40,000 under the 50 percent debt alternative (because interest on debt financing is a tax-deductible expense).

Because the business anticipates being taxed at a 21 percent rate, the expected tax liability is 0.21 × $50,000 = $10,500 under the all-equity alternative and 0.21 × $40,000 = $8,400 for the 50 percent debt alternative. Finally, when taxes are deducted, the business expects to earn $39,500 in profit if it is all-equity financed but only $31,600 if it is 50 percent debt financed.

At first glance, the use of debt financing appears to be the inferior alternative. After all, if 50 percent debt financing is used, the business's projected profitability will fall by $39,500 – $31,600 = $7,900. However, the conclusion that debt financing is bad requires closer examination. What is most important to the owners of Super Health is not the business's dollar profitability but rather the return expected on their equity investment.

The best measure of return to the owners of a business is the **return on equity (ROE)**, which is defined here as projected profit divided by the amount of equity invested. Under all-equity financing, projected ROE is $39,500 ÷ $200,000 = 0.20 = 20%, but with 50 percent debt financing, projected ROE increases to $31,600 ÷ $100,000 = 32%.

Return on equity (ROE)
Net income divided by the book value of equity (net assets), which measures the dollars of earnings per dollar of equity investment. ROE measures the rate of return to the owners of the business.

Exhibit 8.2
Super Health Inc.: Projected P&L Statements

	All-Equity	50% Debt
Revenues	$150,000	$150,000
Operating costs	100,000	100,000
Operating income	$ 50,000	$50,000
Interest expense	0	10,000
Taxable income	$ 50,000	$ 40,000
Taxes (21%)	10,500	8,400
Profit	$ 39,500	$ 31,600
Return on equity	20%	32%

The key to the increased ROE is that although profit decreases when debt financing is used, the amount of equity needed also decreases, and the equity capital requirement decreases more than the profit does. The bottom line is that debt financing can increase owners' expected rate of return. Because the use of debt financing increases, or leverages up, the rate of return to owners, such financing often is called **financial leverage**. Hence, the use of financial leverage is merely the use of debt financing.

Financial leverage
The use of debt financing, which typically increases (leverages up) the rate of return to owners.

At this point, it appears that Super Health's financing decision is straightforward. Given the two financing alternatives, the organization should use 50 percent debt financing because that option promises owners the higher rate of return. However, there *is* a catch. The use of financial leverage increases not only the owners' projected return but also their risk.

Consider what would happen if actual revenues were $25,000 less than expected and actual operating costs were $25,000 higher than expected. In this situation, operating income, and hence ROE, would be zero if all-equity financing is used. This situation would not be good. However, the use of debt financing makes it worse: At 50 percent debt financing, $10,000 in interest must be paid to the bank; with no operating income to pay the interest expense, the owners would either have to put up additional equity capital to pay the interest due or declare the business bankrupt. (The business could theoretically borrow an additional $10,000 to pay the interest, but considering the first year's results, no lenders would likely be interested.) Clearly, the use of 50 percent debt financing has increased the riskiness of the owners' investment.

This simple example illustrates that debt financing can increase both the owners' return and their risk. When risk is considered, the ultimate decision on which financing alternative they should choose is not clear-cut. The zero-debt alternative has a lower expected ROE but lower risk. The 50 percent debt alternative offers a higher expected ROE but carries more risk.

Thus, the decision as to how much debt financing to use is a classic risk–return trade-off: Higher returns can be obtained only by assuming greater risk. What Super Health's founders need to know is whether the higher return is enough to compensate them for the higher risk assumed. To complicate the decision even more, an almost unlimited number of debt-level choices are available, not just the 50/50 mix used in the illustration. This example vividly illustrates that healthcare managers face a difficult task when making the debt-financing decision.

Capital Structure Theory

Trade-off theory
A theory proposing that a business's optimal capital structure balances the costs and benefits associated with debt financing.

At this point, Super Health's founders are left in a quandary because debt financing brings with it both higher returns and higher risk. To help make the decision, academicians have developed several theories of capital structure. The goal of these theories is to determine whether businesses have optimal capital structures.

The most widely accepted idea is the **trade-off theory**, which holds that the capital structure decision involves a trade-off between the costs and benefits of debt financing, where the costs are increasing bankruptcy risk and the benefits are increasing rates of return.

The trade-off theory tells managers that every business has an optimal capital structure that balances the costs and benefits associated with debt financing (see "Critical Concept: Optimal Capital Structure"). In effect, the optimal capital structure is the mix of debt and equity financing that produces the lowest cost of capital for the business. (Cost of capital is discussed in section 8.9 of this chapter.) The key implication of the trade-off theory is that some debt financing is good because owners can capture the benefits of increased return, but too much debt is bad because the increased risk of bankruptcy outweighs the higher expected returns.

> **CRITICAL CONCEPT**
> Optimal Capital Structure
>
> When a business uses debt (as opposed to equity) financing, two consequences arise. First, under most conditions, the expected return to owners increases. (For this reason, debt financing is called financial leverage.) Second, owners' risk increases, and the greater the proportion of debt financing, the greater the impact on return and risk. Thus, the choice as to how much debt financing to use involves a risk–return trade-off. Theory tells us that a business has an optimal capital structure that balances the costs and benefits of debt financing. In essence, some debt financing is good, but too much debt is bad. However, theory cannot identify the optimal structure for any given business, so managers must use qualitative factors to make the decision.

Identifying the Optimal Capital Structure in Practice

The trade-off theory cannot identify the optimal capital structure for any given business because the costs and benefits of debt financing to a specific business, at potential alternative capital structures, cannot be estimated with any precision. Thus, healthcare managers must apply judgment in making the capital structure decision. The following are some important factors that managers must consider:

- *Business risk.* A certain amount of risk, called **business risk**, is inherent in business operations, even when no debt financing is used. This risk is associated with the ability of managers to forecast future profitability. The more uncertainty in the process—say, in forecasting future ROE—the greater the inherent risk of the business. When debt financing is used, owners must bear additional risk above the inherent business risk of the organization. The additional risk to owners (or to the community in the case of not-for-profit organizations) when debt financing is used is called **financial risk**. In general, managers place some limit on the total amount of risk, including business and financial, undertaken by a business. Thus, the greater the inherent business risk, the less room available for the use of financial leverage and hence the lower the proportion of debt financing in the optimal capital structure.

> ***Business risk***
> The risk inherent in the operations of a business, assuming it uses no debt financing.

> ***Financial risk***
> The additional risk placed on the business's owners (or the community) when debt financing is used.

- *Lender and rating agency attitudes.* The attitudes of lenders and rating agencies are important determinants of capital structures. In the majority of situations, managers discuss the business's financial structure with lenders and rating agencies and give a great deal of weight to their advice. In large organizations, managers usually have a target debt rating—say, single A. In small businesses, managers want to restrict debt financing to that readily available from commercial banks. In effect, lenders and rating agencies set a limit on the proportion of debt financing that a business can raise at reasonable interest rates.

- *Reserve borrowing capacity*. Businesses generally maintain a reserve borrowing capacity that preserves their ability to obtain additional debt financing. In essence, managers want to maintain financial flexibility, which includes the ability to survive tough times (should they occur) by taking on additional debt financing. Maintaining the ability to borrow additional funds at reasonable interest rates requires a business to use less debt financing during normal times than other factors may indicate.
- *Industry averages*. Presumably, managers act rationally, so the capital structures of other firms in the industry, particularly the industry leaders, should provide insights about the optimal structure. In general, there is no reason to believe that the managers of one firm are smarter than the managers of other similar firms. Thus, if one business has a capital structure that is significantly different from others in its industry, the managers of that firm should identify the unique circumstances that contribute to the anomaly. If unique circumstances cannot be identified, then it is doubtful that the firm has identified the correct capital structure.
- *Asset structure*. Firms whose assets are suitable as security (collateral) for loans pay lower interest rates on debt financing than do other firms and hence tend to use more debt. Thus, for example, hospitals tend to use more debt than do biotechnology companies. Both the ability to use assets as collateral and low inherent business risk give a firm more **debt capacity**, and hence a target capital structure that includes a relatively high proportion of debt.

Debt capacity
The amount of debt in a business's optimal capital structure. A business with excess debt capacity is operating with less than the optimal amount of debt.

Not-for-Profit Businesses

Do not-for-profit businesses have optimal capital structures? The same general concept we have discussed applies to not-for-profits—namely, some debt financing is good, but too much is bad. In essence, debt financing permits not-for-profits to offer more programs and services than are possible using only equity financing. However, just as with for-profits, not-for-profits that use debt financing bring more risk to the owners (in this case the community), and the greater the proportion of debt, the greater the risk.

In spite of the theoretical similarity in capital structure decisions between for-profit and not-for-profit businesses, not-for-profits have a unique problem: They cannot sell equity to raise new capital and cannot return earnings to equity investors. In contrast, investor-owned firms can easily adjust their capital structures. If they are financially underleveraged (using too little debt), they can simply issue more debt and use the proceeds to repurchase equity from the owners. On the other hand, if they are financially overleveraged (using too much debt), they can issue additional equity and use the proceeds to reduce the amount of debt outstanding.

Because not-for-profit organizations cannot raise equity by merely asking owners to contribute more capital or return equity by issuing dividends or buying back shares, they do not have the same degree of flexibility in adjusting their capital structures as do their for-profit counterparts. Thus, not-for-profits sometimes must delay new programs or services, or temporarily use more than the optimal amount of debt financing because that is the only way that they can provide the services their communities need. Alternately, they may take on low-cost debt financing rather than investing their cash or long-term investments in new services (see "Healthcare in Practice: Capital Structure Decisions in Not-for-Profit Hospitals").

HEALTHCARE IN PRACTICE
Capital Structure Decisions in Not-for-Profit Hospitals

Capital structure decisions in not-for-profit healthcare businesses have never been as clear-cut as they are in for-profit businesses. A great deal of theory-based information is available to for-profit businesses to help them make these decisions. Essentially, for-profits have the goal of maximizing their owners' wealth, and this goal is accomplished by lowering capital costs. However, not-for-profits do not have wealth maximization as a goal, so capital structure theory breaks down in such businesses.

Several studies have been conducted to shed light on how not-for-profit hospitals make capital structure decisions. Although some findings contradict each other, the results are sufficiently consistent to give an idea of what factors drive the decision. To begin, not-for-profit hospitals establish a target capital structure and try to stick to it. Most hospitals have target structures in the 35–40 percent debt range, as measured by the debt-to-financing ratio. (The *debt-to-financing ratio* is defined as long-term debt divided by long-term financing [long-term debt plus equity].) The most important factor in setting the target capital structure is maintaining a sound bond rating (often A). Organizations can do so by using the right amount of debt: Too little debt produces a higher rating, while too much debt produces a lower rating.

(continued)

HEALTHCARE IN PRACTICE
Capital Structure Decisions in Not-for-Profit Hospitals *(continued)*

The focus on bond ratings cannot be overstated. Most not-for-profit hospitals view a high bond rating as an essential element of capital structure policy. The logic here is that not-for-profits are more reliant on debt financing because of their inability to raise capital by selling equity. Note that more reliance on debt does not mean that not-for-profits use more debt than their for-profit counterparts. In fact, not-for-profit hospitals historically have used less debt than for-profit hospitals. However, preserving access to highly rated (low-cost) debt financing, should a critical need arise, is more important for not-for-profits.

In addition to preserving access to additional debt financing, not-for-profit hospitals have other reasons to use modest amounts of debt financing. For one, the fear of lower profitability resulting from recent and expected future reductions in reimbursement rates makes it less desirable to take on large interest payment obligations.

Still, the motivation to limit debt usage is somewhat offset by the fact that not-for-profit hospitals can engage in a practice called tax arbitrage, which involves using low-cost municipal (tax-exempt) financing to invest in higher-return Treasury securities, and hence capture a riskless return. Note, however, that in today's low-interest-rate environment, the value inherent in tax arbitrage is greatly reduced. In addition, laws restrict the ability of not-for-profits to engage in large-scale tax arbitrage, but many hospitals still benefit from the practice by taking on large amounts of debt to fund new facilities that take years to build. Before the funds are actually needed to pay for construction and equipment, they are invested in higher-return securities.

In all, it is clear that not-for-profit hospitals must walk a tightrope regarding the use of debt financing. For most, debt financing is essential to providing the services necessary to meet mission requirements. At the same time, however, the need to ensure access to future debt financing and to keep current interest payments at reasonable levels means that debt-financing usage must be kept under control.

Optimal Capital Structure Implications

Target capital structure
The capital structure that a company strives to achieve and maintain over time. Generally the same as the optimal capital structure.

Once a business estimates its optimal capital structure—say, 30 percent debt financing—it will take the financing actions necessary to attain that structure. Then, as the business needs additional capital to finance asset replacement and growth, it will raise capital over time to maintain its optimal capital structure. Thus, managers will base (target) future financing decisions on the optimal capital structure, so the optimal capital structure often is called the **target capital structure**. Other considerations come into play when raising new capital, but, over the long run, businesses, by their financing decisions, attempt to keep their actual capital structures close to the target.

? SELF-TEST QUESTIONS

1. What is the impact of debt financing on owners' expected return? On owners' risk?
2. Is the capital structure decision mostly objective or subjective? Explain your answer.
3. What is the difference between business and financial risk?
4. What are some of the factors that managers must consider when setting the target capital structure?
5. Is capital structure important to managers of not-for-profit businesses? Explain your answer.
6. Why is a business's optimal capital structure also called its target capital structure?

8.8 THE CHOICE BETWEEN LONG-TERM DEBT AND SHORT-TERM DEBT

Once the optimal mix of debt and equity financing has been identified, the next decision arises: What is the optimal mix of debt maturities? In other words, what is the optimal debt maturity structure? The answer, as with the optimal capital structure, involves a trade-off between risk and return (see "Critical Concept: Optimal Debt Maturity Structure").

In general, the optimal debt maturity structure involves matching the maturities of the debt used with the maturities of the assets being financed. That is, if debt financing is used to increase a business's inventories in preparation for the coming busy season or to pay the salary of a three-month temporary employee, then short-term debt is appropriate. Conversely, if the debt is being used to buy a new scanner or to finance the construction of a new clinic, then long-term debt is appropriate.

The rationale here is that the inventory level and payroll will return to their initial, lower levels when the busy season is over, so the need for financing is temporary (short-term). However, the new diagnostic equipment or clinic will likely be operating for many years, so its financing need is more or less permanent (long-term).

In theory, a business could attempt to match exactly the maturity structure of its assets

> **! CRITICAL CONCEPT**
> **Optimal Debt Maturity Structure**
>
> After a business estimates its optimal mix of debt and equity financing (optimal capital structure), a second decision arises: Should the business's debt financing be all long-term, all short-term, or some combination of the two? In general, a business's debt maturities should match the maturities of the assets being financed with that debt. Thus, if debt financing is being used to build a new facility, the debt should have a long maturity because the facility has a long life. Conversely, if the debt is acquired to undertake a two-month marketing campaign, it should have a short maturity to match the short-term nature of the cash need.

and financing. Inventory expected to be sold in 30 days could be financed with a 30-day bank loan, an X-ray machine expected to last 5 years could be financed by a 5-year term loan, a 20-year building could be financed by a 20-year bond, and so forth. However, two factors make this approach impractical: (1) The duration of assets' lives is uncertain, and (2) some equity capital must be used, and this capital has no maturity.

Self-Test Question

1. What factor most influences a business's debt maturity structure?

8.9 COST OF CAPITAL

Capital suppliers do not provide financing to businesses just for the fun of it. Lenders and owners provide capital with the expectation of earning a return on their investments. Thus, businesses incur a cost for using debt and equity financing, and to make good business decisions, managers must know this cost. The ultimate goal of the cost of capital estimation process is to estimate a business's corporate cost of capital (see "Critical Concept: Corporate Cost of Capital"). This cost, in turn, is used as the required rate of return, or hurdle rate, when evaluating the business's capital investment opportunities. (Capital investment decisions are discussed in detail in chapters 9 and 10.)

The corporate cost of capital is a weighted average of the capital component costs, that is, the costs of debt and equity. After the component costs have been estimated, they are combined to form the corporate cost of capital, with the weights representing the business's target capital structure.

CRITICAL CONCEPT
Corporate Cost of Capital

The corporate cost of capital is the weighted average of the costs of a business's debt and equity financing. The weights used in the calculation are the target (optimal) capital structure weights. Once estimated, the corporate cost of capital sets the minimum acceptable (required) rate of return on new capital investments. For example, assume Bayside Memorial Hospital has a corporate cost of capital of 10 percent. If a new open MRI (magnetic resonance imaging) investment, judged to have average risk, is expected to return at least 10 percent, then it is financially attractive to the hospital. If the open MRI is expected to return less than 10 percent, accepting it will have an adverse impact on the hospital's financial condition.

Cost of Debt

A firm's managers likely will not know at the start of a planning period the exact types and amounts of debt that will be used to finance new asset acquisitions; the type of debt will depend on the specific assets to be financed and on future market conditions. However, a firm's managers do know what types of debt the business usually issues. For example, Puget Sound Family Practice plans to use a bank line of credit to obtain short-term funds to finance temporary needs and a ten-year bank term loan to raise long-term debt capital. Because the practice does not use short-term debt to finance permanent (long-term) assets, its corporate cost of capital estimate will include only long-term debt, which is assumed to be a ten-year loan. (The corporate cost of capital primarily is used to evaluate long-term asset purchases, so it makes sense to base the estimate solely on the cost of long-term financing.)

How should the practice's physicians estimate the component **cost of debt**? For them it is easy; they would discuss their requirements with a loan officer at a commercial bank. The result might be a potential bank loan with an interest rate of 8 percent. If so, that would be the practice's cost of debt when estimating its corporate cost of capital.

Cost of debt
The return (interest rate) required by lenders to furnish debt capital.

For large businesses that use bonds for long-term debt financing, the process is essentially the same, except the call would be to an investment bank, an institution that helps companies sell stocks and bonds. The bottom line is that estimating a business's cost of debt financing is relatively easy. Just talk to the people who arrange the financing and find out the going rate.

Note that the appropriate cost of debt for use in estimating the corporate cost of capital is not the interest rate on debt financing that was obtained in the past. Rather, it is the rate today, which is assumed to be the cost of debt financing throughout the coming planning period.

Cost of Equity

Cost of equity
The return required by owners to furnish equity capital.

The cost of debt is based on the return (interest rate) that lenders require to provide debt financing, and the **cost of equity** to investor-owned businesses can be defined similarly: It is the rate of return that owners require to provide equity financing to a business. Rational investors expect to earn a return on their ownership interest. The return may come in the form of dividends, bonuses, or capital gains (selling the ownership interest for more than its cost). Before the investment is made, equity investors set a minimum required rate of return based on the riskiness of that investment—the higher the risk, the higher the required rate of return. This required rate of return on an ownership investment in a business defines its cost of equity.

Several methods can be used to estimate a business's cost of equity. We will discuss one: the debt cost plus risk premium method. This method operates on the premise that equity investments are riskier than debt investments. Under this assumption, the cost of equity for any business can be thought of as the cost of debt to that business plus a risk premium (see "Critical Concept: Debt Cost Plus Risk Premium Method").

CRITICAL CONCEPT
Debt Cost Plus Risk Premium Method

The debt cost plus risk premium method is used to estimate a business's cost of equity. It is based on the premise that an ownership investment in a business is riskier than a lender's position. Thus, the cost of equity can be estimated by adding a risk premium to the business's cost of debt. The size of the premium varies over time, but generally it is thought to be in the range of 3 to 5 percentage points for large corporations. To illustrate, assume that the current estimate of the risk premium is 4 percentage points. A large business (such as HCA) with a cost of debt of 5 percent would have a cost of equity estimate of 5% + 4% = 9%.

The assumption that an owner's position in a business is riskier than a lender's is based on the following facts. Lenders have a contractually guaranteed return as specified in the debt agreement. If the borrower fails to make the promised payments, lenders have recourse against the business. In fact, if circumstances dictate, lenders can force a business into bankruptcy with the goal of recovering their investment in a court-ordered liquidation.

Conversely, owners have no contractually guaranteed return. If the business succeeds, owners' returns can be high. However, if the business goes under, owners can lose their entire investment. If a company goes bankrupt, lenders typically get some of their principal amount returned, while equity holders typically get nothing back.

Studies suggest that the risk premium for use in the debt cost plus risk premium method has ranged from 3 to 5 percentage points, with an average of 4 percentage points. However, this premium is based on data from large nationwide corporations. Using this premium estimate as a starting point, Puget Sound Family Practice, with a cost of debt of 8 percent, would have a cost of equity estimate of 12.0 percent:

$$\begin{aligned}\text{Cost of equity} &= \text{Cost of debt} + \text{Risk premium}\\ &= 8.0\% + 4.0\% = 12.0\%.\end{aligned}$$

However, we are applying the model to a small business. In such situations, it is typical to add another premium to account for the fact that small businesses are, by nature, riskier than large businesses. Furthermore, the ownership position in a small business cannot easily be sold if the owner wants out. (In large businesses with many shareholders, the stock can easily and quickly be sold at a known price through a stockbroker.)

Thus, owners typically add a premium of about 5 percentage points to account for small business ownership risk and lack of marketability. When Puget Sound Family Practice's physician-owners added this premium to their initial estimate, they concluded that the cost of equity estimate for the practice is 8% + 4% + 5% = 17%.

Even though the cost of equity estimation process is difficult for investor-owned businesses to accomplish in practice, the underlying concept is well accepted. However, the basis for the cost of equity for not-for-profit organizations is controversial. Indeed, viewpoints vary regarding a not-for-profit's cost of equity. For example, some argue that the cost of equity to a not-for-profit business should be the same as for a similar for-profit business. Others argue that the cost of equity should be the return that is required to maintain the desired debt rating. We do not explore the controversy here—suffice it to say that not-for-profits incur a cost of equity that represents the return required on the community's equity investment in the organization.

Combining the Component Costs

The final step in the process is to combine the debt and equity cost estimates to form the corporate cost of capital (CCC). As discussed in a previous section, each business has a target capital structure in mind. Furthermore, when a firm raises new capital, it generally tries to finance it in a way that will keep the actual capital structure reasonably close to its target over time (see "Critical Equation: Corporate Cost of Capital [CCC]"). Following is the general formula for the CCC for all businesses, regardless of ownership:

$$\text{CCC} = [W_d \times \text{Cost of debt} \times (1 - T)] + (W_e \times \text{Cost of equity})$$

where W_d and W_e are the target weights for debt and equity, respectively, and T is the business's tax rate.

For Puget Sound, the cost of debt estimate is 8.0 percent and the cost of equity estimate is 17.0 percent. Furthermore, the business's target capital structure is 30 percent debt and 70 percent equity, and its tax rate is 21 percent. Thus, the practice's CCC estimate is 13.8 percent:

$$\begin{aligned}\text{CCC} &= [W_d \times \text{Cost of debt} \times (1 - T)] + (W_e \times \text{Cost of equity})\\ &= [0.30 \times 8.0\% \times (1 - 0.21)] + (0.70 \times 17.0\%)\\ &= (0.30 \times 6.3\%) + (0.70 \times 17.0\%)\\ &= 1.9\% + 11.9\%\\ &= 13.8\%.\end{aligned}$$

Note that the before-tax cost of debt is reduced by $(1 - T)$ in the formula. This calculation recognizes the fact that the effective cost of debt to a for-profit business is reduced because interest expense is tax deductible. Thus, the effective cost of debt to Puget Sound is not 8.0 percent, but rather 8.0% × (1 – 0.21) = 8.0% × 0.79 = 6.3%. Every dollar of interest expense reduces the practice's taxes by 21 cents, so the effective interest payment is only 79 cents.

As mentioned briefly in our discussion of optimal capital structure, the optimal structure for any business is the mix of debt and equity financing that produces the lowest CCC. Thus, if the capital structure and cost estimates for Puget Sound are correct, 13.8 percent is the lowest CCC attainable. By minimizing the practice's capital costs, the physicians have taken the first step in ensuring financial success.

If the business is not-for-profit, the same equation is used, except that the tax rate entered for T would be zero. This difference might lead to the conclusion that for-profit businesses have a lower CCC because their cost of debt is reduced by taxes. However, the starting cost of debt is lower in not-for-profit businesses because their debt is tax-exempt. The result is an effective cost of debt that is roughly the same whether a provider is for-profit or not-for-profit.

CRITICAL EQUATION
Corporate Cost of Capital (CCC)

The corporate cost of capital is a blend (weighted average) of the costs of a business's debt and equity financing, with the weights being the business's target capital structure. Thus, the CCC estimation can be expressed as:

$$\text{CCC} = [W_d \times \text{Cost of debt} \times (1 - T)] + (W_e \times \text{Cost of equity}),$$

where W_d and W_e are the target weights for debt and equity, respectively, and T is the business's tax rate.

Interpreting the Corporate Cost of Capital

The component cost estimates (the costs of debt and equity) that make up a business's CCC are based on the returns that investors require to supply capital to the business. Thus, if the business cannot earn at least the CCC on its real asset investments, it cannot pay the minimum returns required by its capital suppliers.

From a pure financial perspective, if a business (especially one that is investor owned) cannot earn its CCC on new land, buildings, and equipment investments, no new investments should be made and no new capital should be raised. If existing investments are not earning the CCC, managers should terminate them, liquidate the assets, and return the proceeds to investors for reinvestment elsewhere.

The primary purpose of estimating a business's CCC is to help make capital investment decisions; that is, the cost of capital will be used as the minimum return necessary for a new product or service to be attractive financially. However, the CCC reflects the aggregate risk of the business. Thus, that cost can be applied without modification only to those investments (projects) under consideration that have average risk, where *average* is defined as that risk applicable to the firm's current overall operations. If a project under consideration carries risk that differs significantly from that of the firm's average, then the CCC must be adjusted to account for the differential risk when the project is being evaluated.

To illustrate the impact of project risk, Bayside Memorial Hospital's CCC, 10 percent, is appropriate for use in evaluating a new open MRI (magnetic resonance imaging) facility, which carries risk similar to the hospital's average project. Clearly, it would *not* be appropriate to apply Bayside's 10 percent CCC, without adjustment, to a new project that involves establishing a managed care subsidiary; this project does not carry the same risk as the hospital's average project, which involves the delivery of patient services. (We have much more to say about project risk adjustments in chapter 10.)

? Self-Test Questions

1. What is the equation for the corporate cost of capital (CCC)?
2. What weights should be used in the formula? Why?
3. How is the cost of debt estimated? What about the cost of equity?
4. What is the primary difference between the CCC for investor-owned firms and that for not-for-profit firms?
5. Explain the interpretation of the CCC.
6. Is the CCC the appropriate hurdle rate for all projects that a business evaluates?

Theme Wrap-Up: Starting a New Medical Practice

One of the first tasks undertaken by the six physician-owners of Puget Sound Family Practice was to figure out the business's optimal capital structure (the appropriate financing mix). After looking at national averages for medical practices and discussing the situation with a local banker, the partners decided on an optimal capital structure of 30 percent debt financing and 70 percent equity financing. Thus, their start-up capital of $1.8 million consisted of $1,260,000 in equity put up by the physicians and a $540,000 ten-year term loan from the bank.

Because two of the six physicians were just completing residencies, each of the four practicing physicians put up $315,000 to start the practice. The two new physicians would be paid at a lower rate of compensation for the first five years of employment until they funded their equity portion of the practice. The salaries withheld would be distributed to the four physicians who put up the initial capital, so at the end of five years all six physicians would each have an equity stake in the practice of $210,000.

Because Puget Sound's initial financing requirement was primarily used to purchase assets that have relatively long lives, the business's initial debt structure consisted of all long-term debt. However, at the same time, the practice negotiated a $200,000 line of credit with the bank that could be tapped to meet short-term needs as they occur during the first year of operation.

In addition to identifying the target capital structure, the physicians wanted an estimate of their CCC. The bank loan interest rate was 8.0 percent, so that set the cost of debt to the business. Furthermore, the cost of equity (the return required on the physicians' ownership contributions) was estimated to be 17.0 percent by using the debt cost plus risk premium method and then applying an additional premium to account for the small size of the business. Finally, the component (debt and equity) costs were combined into a weighted average that produced a corporate cost of capital estimate of 13.8 percent.

The 13.8 percent CCC represents Puget Sound's overall cost of financing. Furthermore, the practice is being financed at the lowest possible cost, because it is using the optimal mix of debt and equity. Any future financing needed by the practice will be done in such a way as to keep the business at its target capital structure. If the practice's costs of debt and equity stay constant in the future, any new facilities investments should return at least 13.8 percent to maintain a sound financial position.

Key Concepts

This chapter provides an overview of debt and equity financing, as well as a discussion of optimal capital structure and the cost of capital. Here are the key concepts:

- To operate, any business must have assets; to acquire assets, the business must raise capital. Capital comes in two basic forms: *debt* and *equity*.

- Two fundamental factors affect a loan's interest rate: *risk* and *inflation*.
- *Term loans* and *bonds* are long-term debt contracts under which a borrower agrees to make a series of interest and principal payments on specific dates to the lender. A term loan generally is provided by a single lender, while a bond typically is offered to the public and sold to many different investors.
- In general, bonds are categorized as *Treasury*, which are issued by the federal government; *corporate*, which are issued by taxable businesses; and *municipal*, which are issued by nonfederal governmental entities, including debt issued on behalf of not-for-profit healthcare providers.
- A *debt contract* is a legal document that spells out the rights and obligations of both lenders and borrowers.
- A *trustee* is a person assigned to make sure that the terms of a bond contract are carried out.
- Bond contracts often include *restrictive covenants*, which are provisions designed to protect bondholders against detrimental managerial actions.
- A *call provision* gives the issuer the right to redeem the bonds before maturity under specified terms. A business will call a bond issue and refund it if interest rates fall sufficiently after the bond has been issued.
- Bonds and other forms of debt are assigned ratings that reflect the probability of default. Ratings range from AAA (the highest) to D (the lowest). The higher the rating, and hence the greater the probability of lenders being paid in full, the lower the interest rate.
- The choice between debt and equity financing is a trade-off of risk versus return. The use of debt financing can leverage up the return to owners, but at the same time it increases owners' risk.
- The *optimal*, or *target*, *capital structure* balances the costs and benefits of debt financing and hence minimizes the business's corporate cost of capital.
- The optimal capital structure decision is based on several factors, including business risk, lender and rating agency attitudes, reserve borrowing capacity, national averages, and asset structure.
- Managers of not-for-profit businesses must grapple with the same capital structure decisions faced by managers of investor-owned firms. However, not-for-profit firms do not have the same flexibility in making financing decisions because those firms cannot sell equity to owners.
- In estimating a firm's corporate cost of capital, the *cost of debt* is the interest rate set on new debt.

- The *cost of equity* to investor-owned firms is the return required by its owners. One method for estimating this cost is the *debt cost plus risk premium model*, which adds a premium to the business's cost of debt. A cost of equity is attached to not-for-profit businesses, but its estimation is more challenging.
- A business's *corporate cost of capital (CCC)* is estimated as follows:

$$CCC = [W_d \times \text{Cost of debt} \times (1 - T)] + (W_e \times \text{Cost of equity}),$$

  where W_d is the weight of debt in the target capital structure, W_e is the weight of equity, and T is the tax rate. Note that the effective cost of debt is reduced in for-profit businesses to recognize the tax deductibility of interest payments. In not-for-profit businesses, the starting cost of debt is often lower because the interest on municipal debt is tax-exempt.
- When making capital investment decisions, a business will use the CCC as the hurdle rate for average-risk projects.

From here, our focus turns to how new project proposals are evaluated. In chapters 9 and 10, we discuss the role that the corporate cost of capital estimate plays in the capital investment evaluation process.

End-of-Chapter Questions

8.1 The two primary factors that affect interest rates on debt securities are risk and inflation. Explain the role of each factor.

8.2 Briefly describe the features of the following types of debt:
- a. Term loan
- b. Bond
- c. Line of credit
- d. Municipal bond

8.3 Briefly explain the following debt features:
- a. Loan agreement
- b. Restrictive covenant
- c. Trustee
- d. Call provision

8.4 a. What do bond ratings measure?
- b. How do investors interpret bond ratings?
- c. Why are bond ratings important?
- d. What is credit enhancement?

8.5 Critique this statement: The use of debt financing lowers the profits of the firm, and hence debt financing should be used only as a last resort.

8.6 Discuss some factors that healthcare managers must consider when setting a business's target capital structure.

8.7 How is a business's cost of debt estimated? Its cost of equity?

8.8 Explain the calculation and interpretation of the corporate cost of capital.

End-of-Chapter Problems

8.1 Seattle Health Plans currently uses zero-debt financing. Its operating profit is $1 million, and it pays taxes at a 40 percent rate. It has $5 million in assets and, because it is all-equity financed, $5 million in equity. Suppose the firm is considering replacing half of its equity financing with debt financing that bears an interest rate of 8 percent.

a. What impact would the new capital structure have on the firm's profit, total dollar return to investors, and return on equity?

b. Redo the analysis, but now assume that the debt financing would cost 15 percent.

c. Repeat the analysis required for part a, but now assume that Seattle Health Plans is a not-for-profit corporation and hence pays no taxes. Compare the results with those obtained in part a.

8.2 Calculate the effective (after-tax) cost of debt for Wallace Clinic, a for-profit healthcare provider, assuming that the interest rate set on its debt is 11 percent and its tax rate is set at the following levels:

a. 0 percent

b. 25 percent

c. 40 percent

8.3 St. Vincent's Hospital has a target capital structure of 35 percent debt and 65 percent equity. Its cost of equity estimate is 13 percent and its cost of tax-exempt debt estimate is 7.5 percent. What is the hospital's corporate cost of capital?

8.4 Richmond Clinic has obtained the following estimates for its costs of debt and equity at various capital structures:

Debt (%)	After-Tax Cost of Debt (%)	Cost of Equity (%)
0	—	16.0
20	6.6	17.0
40	7.8	19.0
60	10.2	22.0
80	14.0	27.0

What is the firm's optimal capital structure? (Hint: Calculate its corporate cost of capital at each structure. Also, note that data on component costs at alternative capital structures are not reliable in real-world situations.)

8.5 Morningside Nursing Home, a not-for-profit corporation, is estimating its corporate cost of capital. Its tax-exempt debt currently requires an interest rate of 6.2 percent, and its target capital structure calls for 60 percent debt financing and 40 percent equity (fund capital) financing. Its estimated cost of equity is 15.4 percent. What is Morningside's corporate cost of capital?

CHAPTER 9

CAPITAL INVESTMENT DECISION BASICS

THEME SET-UP: EVALUATING A PROJECT'S FINANCIAL MERIT

Palm Coast Radiology Associates is a group practice affiliated with Bayside Memorial Hospital. In essence, the hospital provides the equipment and technicians necessary to create radiological images, while the radiologists at the practice perform the required readings and interpretations.

At the last scheduled meeting between hospital and group executives, a new MRI (magnetic resonance imaging) system was proposed by Dr. Jamal Fisher, the group's CEO. Although the hospital currently has a conventional MRI system, Dr. Fisher thinks replacing the old one with a new, open system would be beneficial.

MRI technology uses magnets, radio frequencies, and a computer to generate three-dimensional images of organs and structures inside the body. It offers a painless alternative to diagnostic surgeries and can provide early detection and diagnosis of a number of diseases and disabilities, including multiple sclerosis. Bayside's current MRI system requires patients to be surrounded by the scanner, which means that patients must lie in a narrow tube that covers the entire body. The fully enclosed space creates a great amount of patient apprehension and discomfort, and it can be especially uncomfortable for patients who suffer from claustrophobia.

The open system positions the patient in a much less confining imaging space. A receiver coil is placed around the body part that is to be scanned, and then that portion of the body is centered in the machine. An open MRI system greatly reduces the feeling of constraint associated with conventional systems yet produces high-quality images. In addition, the open system can accommodate pediatric patients who need parental support, as well as patients who are too large to fit in a conventional MRI scanner.

During the meeting, all of the radiologists expressed familiarity with and enthusiasm for the new system, but the hospital's chief financial officer, Sergio Obregon, voiced his concern about the cost. "Sure, the new system will be great for patients, but it will cost $2.5 million to buy and install. Can we afford it?" he asked. Dr. Fisher thought about the question for a moment and then replied, "If we can get at least that much in new patient revenue, it should be worth it." Several meeting attendees then became involved in a heated argument about how to assess the financial merits of the potential investment.

By the end of the chapter, you will see how managers can apply discounted cash flow techniques to estimate the financial attractiveness of the proposed MRI system. Then, with all the facts at hand, you can make the final decision.

Learning Objectives

After studying this chapter, you will be able to do the following:

- Explain how managers use project classifications and postaudits in the capital investment decision process.
- Describe the role of financial analysis in healthcare capital investment decisions.
- Discuss the key elements of breakeven analysis.
- Explain why discounted cash flow (DCF) analysis is such an important concept in healthcare finance.
- Perform basic DCF calculations.
- Define the *opportunity cost principle.*
- Measure the financial return on an investment in both dollar and percentage terms.

9.1 INTRODUCTION

Capital investment decision
The business decision involving which long-term assets (e.g., land, buildings, equipment) to buy. Such decisions often are referred to as *capital budgeting decisions.*

This chapter focuses on **capital investment decisions**, which involve the acquisition of land, buildings, and equipment. Capital investment decisions, also called *capital budgeting decisions*, are among the most critical decisions health services managers must make, because they often involve large sums of money and because the results generally affect the business's operations and financial condition for a long time.

Sound capital investment decisions are essential to the success of any business. In this chapter and the next, we discuss many of the concepts that are important to building an effective capital investment analysis system.

9.2 PROJECT CLASSIFICATIONS

Although benefits can be gained from the careful analysis of capital investment proposals, such efforts can be costly. Certain projects may warrant a relatively detailed analysis, along with senior management involvement; for others, simpler procedures should be used. Accordingly, large health services organizations generally classify projects into categories, and by cost in each category, and then analyze each project on the basis of its category and cost.

For example, Bayside Memorial Hospital uses the following classifications:

- *Category 1: Mandatory replacement.* Category 1 consists of expenditures related to replacing worn-out or damaged equipment necessary to the operations of the hospital. In general, these expenditures are mandatory, so organizations usually make decisions relating to them with limited analysis.
- *Category 2: Discretionary replacement.* This category contains expenditures to replace serviceable but technologically obsolete equipment. The purpose of undertaking these projects is to lower costs or to provide more clinically effective services. Because category 2 projects are not mandatory, a detailed decision process is generally required to support these expenditures.
- *Category 3: Expansion of existing services or markets.* Expenditures to increase capacity, or to expand in markets currently served by the hospital, are included here. These decisions are more complex, so a detailed analysis is required, and the final decision is made at a high level in the organization.
- *Category 4: Expansion into new services or markets.* These are projects necessary to provide new services or to expand into geographic areas not currently served. Such projects involve strategic decisions that could change the fundamental nature of the hospital, and they normally require the expenditure of large sums of money over long periods. Invariably, a particularly detailed analysis is required, and the board of trustees generally makes the final decision as part of Bayside Memorial's strategic plan.

- *Category 5: Environmental projects.* This category consists of expenditures for complying with government orders, labor agreements, accreditation requirements, and the like. Unless the expenditures are large, category 5 expenditures are treated like category 1 expenditures.
- *Category 6: Other.* This category is a catchall for projects that do not fit neatly into another category. The primary determinant of how category 6 projects are evaluated is the amount of funds required.

In general, relatively simple analyses and only a few supporting documents are required for replacement decisions and safety or environmental projects, especially those that are mandatory. A detailed analysis is necessary for expansion and other projects.

Note that, in each category, projects are classified by size: Larger projects need more detailed analyses and approval at higher organizational levels. Thus, for example, at Bayside Memorial Hospital, department heads can authorize spending up to $50,000 on discretionary replacement projects, while the full board of trustees must approve expansion projects that cost more than $5 million.

Self-Test Questions

1. What is the primary advantage of classifying capital projects?
2. What are some typical project classifications?
3. What role does project size (cost) play in the classifications?
4. Into what category would the open MRI project be placed?

9.3 THE ROLE OF FINANCIAL ANALYSIS IN CAPITAL INVESTMENT DECISIONS

For investor-owned businesses, the role of financial analysis in capital investment decision-making is clear. If wealth maximization is the goal, investor-owned businesses should undertake projects that contribute to owners' wealth while they ignore those that do not.

However, what about not-for-profit businesses, which do not have wealth maximization as a goal? In such businesses, the appropriate goal typically is to provide quality, cost-effective services to their communities. (A strong argument could be made that this should also be the goal of investor-owned businesses in the healthcare field.) In this situation, capital investment decisions must consider many factors besides a project's financial implications.

Still, good decision-making, and hence the future viability of the business, requires that the financial impact of capital investments be recognized. If a business takes on a series of highly unprofitable projects that meet nonfinancial goals, and such projects are not offset by profitable ones, the firm's financial condition will deteriorate. If this situation persists over time, the business will eventually lose its financial viability and could even be forced into bankruptcy.

Because bankrupt businesses cannot meet a community's needs, even managers of not-for-profit health services organizations must consider a capital investment's potential impact on the organization's financial condition. Managers may make a conscious decision to accept a project with a poor financial prognosis because of its nonfinancial virtues, but they must know the financial impact up front, so that they are not surprised when the project drains the business's financial resources.

Financial analysis provides managers with the relevant information about a capital investment's financial impact and hence helps managers make better decisions, including decisions based primarily on nonfinancial factors. (In section 9.9, we discuss how nonfinancial factors can be formally considered in the capital investment decision process.)

SELF-TEST QUESTIONS

1. What is the role of financial analysis in capital investment decisions in for-profit firms?
2. Why are such analyses important in not-for-profit businesses?

9.4 OVERVIEW OF CAPITAL INVESTMENT FINANCIAL ANALYSIS

The financial analysis of capital investment proposals typically involves the following four steps:

1. *Cash flow estimation.* Estimate the project's cash flows. Usually, this estimation consists of the initial cost, the cash flows that arise from operating the project, and the cash flows associated with closing down the project at the end of its useful life.
2. *Project risk assessment.* Assess the riskiness of the cash flows. (Cash flow estimation and risk assessment are addressed in chapter 10.)
3. *Cost of capital estimation.* Estimate the project cost of capital. As discussed in chapter 8, a business's corporate cost of capital reflects the aggregate risk of the business's assets—that is, the riskiness inherent in the average project. If the project being evaluated does not have average risk, the corporate cost of capital must be adjusted to obtain the project cost of capital.
4. *Financial impact assessment.* Assess the project's financial merit. Several measures can be used for this purpose; we discuss three in this chapter.

? Self-Test Question

1. Explain the four steps in capital investment financial analysis.

9.5 CREATING THE TIME LINE

To illustrate a capital investment financial analysis, consider the situation facing Bayside Memorial Hospital (see the theme set-up). The CEO of the hospital-affiliated radiology group proposed an open MRI project. The system costs $2 million, and Bayside would have to spend another $500,000 for site preparation and installation, for a total initial cost of $2.5 million.

The open MRI system is expected to be in operation for five years, at which time the hospital's strategic plan calls for a new imaging facility. As discussed earlier, the first step in a capital investment financial analysis is to estimate the project's cash flows. Cash flows, basically, are the amounts of money expected to flow into and out of the hospital as a result of acquiring the open MRI system.

We will leave the details of this step for chapter 10, but here is a rough idea of what was done. Bayside's managers, with help from the radiology group physicians, estimated the volume of procedures (scans), the reimbursement amounts expected on each scan, the costs to operate the MRI, and any other cash flows that would result from operating the system.

These flows were then combined with the cost of the system and the flows expected when the system is shut down after five years of operation. The end result is the following set of cash flows, placed on a **time line**:

Time line
A graphical representation of time and cash flows. It may be an actual horizontal line or cells on a spreadsheet.

0	1	2	3	4	5
($2,500,000)	$510,000	$535,500	$562,275	$590,389	$1,369,908

Time lines make it easier to visualize when the cash flows in a particular analysis occur. Time 0 is any starting point (typically the time of the first cash flow in an analysis). In our situation,

- time 0 is when the MRI would be purchased;
- time 1 is one period from the starting point, or the end of period 1; and
- time 2 is two periods from the starting point, or the end of period 2.

The time line goes on until period 5. Thus, the numbers (e.g., 0, 1, 2) represent end-of-period values.

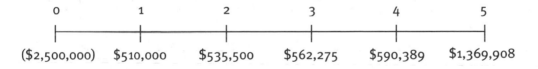

Often, as in this case, the periods are years, but managers can use other time intervals, such as quarters or months, when needed to fit the timing of the cash flows being evaluated. Because, in this example, the periods are years, the interval from 0 to 1 is year 1, and 1 represents both the end of year 1 and the beginning of year 2. (Years are often used in project analyses because the flows are too difficult to forecast with confidence on a more frequent basis.)

Cash flows are shown on a time line directly below the points in time in which they are expected to occur. The $2,500,000 under time 0 is a cost (outflow), so it is set in parentheses. (Outflows are sometimes designated by minus signs rather than by parentheses.) The $510,000 shown under year 1 is an estimate of the net cash inflow resulting from the first year's operation of the open MRI, considering both the system's expected operating revenues and costs. The year 5 net cash flow includes both the net operating cash flow and the cash flow expected from selling the MRI at the end of the project's five-year life.

Time lines play an essential role in capital investment financial analyses because they depict the amount and timing of a project's expected cash flows. The time line may be an actual line, as illustrated earlier, or it may be a series of columns (or rows) on a spreadsheet. Time lines are used extensively in investment analyses, so get into the habit of using them as you work the problems in chapters 9 and 10.

? Self-Test Questions

1. Why are time lines so important in capital investment financial analyses?
2. Draw a three-year time line that illustrates the following situation: An investment of $10,000 at time 0 and inflows of $5,000 at the end of years 1, 2, and 3.

9.6 BREAKEVEN ANALYSIS

Chapter 5 introduced breakeven analysis in conjunction with profit analysis. There, we estimated the volume required for both accounting and economic breakeven.

Here, we apply the breakeven concept in a capital investment setting. In such analyses, one can calculate many types of breakeven. Rather than discuss all the possible types here, we can focus on time breakeven, which is measured by payback (see "Critical Concept: Payback").

The best way to calculate the open MRI's expected payback is to examine the project's cumulative cash flows. (At any point in time, the cumulative cash flow is merely the sum of all the cash flows, with a proper sign indicating an inflow or outflow, that have occurred up to that point.) Payback occurs when the cumulative cash flow turns positive.

Here are the open MRI's annual cash flows and cumulative cash flows:

Year	Annual Cash Flow	Cumulative Cash Flow
0	($2,500,000)	($2,500,000)
1	510,000	(1,990,000)
2	535,500	(1,454,500)
3	562,275	(892,225)
4	590,389	(301,836)
5	1,369,908	1,068,072

We see that the cumulative cash flow at time 0 is –$2,500,000, at year 1 it is –$2,500,000 + $510,000 = –$1,990,000, at year 2 it is –$1,990,000 + $535,500 = –$1,454,500, and so on.

As shown in the far-right column, the $2,500,000 cost of the open MRI project will be recovered at the end of year 5 if the cash flow forecasts are correct, because year 5 is the year that the cumulative flow turns positive. Furthermore, if the cash flows are assumed to come in evenly during the year, breakeven will occur $301,836 ÷ $1,369,908 = 0.22 years (or about 0.2 years) into year 5, so the open MRI project's payback is 4.2 years. (At the end of year 4, $301,836 remains to be recovered, while the cash flow expected in year 5 is $1,369,908. The jump in cash flows in year 5 is the result of salvage value, which we discuss in chapter 10.)

CRITICAL CONCEPT
Payback

Payback is the number of years that it takes to recover the cost of an investment. For example, assume that an EKG (electrocardiogram) machine that costs $2,500 is expected to net $1,000 in cash flow in each of the next five years. If things go as expected, the $2,500 investment will be recovered in three years (with $500 left over), so the payback is three years, or more precisely, two and a half years. The shorter the payback, the better, as the business will more quickly recover its investment in the project.

At one time, payback was used by managers as the sole measure of a project's financial attractiveness: A business might accept all projects with paybacks of five years or less. However, payback has two serious deficiencies when it is used in this way.

First, payback ignores all cash flows that occur after the payback period. To illustrate, Bayside might be evaluating a competing project that has the same cash flows as the open MRI project in periods 0 through 5. However, the alternative project might have a cash inflow of $2 million in year 6. Both projects would have the same payback—4.2 years—and hence be ranked the same, even though the alternative project clearly is better from a financial perspective.

Second, payback ignores the time value of money. (Time value is discussed in the next section.) For these two reasons, payback generally is no longer used as the primary evaluation tool.

Project liquidity
The ability of a project to pay for itself from the cash flows that it generates. Project liquidity is measured by payback; the shorter the payback, the more liquid the project.

In spite of its deficiencies, payback provides useful information to managers as they make capital investment decisions. Payback is a quick measure of **project liquidity**. The shorter the payback, the more quickly the funds invested in a project will become available for other purposes. In addition, cash flows expected in the distant future generally are regarded as riskier than near-term cash flows because they are harder to estimate. Thus, projects with long paybacks that must rely on distant cash flows to achieve profitability are considered to be more risky than projects with short paybacks. Considering both these factors, shorter payback projects typically are considered to be more financially attractive than longer payback projects.

(?) Self-Test Questions

1. What is payback?
2. What are the benefits of payback?
3. What are its deficiencies?

9.7 DISCOUNTED CASH FLOW ANALYSIS

Up to this point, our financial analysis of the open MRI investment has been limited to breakeven analysis. We have laid out the expected cash flows from the project on a time line and estimated that it would take 4.2 years for Bayside to recover its investment, assuming that everything occurs as expected. If we were whizzes at processing information, we might be able to merely look at the cash flows and make a complete judgment about the project's financial attractiveness. However, most people cannot do this, so summarizing the information contained in the project's cash flows would be useful.

Discounted cash flow (DCF) analysis
The use of time value of money techniques to estimate the value of an investment.

The process of assigning appropriate values to cash flows that occur at different points in time and then summarizing this information in a single value is called **discounted cash flow (DCF) analysis**. DCF analysis is an important part of healthcare finance because most financial analyses involve future cash flows. In fact, of all the investment analysis techniques, none is more important than DCF analysis. The concepts presented here are the cornerstones of all investment analyses, so an understanding of DCF concepts is essential to good capital investment decision-making.

The economic principle that underlies DCF analysis is the time value of money. This principle is based on the fact that a dollar to be received in the future is worth less than a current dollar; a dollar in hand today can be invested in an interest-bearing account and hence can be worth more than one dollar received in the future (see "Critical Concept: Time Value of Money"). Because current dollars are worth more than future dollars, capital investment decisions must account for both the magnitude and the timing of the forecasted cash flows.

Future Value (Compounding)

We start our discussion of DCF analysis by examining how money invested today grows over time. The process of moving from today's value to a future value is called **compounding** because the value increases, or compounds, over time.

Although compounding is not used a great deal in capital investment analyses, it is the best starting point for learning DCF concepts. To illustrate compounding, suppose you deposit \$100 in a bank account that pays 5 percent annual interest (when interest is earned annually, it is credited to the account at the end of each year). How much would be in the account at the end of one year?

CRITICAL CONCEPT
Time Value of Money

The time value of money principle is based on the fact that money in hand is worth more than funds expected to be received in the future. For example, consider \$100 in hand today versus \$100 to be received in one year. If the \$100 in hand today is invested in a bank account that pays 5 percent interest, it will earn \$5 in interest and be worth \$105 at the end of one year. However, the \$100 to be obtained at the end of the year is only worth \$100 when received. Discounted cash flow (DCF) analysis is used to account for the time value of money.

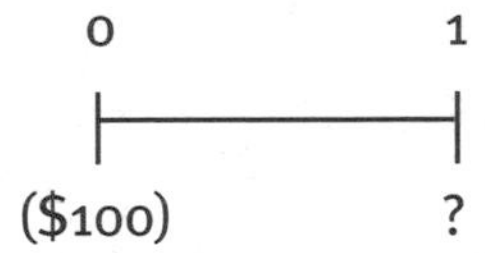

Compounding
The process of finding the future value of a current (starting) amount or series of cash flows.

To put the analysis on a time line, note that the account is opened with a deposit of \$100 at time 0. The amount is shown as an outflow, because you will be turning the money over to the bank. The question mark at year 1 signifies that you want to know the value of the account at that time, after being on deposit for one year.

During one year's time, you will earn 5 percent interest on the initial \$100, so the interest earned is \$100 × 0.05 = \$5. Thus, at the end of one year the amount in the account is \$100 + \$5 = \$105. Note that the balance in the account at year 1 can be calculated directly by multiplying the starting amount, \$100, by 1 + Interest rate (expressed as a decimal). Thus, the ending amount after one year is \$100 × (1 + 0.05) = \$100 × 1.05 = \$105.

What would be the value of the \$100 if you left the money in the account for two years? At the start of the second year, the account balance is \$105. Interest of \$105 × 0.05 = \$5.25 is earned on the now larger beginning amount during the second year, so the account balance at the end of year 2 is \$105 + \$5.25 = \$110.25.

The year 2 interest, \$5.25, is higher than the first year's interest, \$5, because \$5 × 0.05 = \$0.25 in interest was earned during the second year on the first year's interest. Again, we could calculate the balance after two years as \$105 × 1.05 = \$110.25. In addition, we could calculate the balance at the end of year 2 directly from the initial starting amount, \$100, as follows: \$100 × 1.05 × 1.05 = \$100 × $(1.05)^2$ = \$110.25. By multiplying by 1.05 two times, we recognize that the initial deposit is compounded at a 5 percent rate over two years.

What about the balance after five years? The compounding process continues, and because the beginning balance is higher at the beginning of each succeeding year, the annual interest earned increases in each year. At the end of year 5, the balance would be $\$100 \times (1.05)^5 = \$127.63$. Thus, after five years, you would earn \$27.63 in total interest on your initial \$100 investment.

These calculations demonstrate that a pattern exists in future value calculations. In general, the future value of a single starting amount at the end of *N* years can be found by applying this equation:

$$FV_N = PV \times (1 + I)^N,$$

where

- FV_N is the future value at the end of *N* years,
- *PV* is the initial starting amount (present value), and
- *I* is the interest rate (expressed in decimal form).

Future values, as well as most other DCF calculations, can be performed using three methods: regular calculator (calculator without financial functions), financial calculator (calculator with financial functions), or spreadsheet. We include the regular calculator solution in our discussions (when applicable). Financial calculator and spreadsheet solutions are presented in boxes (see "Solution Technique: Future Value").

To use a regular calculator to solve compounding problems, multiply the PV by (1 + I) for *N* times or use the exponential function to raise (1 + I) to the *N*th power and then multiply the result by the PV. Perhaps the easiest way to find the future value of \$100 after five years when compounded at 5 percent is to enter \$100, then multiply this amount by 1.05 five times. If the calculator is set to display two decimal places, the answer would be \$127.63:

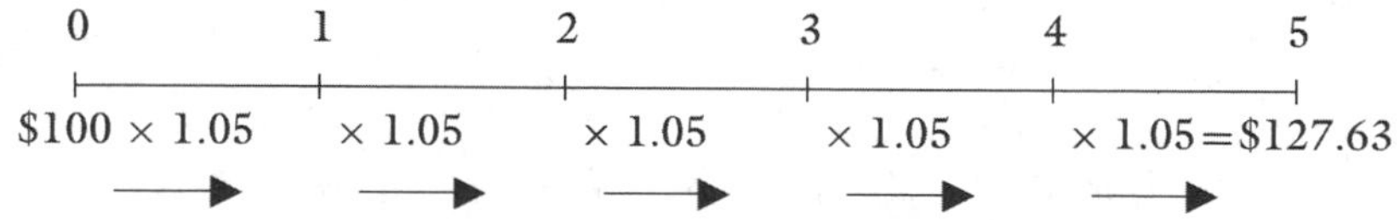

As denoted by the arrows, compounding involves moving to the right along the time line.

SOLUTION TECHNIQUE
Future Value

Financial Calculator

Financial calculators have been preprogrammed to solve many types of time value analyses, including the future value of a single starting amount. In effect, the future value equation is programmed directly into the calculator. With a financial calculator, the future value is found using three of the following five time value input keys:

To find the future value of $100 after five years at 5 percent interest using a financial calculator, just enter PV = 100, I = 5, and N = 5, then press the FV key. The answer, $127.63 (rounded to two decimal places), will appear.

Some financial calculators require that cash flows be designated as either inflows or outflows (entered as either positive or negative values). Applying this logic to the illustration, you deposit the initial amount, which is an outflow to you, and take out, or receive, the ending amount, which is an inflow to you. If the calculator requires a sign convention, the PV would be entered as –100. (If the PV were entered as 100, a positive value, the calculator would display –127.63 as the answer.) The calculator solution can be shown pictorially as follows:

Inputs 5 5 – 100

Output = 127.63

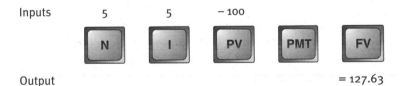

Different financial calculators require slight changes to the procedures given here. For example, sometimes the time value buttons are keys on the calculator, whereas on other calculators the time value variables appear on a screen. Also, some calculators

(continued)

SOLUTION TECHNIQUE
Future Value *(continued)*

require that the compute (CPT) button be pressed before pressing FV. Thus, if you are using a financial calculator to perform DCF calculations, be sure to read the user's manual.

Spreadsheet

Spreadsheet programs are ideally suited for time value analyses. For simple time value calculations, it is easy to enter the appropriate formula directly into the spreadsheet. For example, you could enter the spreadsheet version of the future value equation into cell A6: =100*(1.05)^5. Here, = tells the spreadsheet that a formula is being entered into the cell; * is the spreadsheet multiplication sign; and ^ is the spreadsheet exponential, or power, sign.

	A	B	C	D
1				
2	5	Nper	Number of periods	
3	$ 100.00	Pv	Present value	
4	5.0%	Rate	Interest rate	
5				
6	$ 127.63	=100*(1.05)^5 (entered into cell A6)		
7				
8	$ 127.63	=A3*(1+A4)^A2 (entered into cell A8)		
9				
10	$ 127.63	=FV(A4,A2,–A3) (entered into cell A10)		

When this formula is entered into cell A6, the value $127.63 appears in the cell (when formatted with a dollar sign to two decimal places). Note that different spreadsheet programs use a slightly different syntax in their time value analyses. The examples presented here use the Excel syntax.

In most situations, it is more useful to enter a formula that can accommodate changing input values than to embed these values directly in the formula, so it would be better to solve this future value problem with this formula: =A3*(1+A4)^A2, as done in cell A8. Here, the present value ($100) is contained in cell A3, the interest rate (0.05, which is displayed as 5 percent) in cell A4, and the number of periods (5) in cell A2. With this formula, future values can be easily calculated with different starting amounts, interest rates, or number of years by changing the values in the input cells.

SOLUTION TECHNIQUE
Future Value *(continued)*

In addition to entering the appropriate formula, many DCF calculations are preprogrammed by the spreadsheet software. Preprogrammed formulas consist of a number of arithmetic calculations combined into one statement; thus, spreadsheet users can save the time and tedium of building formulas from scratch.

Each formula begins with a unique name that identifies the calculation to be performed, along with one or more arguments (the input values for the calculation) enclosed in parentheses. The best way to access the time value formulas is to use the spreadsheet's formulas tab.

For this future value problem, first move the cursor to cell A10 (the cell where you want the answer to appear). Then, click on the formulas tab; select financial for the category and FV (future value) for the name; and enter A4 for Rate, A2 for Nper (number of periods), and –A3 for PV. (Note that the Pmt and Type entries are left blank for this problem. These entries are used for solving different types of problems. Also, note that the cell address entered for PV has a minus sign. This operator is necessary for the answer to be displayed as a positive number.) Finally, press OK, and the result, $127.63, appears in cell A10.

Present Value (Discounting)

Suppose you have been offered the opportunity to make an investment (perhaps buy a low-risk security) that promises to pay $127.63 at the end of five years. How much would you be willing to pay for that investment? In other words, what is the investment worth today? To answer that question, you need another piece of information: the interest rate you could earn on other investments of similar risk to the one being offered. If similar investments offer a 5 percent annual rate of return (interest rate), then use 5 percent to value the offer.

The compounding example presented in the previous section shows that an initial amount of $100 invested at 5 percent per year would be worth $127.63 at the end of five years. Thus, you should be indifferent to the choice between $100 today and $127.63 at the end of five years. Today's $100 is defined as the present value of $127.63 due in five years when 5 percent is the comparison rate of return. If the price of the investment being offered is exactly $100, you could buy it or turn it down because that is its fair value. If the price is less than $100, you should buy it. However, if the price is greater than $100, you should decline the offer.

Conceptually, the present value of a cash flow due *N* years in the future is the amount that, if it were on hand today, would grow to equal the future amount when compounded at the appropriate comparison rate. In effect, the present value tells us what amount would have to be invested to earn the return available on similar alternative investments. If the investment can be obtained for a lesser amount, a higher rate will be earned. If the investment costs more than the present value, the rate earned will be less than that available on similar alternatives.

Discounting
The process of finding the present value of an amount or series of cash flows expected to be received in the future.

Finding present values is called **discounting**, because the amount you are calculating (the present value) is smaller than the starting amount (the future value). Discounting is simply the reverse of compounding: If the PV is known, compound to find the FV; if the FV is known, discount to find the PV.

Here is the time line for calculating the security's present (current) value:

0	5%	1	2	3	4	5
?						\$127.63

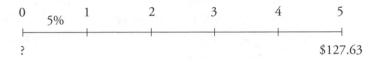

To develop the discounting equation for a single ending amount, solve the compounding equation for PV:

$$\text{Compounding: } FV_N = PV \times (1 + I)^N.$$
$$\text{Discounting: } PV = FV_N \div (1 + I)^N.$$

The equations show us that compounding problems are solved by multiplication, while discounting problems are solved by division.

To solve this problem using a regular calculator, enter \$127.63 and divide it five times by 1.05:

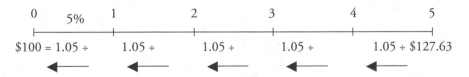

0 (5%)	1	2	3	4	5
\$100 = 1.05 ÷	1.05 ÷	1.05 ÷	1.05 ÷	1.05 ÷ \$127.63	
←	←	←	←	←	

As shown by the arrows, discounting is moving left along the time line. For financial calculator and spreadsheet solutions, see "Solution Technique: Present Value." For additional information about time value of money, see online chapter 18, "Time Value Analysis," which is available at ache.org/books/FinanceFundamentals3.

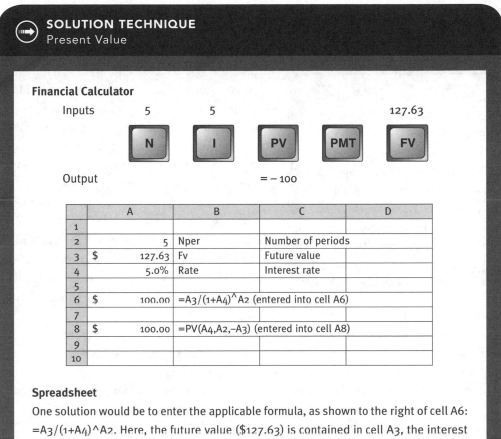

SOLUTION TECHNIQUE
Present Value

Financial Calculator

	N	I	PV	PMT	FV
Inputs	5	5			127.63
Output			= – 100		

	A	B	C	D
1				
2	5	Nper	Number of periods	
3	$ 127.63	Fv	Future value	
4	5.0%	Rate	Interest rate	
5				
6	$ 100.00	=A3/(1+A4)^A2 (entered into cell A6)		
7				
8	$ 100.00	=PV(A4,A2,–A3) (entered into cell A8)		
9				
10				

Spreadsheet

One solution would be to enter the applicable formula, as shown to the right of cell A6: =A3/(1+A4)^A2. Here, the future value ($127.63) is contained in cell A3, the interest rate (0.05, which is displayed as 5 percent) in cell A4, and the number of periods (5) in cell A2. With this formula, present values easily can be calculated with different starting future amounts, interest rates, or number of years.

Cell A8 illustrates the preprogrammed formula. First, move the cursor to that cell (the cell where you want the answer to appear). Then, click on the formulas tab; select financial for the category and PV (present value) for the formula name; and enter A4 for Rate, A2 for Nper (number of periods), and –A3 for Fv. (Note that the Pmt and Type entries are left blank for this problem. Also, note that the cell address entered for Fv has a minus sign. This operator is necessary for the answer to be displayed as a positive number.) Finally, press OK, and the result, $100.00, appears in cell A8.

Opportunity Cost of Capital

In the last section, we chose an interest (discount) rate to value the proposed investment. We used 5 percent, the interest rate offered on alternative investments of similar risk. In doing this, we implemented a concept called the *opportunity cost of capital* (see "Critical Concept: Opportunity Cost of Capital").

CRITICAL CONCEPT
Opportunity Cost of Capital

The opportunity cost of capital (money) is a tried-and-true economic principle. If you invest $100 in investment A, those funds will not be available for any other purpose. Thus, you should require that the return on investment A be at least as good as the return on similar alternative investments. If investment A is not as good as similar investment B, then the $100 should be invested in B rather than in A. In other words, investment A has an opportunity cost, and that cost is the return that one would expect to earn on alternative investments with similar risk.

The opportunity cost of capital plays a crucial role in DCF analysis. To illustrate, suppose you bought the winning ticket for the Florida lottery and now have $1 million to invest. Should you assign some cost to these funds? At first blush, it might appear that this money has zero cost because its acquisition was purely a matter of luck. However, as soon as you think about what to do with the $1 million, you must think in terms of the opportunity costs involved.

By using the money to invest in one alternative (e.g., in the stock of Health Management Associates), you forgo the opportunity to make some other investment with the same funds (e.g., buying US Treasury securities). Thus, an opportunity cost is associated with any investment planned for the $1 million, even though the lottery winnings were free.

Because one investment decision automatically negates all other possible investments with the same funds, the cash flows expected to be earned from any investment must be discounted at a rate that reflects the return that could be earned on forgone investment opportunities. The problem is that the number of forgone investment opportunities is virtually infinite, so which one should be chosen to establish the opportunity cost discount rate?

The opportunity cost rate to be applied in DCF analyses is the rate that could be earned on alternative investments of similar risk. It is not logical to assign a low opportunity cost rate to a series of risky cash flows, or vice versa. This concept is important, so it is worth repeating: The opportunity cost rate (i.e., the discount rate) applied to investment cash flows is the rate that could be earned on alternative investments with similar risk.

In addition, it is essential to recognize that the discounting process itself accounts for the opportunity cost of capital (i.e., the loss of use of the funds for other purposes) (see "For Your Consideration: Discounted Payback"). In effect, discounting a potential investment at, say, 10 percent produces a present value that provides a 10 percent return. Thus, if the investment can be obtained for less than its present value, it will earn more than its opportunity cost of capital and hence is a good investment. Alternately, if the cost of the investment is greater than its present value, it will earn less than its opportunity cost of capital and hence is a bad investment.

Finally, note that the opportunity cost rate does not depend on the source of the funds to be invested. Rather, the primary determinant of this rate is the riskiness of the cash flows being discounted. Thus, the same opportunity cost rate would be applied to a potential investment regardless of whether the funds to be used for the investment were won in a lottery, taken out of petty cash, or obtained by selling securities.

FOR YOUR CONSIDERATION
Discounted Payback

When we discussed payback, which measures time breakeven, we noted that it has two deficiencies: It ignores all cash flows beyond the payback period, and it does not consider the time value of money.

Discounted payback is a breakeven measure similar to the conventional payback, except that the cash flows in each year are discounted to time 0 by the project's cost of capital, but they are kept at their original positions on the time line. Then, these discounted dollar amounts are used to calculate payback. With this approach to the calculation, the discounted payback solves the conventional payback's problem of not considering the project's cost of capital in the payback calculation. In other words, discounted payback takes into consideration the time value of money. Applied to Bayside's open MRI project, the discounted payback is 4.9 years, compared to a conventional payback of 4.2 years.

What is your opinion of discounted payback? Does it make sense that the discounted payback is longer than the conventional payback? Is it a better measure of project liquidity than the conventional payback?

At this point, you may question the ability of analysts to assess the riskiness of a set of cash flows or to choose an opportunity cost rate with any confidence. Fortunately, the process is not as difficult as it may appear here. We discuss risk assessment in more detail in chapter 10. Furthermore, businesses have a benchmark discount rate that can be used as a starting point when making capital investment decisions—the corporate cost of capital, which is covered in chapter 8.

Self-Test Questions

1. What is compounding?
2. What is discounting? How is it related to compounding?
3. What are the three primary methods used to perform DCF calculations?
4. Why does an investment have an opportunity cost of capital even when the funds employed have no explicit cost?
5. How are opportunity cost rates established?

9.8 RETURN ON INVESTMENT

Now that you have a basic understanding of DCF analysis, we can continue with Bayside's open MRI analysis. With any investment, the most important financial question is, Do you expect to make any money? Thus, the key measure of a project's financial attractiveness is its expected profitability, or **return on investment (ROI)**. In this section, we discuss two ROI measures that healthcare organizations use to answer the profitability question (see "Healthcare in Practice: Capital Investment Analysis in Healthcare Organizations").

Return on investment (ROI)
The profitability of an investment, measured in either dollars or percentage (rate of) return.

HEALTHCARE IN PRACTICE
Capital Investment Analysis in Healthcare Organizations

Over the last 20 years, several surveys have been conducted to assess how healthcare organizations analyze and make capital investment decisions. In the 1980s, approximately half of surveyed hospitals used return on investment (ROI) measures to assess financial attractiveness, while about 40 percent used the payback method. ROI measures include net present value (NPV) and internal rate of return (IRR).

Fast forward to today. Now, virtually all large healthcare organizations use ROI measures to assess financial impact. NPV is the most common measure, but many systems use multiple financial measures rather than just one. The most frequently used are NPV, IRR, and payback. Large businesses do not seem to place complete faith in one measure but prefer to paint a complete picture of the expected financial consequences of a proposed capital investment.

For example, NPV provides information about the expected dollar contribution to an organization's financial value. IRR gives some information about the safety margin inherent in the project, because an IRR much higher than the cost of capital means that the project's cash flows could fall short of predictions, yet the project would still be profitable. Finally, payback is useful in screening capital investments in changing technologies, where continuous innovation can make the investment obsolete in a short time.

Little difference appears in the financial analysis techniques used by for-profit and not-for-profit businesses. Both types realize that financial soundness is important in meeting organizational goals.

In addition to financial factors, most large healthcare organizations recognize that nonfinancial factors play an important role in the decision process. For example, contribution to the mission and fit with the organization's long-term strategic vision are commonly mentioned as important decision factors.

HEALTHCARE IN PRACTICE
Capital Investment Analysis in Healthcare Organizations *(continued)*

Furthermore, many healthcare organizations have a formal system for incorporating physician input into the decision process. All organizations reported undertaking projects with poor financial prospects because of "mission virtues." Such projects were viewed as paying healthcare dividends to the community as opposed to paying financial dividends to the business.

Although little information is available regarding the capital investment policies of small healthcare businesses (such as small medical practices), evidence from other industries suggests that such businesses are less sophisticated than their larger counterparts. Indeed, most capital investment decisions at small businesses appear to be made on the sole basis of need as opposed to financial attractiveness. If the owners perform some type of financial analysis, it is more likely to be a back-of-the-envelope calculation as opposed to a detailed analysis. That said, as reimbursement rates tighten and as sophisticated business practices filter down to smaller businesses, the use of ROI measures is expected to become as widespread in small businesses as it is in large businesses.

Note: This Healthcare in Practice is based on information in K. L. Reiter, D. G. Smith, J. R. C. Wheeler, and H. L. Rivenson, 2000, "Capital Investment Strategies in Health Care Systems," *Journal of Health Care Finance* (Summer): 31–41. Though this source is from 2000, the information is still relevant today.

Net Present Value

Net present value (NPV) is a dollar ROI measure that uses DCF analysis, so it is often referred to as a DCF profitability measure (see "Critical Concept: Net Present Value"). NPV is calculated and interpreted as follows:

- *Find the present values.* Find the present (time 0) value of each cash flow, including both inflows and outflows, when discounted at the opportunity cost of capital.
- *Sum the present values.* The resulting sum is defined as the project's NPV. (The term *NPV* is used because it is the sum, or net, of the present values of an investment's expected cash flows.)

CRITICAL CONCEPT
Net Present Value

Net present value (NPV) measures the dollar value of an investment on the basis of its opportunity cost of capital. To illustrate, assume a $100 investment is expected to return $120 after one year. Furthermore, the return available on alternative investments of similar risk (opportunity cost of capital) is 5 percent. The NPV of this investment is $\$120 \div (1.05)^1 - \$100 = \$114.29 - \$100 = \$14.29$. Thus, the investment is expected to (1) return the $100 initial investment, (2) provide a 5 percent return on those funds, and (3) create $14.29 of additional value (on a present value basis). An NPV of zero means that the investment just breaks even in the sense that it earns its opportunity cost of capital but no more.

- *Interpret the NPV.* If the NPV is positive, the project is expected to be profitable; the higher the NPV, the more profitable the project. If the NPV is zero, the project just breaks even in an economic sense. If the NPV is negative, the project is expected to be unprofitable.

To calculate the NPV of Bayside's open MRI project, we first need a discount rate (opportunity cost of capital). Bayside's corporate cost of capital is 10 percent, so if we assume that the project has average risk (the same risk as Bayside's average project), then 10 percent can be used to calculate this project's NPV. (In chapter 10, we assess the riskiness of the project. If the riskiness of the project is more than or less than the average risk for Bayside, the discount rate will have to be adjusted.)

Using a 10 percent discount rate, the NPV of Bayside's open MRI project is calculated as follows:

0	1	2	3	4	5
($2,500,000)	$510,000	$535,500	$562,275	$590,389	$1,369,908

463,636 ← (year 1)
442,562 ← (year 2)
422,446 ← (year 3)
403,244 ← (year 4)
850,605 ← (year 5)

$ 82,493 = NPV

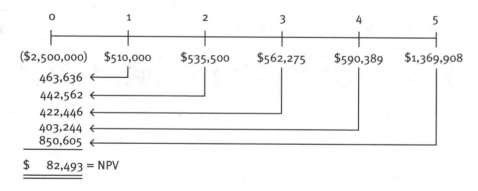

Financial calculators and spreadsheets have NPV formulas that easily perform the mathematics, given the cash flows and opportunity cost of capital (see "Solution Technique: Net Present Value").

The rationale behind the NPV method is straightforward. An NPV of zero signifies that the project's cash inflows are just sufficient to (1) return the capital invested in the project and (2) provide the required rate of return on that capital (meet the opportunity cost of capital). If a project has a positive NPV, it is generating excess cash flows, which are available to management to reinvest in the business and, for investor-owned firms, to pay bonuses (if a proprietorship or partnership) or dividends.

SOLUTION TECHNIQUE
Net Present Value

Financial Calculator

The present value of an uneven cash flow stream can be solved with most financial calculators by using the following steps:

- *Enter the cash flows.* Input the individual cash flows, in chronological order, into the cash flow register, where they usually are designated as CF_0 and CF_j (CF_1, CF_2, CF_3, and so on). For the open MRI project, enter $2,500,000, $510,000, $535,500, $562,275, $590,389, and $1,369,908 in that order into the cash flow register.
- *Enter the discount rate.* In this case, enter I = 10.
- *Push the NPV key.* The answer, $82,493, will appear.

Note that amounts entered into the cash flow register remain there until the register is cleared. Thus, if a problem with eight cash flows had been previously worked, and the new problem with only four cash flows is entered, the calculator assumes that the final four cash flows from the first calculation belong to the second calculation. Be sure to clear the register before starting a new time value analysis.

Spreadsheet

The solution can also be found with a spreadsheet, as the following exhibit shows.

	A	B	C	D
1				
2	10.0%		Project cost of capital	
3	$ (2,500,000)		Cash flow 0	
4	$ 510,000		Cash flow 1	
5	$ 535,500		Cash flow 2	
6	$ 562,275		Cash flow 3	
7	$ 590,389		Cash flow 4	
8	$ 1,369,908		Cash flow 5	
9				
10	$82, 493	=NPV(A2,A4:A8)+A3 (entered into cell A10)		

In this example, we have merely entered the net cash flows into the spreadsheet. In a typical capital investment analysis, the spreadsheet would be used to calculate the net cash flows (chapter 10 discusses cash flow analysis).

The project's NPV is calculated in cell A10 using the NPV formula. The first entry in the formula (A2) is the discount rate (opportunity cost of capital), while the second entry (A4:A8)

(continued)

SOLUTION TECHNIQUE
Net Present Value *(continued)*

designates the range of cash inflows from years 1 through 5. Because the NPV formula calculates NPV one period before the first cash flow entered in the range, it is necessary to start the range with year 1 rather than time 0. Finally, to complete the calculation in cell A10, A3 (the initial outlay) is added to the NPV formula. The result, $82,493, is displayed in cell A10.

If a project has a negative NPV, its cash inflows are insufficient to compensate the organization for the capital invested, or perhaps even insufficient to recover the initial investment. Thus, the project is unprofitable, and its acceptance would cause the financial condition of the firm to deteriorate. For investor-owned businesses, NPV is a direct measure of the contribution of the project to owners' wealth, so NPV is considered by many people to be the best measure of project profitability. While NPV is most often applied to capital investment decisions, the same method can be used to assess the expected financial return on clinical or quality improvement projects (see "For Your Consideration: The Business Case for Quality").

FOR YOUR CONSIDERATION
The Business Case for Quality

Thus far, we have applied capital investment analysis techniques to assess the ROI on the acquisition of fixed assets, such as land, buildings, and equipment. Increasingly, healthcare managers apply this analytic approach to evaluating investment in noncapital opportunities, such as quality improvement initiatives. Because organizations are resource constrained, the absence of a "business case," or financial return on investment, for quality is often cited as a reason healthcare organizations do not implement quality improvement interventions, despite strong evidence that supports their effectiveness.

The principles of capital investment analysis are reflected in the most widely accepted definition of the business case for quality, which states that "a *business case* for a health care improvement intervention exists if the entity that invests in the intervention realizes a financial return on its investment in a reasonable time frame, using a reasonable rate of discounting. This may be realized as 'bankable dollars' (profit), a reduction in losses for a given program or population, or avoided costs. In addition, a *business case* may exist if the investing entity believes that a positive indirect effect on organizational function and sustainability will accrue within a reasonable time frame" (Leatherman et al. 2003).

FOR YOUR CONSIDERATION
The Business Case for Quality *(continued)*

Estimating cash flows (discussed in chapter 10) is an important, yet difficult, step in capital investment analysis. Similarly, estimating the cash flows from quality improvement programs is challenging, as many of these programs generate little to no revenue that can be directly attributed to the initiative. In this case, as the earlier definition suggests, the business case may be largely driven by either identifying indirect financial benefits or identifying the cash flows that occur incidentally to the initiative but cannot be directly traced to the program. For example, improved quality may increase the organization's market share or its ability to recruit and retain clinicians. Once the relevant cash flows from the quality improvement initiative are identified, the business case can be assessed by calculating the ROI, measured by the NPV or IRR.

What is your opinion about the business case for quality? Should quality improvement initiatives be held to the same ROI criterion as traditional capital investment decisions?

Note: The business case definition is based on information in S. Leatherman, D. Berwick, D. Iles, L. S. Lewin, F. Davidoff, T. Nolan, and M. Bisognano, 2003, "The Business Case for Quality: Case Studies and an Analysis," *Health Affairs* 22 (2): 17–30.

The NPV of Bayside's open MRI project is $82,493, so on a present value basis, the project is expected to generate a value of more than $80,000 after all costs, including the opportunity cost of capital, have been considered. Thus, the project is profitable, and its acceptance would have a positive impact on Bayside's financial condition. Note that NPV is, in reality, an expected value, although it typically is not called *expected NPV*. Thus, the actual (realized) profitability of the MRI project may be greater than or less than the (expected) NPV of $82,493, depending on whether the realized cash flows are greater than or less than those expected when the project is analyzed.

CRITICAL CONCEPT
Internal Rate of Return (IRR)

Internal rate of return measures the expected rate (percentage) of return on an investment. Assume that a $100 investment is expected to return $120 after one year. The discount rate that equates the present value of the expected $120 cash inflow to the $100 cost is 20 percent: $120 ÷ 1.20 = $100. Thus, the IRR of this investment is 20 percent. In other words, the $100 investment is expected to earn a 20 percent return: $100 × 1.20 = $120. If the opportunity cost of capital (the return available on alternative investments of similar risk) is 10 percent, this investment is expected to provide a return above those available on comparable alternatives, and hence the investment is financially attractive.

Internal Rate of Return

Like NPV, internal rate of return (IRR) is a DCF ROI measure (see "Critical Concept: Internal Rate of Return [IRR])"). However, whereas NPV measures a project's dollar profitability, IRR measures a project's percentage profitability (i.e., its expected rate of return).

Mathematically, IRR is defined as the discount rate that equates the present value of the project's expected cash inflows to the investment outlay. (In other words, IRR is the discount rate that forces the NPV of the project to be zero.) A financial calculator or a spreadsheet can be used to solve for IRR (see "Solution Technique: Internal Rate of Return").

For Bayside's open MRI project, the rate that causes the sum of the present values of the cash inflows to equal the $2,500,000 cost of the project is about 11.1 percent:

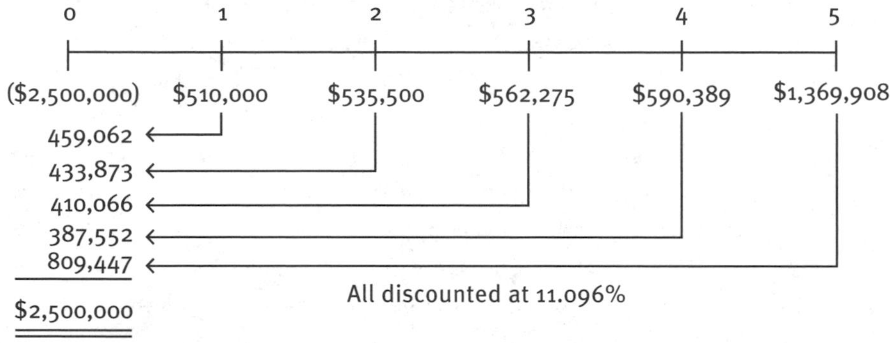

SOLUTION TECHNIQUE
Internal Rate of Return

Financial Calculator

To solve for the IRR using a financial calculator, use the same cash flows that were entered to solve for NPV. Now push the IRR button to obtain the answer: 11.1 percent.

Spreadsheet

To solve for the IRR using a spreadsheet, go to the formulas tab, choose financial as the category, and select the IRR formula. Note that we have placed the IRR formula in cell A10. The first entry in the formula (A3:A8) specifies the range of cash flows to be used in the calculation, while the next entry (A2) gives a starting value for the spreadsheet calculation. The answer, 11.1 percent, is displayed in cell A10.

	A	B	C	D
1				
2	10.0%		Project cost of capital	
3	$ (2,500,000)		Cash flow 0	
4	510,000		Cash flow 1	
5	535,500		Cash flow 2	
6	562,275		Cash flow 3	
7	590,389		Cash flow 4	
8	1,369,908		Cash flow 5	
9				
10	11.1%	= IRR(A3:A8,A2) (entered into cell A10)		

Thus, the MRI project's IRR is 11.1 percent. Put another way, the project is expected to generate an 11.1 percent rate of return on its $2,500,000 investment. The IRR is the rate of return expected on the investment, assuming all the cash flows anticipated actually occur.

If the IRR exceeds the project cost of capital (opportunity cost rate), a surplus is expected to remain after recovering the invested capital and earning its opportunity cost. If the IRR is less than the project cost of capital, however, taking on the project imposes an expected financial cost on the firm's shareholders or stakeholders.

The open MRI project's 11.1 percent IRR exceeds its 10 percent project cost of capital. Thus, as measured by IRR, the MRI project is profitable, and its acceptance would enhance Bayside's financial condition. As in our discussion of NPV, a project's IRR actually represents its expected rate of return. After the project is terminated, the actual (realized) rate of return may be higher than or lower than that expected.

Comparison of the NPV and IRR Methods

Consider a project with a zero NPV. In this situation, the project's IRR must equal its opportunity cost of capital. The project only earns its opportunity cost of capital, so acceptance would neither enhance nor diminish the firm's financial condition. To have a positive NPV, the project's IRR must be greater than its cost of capital, and a negative NPV signifies a project with an IRR that is less than its cost of capital. Thus, projects that are deemed profitable by the NPV method will also be deemed profitable by the IRR method.

In our open MRI analysis, the project would have a positive NPV for all costs of capital less than 11.1 percent. If the cost of capital were greater than 11.1 percent, the project would have a negative NPV. In effect, the NPV and IRR are perfect substitutes for one another in measuring whether a project is profitable. Although NPV and IRR are common, other measures of return on investment also exist (see "For Your Consideration: Accounting Rate of Return").

FOR YOUR CONSIDERATION
Accounting Rate of Return

The accounting rate of return (ARR) uses accounting information to measure the profitability of an investment. Although the calculation can be performed in several ways, the generic formula is

Accounting rate of return = Average net profit ÷ Average investment,

where both profit and investment are measured in accounting (profit and loss statement) terms and averaged over the life of the project.

(continued)

FOR YOUR CONSIDERATION
Accounting Rate of Return *(continued)*

For example, a five-year project that costs $100,000 would have an average annual investment of $100,000 ÷ 5 = $20,000. If the aggregate (total) profit over the five years was forecasted to be $25,000, the average annual net profit would be $5,000. Thus, the project's ARR would be $5,000 ÷ $20,000 = 25%.

Proponents of ARR cite the following advantages: (1) It is simple to use and understand; (2) it can be readily calculated from accounting data, unlike NPV and IRR; and (3) it incorporates the average of the entire stream of income as opposed to looking at individual years. What is your opinion of the ARR? Does it have any weaknesses compared to NPV and IRR? Should healthcare organizations use ARR to make capital investment decisions?

SELF-TEST QUESTIONS

1. What is the difference between return on investment and profitability?
2. Briefly describe how to calculate net present value (NPV) and internal rate of return (IRR).
3. How are NPV and IRR interpreted?
4. Can NPV and IRR lead to different conclusions about a project's financial attractiveness?
5. Evaluate the following statement: "NPV and IRR are expected values."

9.9 PROJECT SCORING

Many other factors, beside financial, must be considered in a complete capital investment analysis. To incorporate multiple factors into the decision, many businesses use a quasi-subjective project scoring approach that attempts to capture both financial and nonfinancial factors (see "Critical Concept: Project Scoring"). Exhibit 9.1, used by Bayside Memorial Hospital, illustrates one such approach.

Bayside ranks projects on three dimensions: stakeholder, operational, and financial. In each dimension, multiple factors are examined and assigned scores that range from two points for very favorable impact to minus one point for negative impact. The scores in each dimension are added to obtain scores for each of the three dimensions, and then the dimension scores are summed to obtain a total score for the project. The total score gives Bayside's managers a feel for the relative values of projects under consideration when all factors, including financial, are taken into account. Exhibit 9.2 contains the scores assigned by Bayside's managers for the open MRI project. By their judgment, the project has a score of 6, which can be compared with scores of other current projects or with the average score of past projects.

Note that the scoring system is completely arbitrary, so the open MRI project with a score of 6, for example, is not necessarily twice as good as a project with a score of 3 or half as good as a

CRITICAL CONCEPT
Project Scoring

Project scoring is a technique for incorporating both financial and nonfinancial factors in capital investment decisions. The various factors, such as IRR (a financial factor) and impact on patients (a nonfinancial factor), are graded on a numerical scale. These grades are then added, and the total score reflects the overall attractiveness of the project. The higher the score, the more attractive the project, considering both financial and nonfinancial factors.

Exhibit 9.1
Bayside Memorial Hospital: Project Scoring Exhibit

	Relative Score			
Criteria	**2**	**1**	**0**	**−1**
Stakeholder Factors				
Physicians	Strongly supports	Supports	Neutral	Opposed
Employees	Greatly helps morale	Helps morale	No effect	Hurts morale
Visitors	Greatly enhances visit	Enhances visit	No effect	Hurts image
Patients	High	Moderate	None	Negative
Operational Factors				
Outcomes	Greatly improves	Improves	No effect	Hurts outcomes
Length of stay	Documented decrease	Anecdotal decrease	No effect	Increase
Technology	Breakthrough	Improves current	Adds to current	Lowers
Productivity	Large decrease in FTEs*	Decrease in FTEs	No change in FTEs	Adds FTEs
Financial Factors				
Payback	Less than 2 years	2–4 years	4–6 years	Over 6 years
IRR	Over 20%	15–20%	10–15%	Less than 10%
Stakeholder factor score	___			
Operational factor score	___			
Financial factor score	___			
Total score	═══			

*Full-time equivalent

EXHIBIT 9.2
Bayside Memorial Hospital: Project Score for the Open MRI

Stakeholder Factors	
Physicians	2
Employees	0
Visitors	0
Patients	2
Total stakeholder	4
Operational Factors	
Outcomes	1
Length of stay	0
Technology	1
Productivity	0
Total operational	2
Financial Factors	
Payback	0
IRR	0
Total financial	0
Total score	6

project with a score of 12. Nevertheless, Bayside's project scoring system forces its managers to address multiple issues when making capital investment decisions, and the system does provide a relative ranking of projects under consideration.

SELF-TEST QUESTION

1. Describe the concept and use of a project scoring system.

9.10 THE POSTAUDIT

Capital budgeting is not a static process. If a long lag occurs between a project's acceptance and its implementation, any new information concerning either capital costs or the project's cash flows should be analyzed before the final start-up occurs. Furthermore, the performance of each project should be monitored throughout the project's life.

The process of formally monitoring project performance over time is called the **postaudit**. It involves comparing actual results with those projected; explaining why differences occur; and analyzing potential changes to the project's operations, including replacement or termination.

Postaudit
The feedback process in which the performance of projects previously accepted is reviewed and necessary changes are made.

The postaudit serves several purposes, including the following:

- *Improve forecasts.* When managers systematically compare forecasts to actual outcomes, estimates tend to improve. Conscious or unconscious biases that occur can be identified and, one hopes, eliminated; new forecasting methods are sought as the need for them becomes apparent; and managers tend to do everything better, including forecasting, if they know that their actions are being monitored.
- *Develop historical risk data.* Postaudits permit managers to develop historical risk and expected-rates-of-return data on new project proposals. These data can then be used to make judgments about the relative risk and profitability of future projects as they are evaluated.
- *Improve operations.* Managers run organizations, and they can perform at higher or lower levels of efficiency. When a forecast is made, for example, by the surgery department, the department director and medical staff are, in a sense, putting their reputations on the line. If costs are above predicted levels and volume is below expectations, the managers involved will strive, within ethical bounds, to improve the situation and to bring results into line with forecasts. As one hospital CEO put it: "You academics worry only about making good decisions. In the healthcare industry, we also have to worry about making decisions good."
- *Reduce losses.* Postaudits monitor the performance of projects over time, so the first indication that termination or replacement should be considered often arises when the postaudit indicates that a project is performing poorly.

? Self-Test Questions

1. What is a postaudit?
2. Why are postaudits important to the financial effectiveness of a business?

Theme Wrap-Up: Evaluating a Project's Financial Merit

Bayside's managers began their capital investment analysis of the proposed open MRI project by performing three steps.

First, they laid out the net cash flows expected from the project, which include both costs and revenues, on a time line. This step enabled them to see the amounts and timing of the flows expected if the open MRI is purchased. Then, they used those cash flows to estimate the payback, 4.2 years, which is the expected time required to recover the initial $2.5 million investment.

Second, they applied DCF analysis, which accounts for the time value of money, to assess the profitability, or ROI, of the proposal. To perform ROI analyses, it is necessary to apply an opportunity cost of capital—the return that could be earned on alternative investments of similar risk to the project being analyzed. Bayside's managers used the corporate cost of capital, 10 percent, as the opportunity cost of capital in their initial analysis.

The ROI analysis determined that the NPV of the project was $82,493 and the IRR was 11.1 percent. NPV measures dollar profitability, and the positive amount signifies that the project is expected to add financial value to the hospital. IRR measures the expected rate of return on the project, and because the 11.1 percent IRR was greater than the 10 percent opportunity cost of capital, IRR confirmed that the project was financially attractive.

Third, Bayside's managers used a project scoring system to incorporate nonfinancial factors into the decision process.

At this point, the open MRI proposal appears financially attractive. However, the analysis is not yet complete. In chapter 10, we find out how Bayside's managers estimated the project's net cash flows and, more important, how they assessed the project's riskiness. If the open MRI project turns out to have either more or less risk than Bayside's average project, the ROI analysis has to be revised, which could change the conclusions about the project's financial attractiveness.

Key Concepts

This chapter covers the basics of capital investment analysis. Here are the key concepts:

- *Capital investment analysis* involves analyzing potential expenditures on land, buildings, and equipment and deciding whether the organization should undertake those investments.
- A capital investment analysis consists of four steps: (1) Estimate the expected cash flows, (2) assess the riskiness of those flows, (3) estimate the appropriate opportunity cost of capital, and (4) determine the project's profitability and breakeven characteristics.
- *Time breakeven*, which is measured by *payback*, provides managers with insights into a project's liquidity and risk.

- *Discounted cash flow analysis* uses time value of money techniques to estimate the value of an investment's expected cash flows.
- *Compounding* is the process of determining the future value of a current cash flow or series of flows.
- *Discounting* is the process of finding the present value of a future cash flow or series of flows.
- Project profitability is assessed by *return on investment (ROI)* measures. The two most commonly used ROI measures are net present value and internal rate of return.
- *Net present value (NPV)*, which is simply the sum of the present values of all the project's cash flows when discounted at the project's opportunity cost of capital, measures a project's expected dollar profitability. An NPV greater than zero indicates that the project is expected to be profitable after all costs, including the opportunity cost of capital, have been considered. Furthermore, the higher the NPV, the more profitable the project.
- *Internal rate of return (IRR)*, which is the discount rate that forces a project's NPV to equal zero, measures a project's expected rate of return. If a project's IRR is greater than its opportunity cost of capital, the project is expected to be profitable, and the higher the IRR, the more profitable the project.
- Firms often use *project scoring* to incorporate a large number of factors subjectively, including financial and nonfinancial elements, into the capital investment decision process.
- The *postaudit* is a key element in capital budgeting. By comparing actual results with predicted results, managers can improve both operations and the cash flow estimation process.

Our discussion of capital investment decisions continues in chapter 10, which focuses on cash flow estimation and risk assessment.

End-of-Chapter Questions

9.1 a. What is capital investment analysis? Why are capital investment decisions so important to businesses?

b. What is the purpose of placing capital investments in categories, such as mandatory replacement or expansion of existing products, services, or markets?

c. Should financial analysis play the dominant role in capital investment decisions? Explain your answer.

d. What are the four steps of capital investment financial analysis?

9.2 a. What is the opportunity cost of capital?
b. How is this rate used in discounted cash flow (DCF) analysis?
c. Is this rate a single number that is used in all situations?

9.3 Describe the following project breakeven and profitability measures. Be sure to include each measure's economic interpretation.
a. Payback
b. Net present value (NPV)
c. Internal rate of return (IRR)

9.4 Describe a project scoring system.

9.5 What is a postaudit? Why is the postaudit critical to good investment decision-making?

End-of-Chapter Problems

9.1 Find the following values for a single cash flow:
a. The future value of $500 invested at 8 percent for one year
b. The future value of $500 invested at 8 percent for five years
c. The present value of $500 to be received in one year when the opportunity cost rate is 8 percent
d. The present value of $500 to be received in five years when the opportunity cost rate is 8 percent

9.2 Consider the following net cash flows:

Year	Cash Flow ($)
0	0
1	250
2	400
3	500
4	600
5	600

a. What is the net present value if the opportunity cost of capital (discount rate) is 10 percent?
b. Add an outflow (or cost) of $1,000 at time 0. Now, what is the net present value?

9.3 Consider another set of net cash flows:

Year	Cash Flow ($)
0	2,000
1	2,000
2	0
3	1,500
4	2,500
5	4,000

a. What is the net present value of the stream if the opportunity cost of capital is 10 percent?
b. What is the value of the stream at the end of year 5 if the cash flows are invested in an account that pays 10 percent annually?
c. What cash flow today (time 0), in lieu of the $2,000 cash flow, would be needed to accumulate $20,000 at the end of year 5? (Assume that the cash flows for years 1 through 5 remain the same.)

9.4 Better Health Inc. is evaluating two capital investments, each of which requires an up-front (time 0) expenditure of $1.5 million. The projects are expected to produce the following net cash inflows:

Year	Project A ($)	Project B ($)
1	500,000	2,000,000
2	1,000,000	1,000,000
3	2,000,000	600,000

a. What is each project's IRR?
b. What is each project's NPV if the opportunity cost of capital is 10 percent? 5 percent? 15 percent?

9.5 Capital Healthplans Inc. is evaluating two different methods for providing home health services to its members. Both methods involve contracting out for services, and the health outcomes and revenues are not affected by the method chosen. Therefore, the net cash flows for the decision are all outflows. Here are the projected flows:

Year	Method A ($)	Method B ($)
0	(300,000)	(120,000)
1	(66,000)	(96,000)
2	(66,000)	(96,000)
3	(66,000)	(96,000)
4	(66,000)	(96,000)
5	(66,000)	(96,000)

a. What is each alternative's IRR?

b. If the opportunity cost of capital for both methods is 9 percent, which method should be chosen? Why?

9.6 Assume that you are the chief financial officer at Porter Memorial Hospital. The CEO has asked you to analyze two proposed capital investments—project X and project Y. Each project requires a net investment outlay of $10,000, and the opportunity cost of capital for each project is 12 percent. The projects' expected net cash flows are as follows:

Year	Project X ($)	Project Y ($)
0	(10,000)	(10,000)
1	6,500	3,000
2	3,000	3,000
3	3,000	3,000
4	1,000	3,000

a. Calculate each project's payback, NPV, and IRR.

b. Which project (or projects) is financially acceptable? Explain your answer.

9.7 The director of capital budgeting for Big River Health Systems Inc. has estimated the following cash flows (in thousands of dollars) for a proposed new service:

Year	Expected Net Cash Flow ($)
0	(100)
1	70
2	50
3	20

The project's opportunity cost of capital is 10 percent.

a. What is the project's payback period?

b. What is the project's NPV?

c. What is the project's IRR?

CHAPTER 10

PROJECT CASH FLOW ESTIMATION AND RISK ANALYSIS

THEME SET-UP: ESTIMATING A PROJECT'S CASH FLOWS AND ASSESSING RISK

In chapter 9, we explored the financial implications of Bayside Memorial Hospital's potential purchase of an open MRI (magnetic resonance imaging) system. The new MRI system greatly reduces the feeling of constraint associated with conventional MRI technology and produces high-quality images. In addition, the open MRI system can accommodate pediatric patients who need parental support and patients who are too large to fit in a conventional MRI machine.

Bayside's initial analysis used various techniques to assess the payback and profitability of the project. However, in their discounted cash flow (DCF) analysis, Bayside's managers assumed that the project had average risk, so they used the corporate cost of capital, 10 percent, as the opportunity cost of capital. The results so far indicate a payback of 4.2 years, a net present value (NPV) of $82,493, and an internal rate of return (IRR) of 11.1 percent. In addition, Bayside's managers used a project scoring system to incorporate nonfinancial factors into the decision process. At this point, the open MRI project seems attractive. However, the managers have not finished their analysis.

Now, they must assess the project's riskiness. If the proposal is found to have either more or less risk than Bayside's average project, the managers will have to modify the financial analysis. In addition, Dr. Fisher, the radiology group CEO who proposed the project, was not sure of the process that Bayside's managers used to estimate the project's net cash flows. Thus, he asked the managers to explain how the cash flows were developed.

By the end of the chapter, you will learn how project cash flows are estimated. Furthermore, you will understand what investment risk is, how it is assessed, and what impact it has on capital investment decisions.

Learning Objectives

After studying this chapter, you will be able to do the following:

- Define the key elements of cash flow estimation.
- Conduct a basic project cash flow analysis.
- Explain the concept of investment risk.
- Discuss the techniques used in project risk assessment.
- Conduct a project risk assessment.
- Incorporate risk into the capital investment decision process.

10.1 INTRODUCTION

Chapter 9 covers the basics of capital investment decisions, including discounted cash flow analysis, breakeven analysis, and return on investment (profitability) measures. This chapter extends this discussion to include cash flow estimation and risk analysis.

Both cash flow estimation and risk analysis are critical to good capital investment decisions. If the cash flow estimates are wrong, the entire financial analysis is of little, or no, value. Furthermore, if risk is ignored, the financial analysis could lead to improper capital investment decisions.

10.2 CASH FLOW ESTIMATION

The most difficult, yet most important, step in evaluating capital investment proposals is cash flow estimation. This step involves estimating the investment outlays, annual net operating flows, and cash flows associated with project termination. Many separate (component) cash flows are involved, and many individuals typically participate in the process.

Often, historical data can be used to help make the cash flow estimates. However, for projects that involve new services, scant data are available. Thus, often, forecasts are not much better than rough estimates. Making accurate forecasts of the costs and revenues associated with many projects is difficult, so forecast errors can be quite large (see "For Your Consideration: Cash Flow Estimation Bias"). For this reason, risk analyses must be performed on prospective projects.

FOR YOUR CONSIDERATION
Cash Flow Estimation Bias

As you know, cash flow estimation is the most critical and most difficult part of the capital investment analysis process. Cash flows often must be forecasted many years into the future, and estimation errors (some of which can be large) are bound to occur. However, as long as cash flow estimates are unbiased and the errors are random, they will tend to offset one another from project to project and, when many projects are considered, realized aggregate profitability will be close to that expected.

However, some managers tend to overstate revenues and understate costs on most projects, which results in an upward bias in estimated profitability. If this occurs, more projects will be accepted than would be if no bias existed. Several potential reasons may explain cash flow estimation bias. Perhaps managers have an incentive to maximize department size rather than profitability. Perhaps managers may become emotionally attached to their project proposals and are unable to make objective estimates.

Do you think that cash flow estimation bias exists in health services organizations? If so, why might that be the case? What steps could senior management take to eliminate the bias?

> **CRITICAL CONCEPT**
> Incremental Cash Flow
>
> Incremental cash flows are flows that are properly included in a capital investment analysis. The term *incremental* means that the flows arise solely because of project acceptance—if the project is accepted, and only if the project is accepted, these cash flows will result. The term *cash flow* means that these are the amounts of cash that actually flow into or out of the business. Some flows might appear to be incremental flows, but if they occur whether or not the project is undertaken, they are nonincremental to the decision and hence should not be included in the analysis. Conversely, flows that might not be directly related to the project may still be incremental. One example is the loss of revenues on an existing project that results if a new, but similar, project is undertaken.

Neither the difficulty nor the importance of cash flow estimation can be overstated. However, the following guiding principles can help healthcare managers eliminate most of the common errors that arise.

Focus on Incremental Cash Flows

The relevant cash flows to consider when evaluating a new capital investment are the project's incremental cash flows, which are formally defined as the firm's cash flows in each period if the project is undertaken, minus the firm's cash flows in each period if the project is not undertaken (see "Critical Concept: Incremental Cash Flow"). In capital investment decisions, the decision must be based on the actual dollars that flow into and out of the business rather than on revenues and expenses defined by accountants for other purposes. After all, it is cash flow that creates value. The focus on cash flow actually makes the estimation process easier, because applying a set of sometimes complicated accounting rules is not necessary when analyzing capital investments.

In theory, project cash flows should be analyzed exactly as they are expected to occur. Of course, there must be a compromise between accuracy and simplicity. A time line with daily cash flows would, in theory, provide the most accuracy, but daily cash flow estimates would be costly to construct, unwieldy to use, and probably no more accurate than annual cash flow estimates. Thus, in most situations, analysts simply assume that all cash flows occur at the end of each year, so the typical time line for a capital investment analysis uses years as periods.

Estimating Project Life

Perhaps the first decision that must be made in forecasting a project's cash flows is the life of the project. Does the cash flow forecast need to be for 20 years, or is 5 years sufficient? Many projects, such as a new hospital wing or an ambulatory surgery center, have long, productive lives. In theory, the cash flow forecast should extend for the full life of the project, yet most managers would have little confidence in estimates for cash flows beyond the near term.

Thus, healthcare organizations often set an arbitrary limit on project life—say, five or ten years. If the forecasted life is less than the arbitrary limit, the forecasted life is used to develop the cash flows. If the forecasted life exceeds the limit, project life is truncated and the cash flows beyond the limit do not appear on the time line.

If truncation occurs, it is important to recognize that some of the project's value is being ignored, because the cash flows omitted from the analysis typically consist of inflows. The recognition of lost value can be quantitative (by assigning a **terminal value** to the project) or qualitative (by merely noting that the NPV of the project understates its true value).

Conversely, many projects have short lives, and hence the analysis will extend over the project's entire life. In such situations, the assets associated with the project may still have some value remaining when the project is terminated. The cash flow expected to be realized from selling the project's assets at termination is called **salvage value**. Even if a project is being terminated for old age, any cash flows that will arise by virtue of scrap value must be included in the analysis. Note that the net cash flow at termination can be negative if the cost of dismantling the project is greater than the market value of the assets to be sold.

Terminal value
The cash flow assigned to the last year on the time line of a long-life project to account for the value lost because the cash flows were truncated.

Salvage value
The estimated value of an asset at the end of its useful life.

Ignore Sunk Costs

A **sunk cost** is an outlay that has already occurred or has been irrevocably committed, so it is unaffected by the current decision to accept or reject a project. To illustrate, suppose that in 2020, Gold Coast Surgery Center is evaluating the purchase of a robotic surgery system. To help in the decision, in 2019 the center hired and paid $10,000 to a consultant to conduct a feasibility study.

This cash flow is *not* relevant and hence nonincremental to the capital investment decision—it is not contingent on the equipment purchase; it has already occurred. Sometimes a project will appear to be unprofitable when all of its associated costs, including sunk costs, are considered. However, on an incremental basis, the project may be profitable and managers should undertake it. Thus, the correct treatment of sunk costs can be critical to the decision.

Sunk cost
A cost that has already occurred or is irrevocably committed. Sunk costs are nonincremental to capital investment analyses and hence should not be included.

Include Opportunity Costs

All relevant **opportunity costs** must be included in a capital investment analysis. To illustrate, one opportunity cost involves the use of the capital required to finance the project. If a business uses its money to invest in project A, it cannot use the capital to invest in project B, or for any other purpose.

The opportunity cost associated with the use of capital is accounted for in the discount rate, which represents the return that the business could earn by investing the funds in alternative investments of similar risk (the opportunity cost of capital). Thus, the discounting process used to calculate NPV forces the opportunity cost of capital to be considered in the analysis. (Similarly, the opportunity cost of capital is considered when a project's IRR is compared to its cost of capital.)

Opportunity cost
The cost associated with alternative uses of the same asset. For example, if land is used for one project, it is no longer available for other uses, and hence an opportunity cost arises.

In addition to the opportunity cost of capital, other types of opportunity costs arise in capital investment analyses. For example, assume that Gold Coast's robotic surgery system would be installed in a separate freestanding facility and that Gold Coast currently owns the land on which the facility would be built.

When analyzing this project, the value of the land cannot be disregarded merely because no cash outlay is required. An opportunity cost is inherent in the use of the land because using it for the robotic surgery facility deprives Gold Coast of its use for other purposes. The property might be used for conventional surgical suites or a parking garage rather than sold. However, the best measure of the land's value, and hence the opportunity cost inherent in its use, is the cash flow that could be realized from selling the property.

Gold Coast purchased the land ten years ago at a cost of $50,000, but the current market value of the property is $130,000, after subtracting all legal and real estate costs, taxes, and other fees required to sell the land. Thus, the robotic surgery system project should have a $130,000 opportunity cost charged against it. After all, if not used for the project, the land could be sold, resulting in a $130,000 net cash inflow to the center.

Include Impact on Existing Business Lines

Capital investment analyses must consider the effects of the project under consideration on the organization's existing business lines. Such effects can be either positive or negative. To illustrate a negative effect, assume that some of the patients who are expected to undergo robotic surgery would have been treated by conventional surgery at the center, so these conventional revenues will be lost if the robotic facility goes into operation. Thus, the incremental cash flows to Gold Coast are the flows attributable to the robotic surgery facility, minus those flows lost from forgone conventional surgery services. Note that the forgone cash flows include not only revenues but also the costs inherent in providing these conventional surgery services. In essence, the forgone revenue and cost flows, when combined, represent the profits lost from conventional surgery services.

On the other hand, new patients that come to Gold Coast because of the new robotic surgery capability may use other services provided by the center. In this situation, the incremental cash flows generated by these patients' use of other services should be credited to the robotic project. If possible, both positive and negative effects on other projects should be quantified, but at a minimum they should be noted so that these effects are subjectively considered when the final decision regarding the project is made.

Include Inflation Effects

Because inflation can have a considerable influence on a project's profitability, it must be considered in all capital investment analyses. As we discuss in chapter 8, a business's corporate cost of capital is a weighted average of its costs of debt and equity. These costs are estimated on the basis of investors' required rates of return, and investors incorporate an inflation premium into such estimates.

For example, a lender might require a 3 percent return on a ten-year loan in the absence of inflation. However, if inflation is expected to average 4 percent over the coming ten years, the investor would require a 7 percent return. Thus, investors add an inflation premium to their required rates of return to help protect against the loss of purchasing power that stems from inflation.

Because inflation effects are already embedded in the corporate cost of capital, and because this cost will be used to set the opportunity cost (discount) rate used in the analysis, inflation effects must also be built into the project's cash flow estimates. If the cash flow estimates do not include inflation effects, but a discount rate is used that does include inflation, the profitability of the project will be understated (the NPV will be too low).

The best way to deal with inflation is to apply inflation effects to each component cash flow using the best available information about how each component will be affected. For example, labor costs would be increased by the wage inflation rate, inventory costs would be adjusted by the supplies inflation rate, revenues would be adjusted by price (reimbursement rate) inflation, and so on. Because it is impossible to estimate future inflation rates with much precision, errors are bound to occur.

Sometimes inflation is assumed to be neutral—that is, it is assumed to affect all revenue and cost components equally. However, this assumption has little merit—in most years it is unlikely that both revenues and costs would inflate at the same rate. Inflation adds to the uncertainty, and hence risk, of a project under consideration as well as to the complexity of a capital investment cash flow estimation.

Include Any Strategic Value

Sometimes a project will have value, called **strategic value**, that stems from future investment opportunities that can be undertaken only if the project currently under consideration is accepted. Typically, such value is not captured by a project's cash flow estimates. To illustrate, consider University Hospital's decision to start a kidney transplant program. The financial analysis of this project showed the program to be unprofitable, but the hospital's managers considered kidney transplants to be the first step in an aggressive program that would include liver, heart, and lung transplants. Not only would the entire transplant program be profitable, but it would also enhance the hospital's reputation for technological and clinical excellence and hence increase the hospital's ability to attract new patients.

> ***Strategic value***
> The value inherent in a capital investment that is not captured in its cash flow estimates. For example, a project may provide a foot in the door in a new service area that could lead to other profitable investments.

In theory, the best approach to dealing with strategic value is to forecast the cash flows from the follow-on projects, estimate their probabilities of occurrence, and then add the expected cash flows from the follow-on projects to the cash flows of the project under consideration.

In practice, this ideal is usually impossible to achieve, because either the follow-on cash flows are too nebulous to forecast or the potential follow-on projects are too numerous to quantify. At a minimum, decision makers must recognize that some projects have strategic value, and this value should be qualitatively considered when making capital investment decisions.

? Self-Test Questions

1. Briefly discuss the following concepts associated with cash flow estimation:
   - Incremental cash flow
   - Project life
   - Cash flow timing
   - Terminal value
   - Salvage value
   - Sunk costs
   - Opportunity costs
   - Effects on current projects
   - Inflation effects
   - Strategic value
2. Evaluate the following statement: "Ignoring inflation effects and strategic value can result in overstating a project's financial attractiveness."

10.3 ESTIMATING THE CASH FLOWS FOR BAYSIDE'S OPEN MRI PROJECT

In the previous chapter, we used the net cash flows for the open MRI project to illustrate several measures of project financial attractiveness. However, we did not include the details of how the net cash flows were estimated. In this section, we discuss the specifics of the cash flow estimation process. Along the way, we review some of the concepts discussed in the previous section and introduce several others that are important to good cash flow estimation.

The Basic Data

Managers at Bayside Memorial Hospital, in collaboration with physicians from the radiology group, developed the required component cash flows (basic input data). The system costs $2 million, and the hospital would have to spend another $500,000 for site preparation, delivery, and installation. Because the system would be installed in the hospital, the space to be used has a very low, or zero, market value to outsiders. Furthermore, its value to Bayside for alternative uses is very difficult to estimate, so no opportunity cost was assigned to account for the value of the site.

Bayside's managers developed the project's forecasted revenues by conducting the analysis contained in exhibit 10.1. The estimated average charge per scan is $1,000, but

Exhibit 10.1
Bayside Memorial Hospital: Open MRI System Revenue Analysis

Payer	Number of Scans per Week	Charge per Scan	Total Charges	Basis of Payment	Net Payment per Scan	Total Payments
Medicare	5	$1,000	$ 5,000	Fixed fee	$740	$ 3,700
Medicaid	2	1,000	2,000	Fixed fee	700	1,400
Private insurance	5	1,000	5,000	Full charge	1,000	5,000
Blue Cross	2	1,000	2,000	Percent of charge	840	1,680
Managed care	4	1,000	4,000	Percent of charge	750	3,000
Self-pay	2	1,000	2,000	Full charge	110	220
Total	20		$20,000			$15,000
Average			$ 1,000			$ 750

25 percent of this amount is expected to be lost on discounts to payers, charity care, and bad debt losses. Thus, the actual reimbursement expected, on average, is $750 per scan.

The open MRI system is estimated to have a weekly utilization (volume) of 20 scans, and each scan will cost the hospital $30 in supplies. The system is expected to operate 50 weeks a year, with the remaining two weeks devoted to maintenance. The MRI system would require 1.5 full-time equivalent technicians, resulting in an incremental increase in annual labor costs of $60,000, including fringe benefits.

No increase in overhead costs is associated with the new open MRI. (Additional existing overhead may be allocated to the new system, but such a reallocation is not an incremental cash flow—that is, it is not a new cash cost to Bayside.) The open MRI would require maintenance, which would be furnished by the manufacturer for an annual fee of $150,000, payable at the end of each year of operation.

The MRI system is expected to be in operation for five years, at which time the hospital's master plan calls for a new imaging facility. The hospital plans to sell the MRI at that time for an estimated $750,000 salvage value, net of removal costs. The inflation rate is estimated to average 5 percent over the period, and this rate is expected to affect all revenues and costs equally.

Cash Flow Analysis

The next step in the analysis is to convert the basic cash flow data into the project's net cash flows. This analysis is presented in exhibit 10.2. Here are the key points of the analysis by line number:

- *Line 1.* Line 1 contains the estimated cost (price) of the open MRI system—$2,000,000. In general, capital investment analyses assume that the first cash flow, normally an outflow, occurs at time 0, the starting point of the analysis. Note that cash outflows are shown in parentheses.
- *Line 2.* The related site-preparation expense, including shipping and installation costs—$500,000—is also assumed to occur at time 0.
- *Line 3.* Line 3 adds the two initial cost components to obtain the project's total cost—$2,500,000.
- *Line 4.* Annual net revenues = Weekly volume × Weeks of operation per year × Average reimbursement per scan = 20 × 50 × $750 = $750,000 in year 1. The 5 percent inflation rate is applied to all revenues and costs that would likely be affected by inflation, so the net revenue amounts shown on line 4 increase by 5 percent over time.
- *Line 5.* Labor costs are forecasted to be $60,000 during the first year, and these costs are assumed to increase over time at the 5 percent inflation rate. Although most of the operating revenues and costs would occur more or less evenly over the year, it is difficult to forecast exactly when the flows would occur. Furthermore, the potential for large errors in cash flow estimation is significant. For these reasons, operating cash flows are assumed to occur at the end of each year. Also, the assumption is that the open MRI system could be placed in operation quickly. If this were not the case, then year 1's operating flows would be reduced. In some situations, it might take several years from the first cash outflow to the point when the project is operational and begins to generate net revenues and hence cash inflows.
- *Line 6.* Maintenance fees—$150,000 for year 1—must be paid to the manufacturer at the end of each year of operation. These fees are assumed to increase at the 5 percent inflation rate.
- *Line 7.* Each scan uses $30 of supplies, so supply costs in year 1 total 20 × 50 × $30 = $30,000, and they are expected to increase each year by the inflation rate.
- *Line 8.* Line 8 shows the project's net operating income in each year, which is merely net revenues minus all operating expenses. For year 1, the value is $510,000.
- *Line 9.* The project is expected to be terminated after five years, at which time the MRI system would be sold for an estimated $750,000, net of removal and other project shutdown costs. This salvage value cash flow is shown as an inflow at the end of year 5.

EXHIBIT 10.2
Bayside Memorial Hospital: Open MRI System Cash Flow Analysis

	Cash Revenues and Costs					
	Time 0	Year 1	Year 2	Year 3	Year 4	Year 5
1. System cost	($2,000,000)					
2. Installation expenses	(500,000)					
3. Total cost	($2,500,000)					
4. Net revenues		$750,000	$787,500	$826,875	$868,219	$ 911,630
5. Labor costs		(60,000)	(63,000)	(66,150)	(69,457)	(72,930)
6. Maintenance cost		(150,000)	(157,500)	(165,375)	(173,644)	(182,326)
7. Supplies		(30,000)	(31,500)	(33,075)	(34,729)	(36,465)
8. Net operating income		$510,000	$535,500	$562,275	$590,389	$ 619,908
9. Salvage value						750,000
10. Net cash flow	($2,500,000)	$510,000	$535,500	$562,275	$590,389	$1,369,908

Profitability measures (from chapter 9):
Net present value = $82,493.
Internal rate of return = 11.1%.

Note: Some rounding occurs in this exhibit.

- *Line 10.* The project's net cash flows are shown on line 10. The project requires a $2,500,000 investment at time 0 but then generates cash inflows over its five-year operating life.

The bottom of the exhibit contains the results of the profitability (return on investment [ROI]) analysis performed in chapter 9. In chapter 9, we estimated the project's NPV to be $82,493, when the opportunity cost of capital was assumed to be Bayside's corporate cost of capital, 10 percent. In addition, the project's IRR was found to be 11.1 percent.

Note that the cash flows in exhibit 10.2 do not include any allowance for interest expense on any debt capital used to acquire the MRI system. On average, Bayside will finance new projects in accordance with its target capital structure, which consists of 35 percent debt financing and 65 percent equity financing. The costs associated with this financing mix, including both interest costs and the cost of equity capital, are incorporated into the firm's 10 percent corporate cost of capital. Because the cost of debt financing is included in the discount rate that is applied to the net cash flows to obtain ROI, recognition of interest expense in the cash flows would be double counting.

If the project were being analyzed by a for-profit provider, some adjustments would have to be made to the cash flows to account for tax effects. Although these adjustments are not complicated, a thorough discussion at this point is not warranted.

Finally, note that this project is a replacement project in the sense that the open MRI system will be replacing the current conventional MRI system. Replacement projects typically have a somewhat more complicated cash flow structure than do entirely new projects. For example, the current revenues and costs are lost to the business. In addition, the old MRI could be sold if it is replaced.

Bayside's managers believed that these cash flows were either not material or not relevant to the analysis because (1) the current system is leased and hence will merely be returned to the owner, and (2) a competing outpatient imaging center may soon have its own open MRI system, so Bayside patients seeking an open system would be lost whether or not the hospital buys one. Thus, the cash flows were treated as if the project were a new, as opposed to a replacement, project.

? SELF-TEST QUESTIONS

1. Briefly, how is a project cash flow analysis constructed?
2. What are the key differences in cash flow analyses performed by investor-owned and not-for-profit businesses?
3. What is the difference between a new and a replacement project?

10.4 RISK ANALYSIS

The higher the risk associated with any investment, the higher its required rate of return. Thus, the ultimate goal in project risk analysis is to ensure that the opportunity cost of capital used as the discount rate in a project's ROI analysis properly reflects the riskiness of that project.

Generically, *risk* is defined as "a hazard; a peril; exposure to loss or injury." Thus, risk refers to the chance that an unfavorable event will occur. If a person engages in skydiving, she is taking a chance with injury or death; skydiving is risky. If a person gambles at roulette, he is not risking injury or death but is taking a financial risk. Even when a person invests in stocks or bonds, she is taking a risk in the hope of earning a positive rate of return. Similarly, when Bayside invests in new assets, such as an open MRI system, it is taking a financial risk.

Risk-free investment
An investment that has a guaranteed (sure) return. In other words, the probability of earning the return expected is 100 percent.

To illustrate financial risk, consider two potential personal investments. The first investment consists of a one-year, $1,000 investment in a bank certificate of deposit (CD). The interest rate on the CD is 5.0 percent, so the expected interest earned at the end of one year is $1,000 × 0.050 = $50. The return on the CD is fixed by contract and, furthermore, is insured by a governmental agency. Thus, there is virtually a 100 percent probability that the investment will actually earn the 5.0 percent rate of return that is expected. In this situation, the investment is described as a **risk-free investment**.

Now, assume that the $1,000 is invested in a biotechnology partnership that will be terminated in one year. If the partnership develops a new commercially valuable product, its rights will be sold for $2,000, producing a rate of return of 100 percent. But if nothing worthwhile is developed, the partnership will be worthless and no money will be received. The investor may expect to earn $2,000 from the partnership, but she also faces the chance of losing the entire $1,000 investment. Because there is some possibility of earning a return that is far less than expected, the partnership investment is described as risky.

Thus, financial risk is related to the probability of earning a return less than expected. The greater the chance of earning a return far below that expected, the greater the amount of financial risk.

Now we will apply the concept of financial risk to Bayside's open MRI system project (see "Critical Concept: Financial Risk"). Exhibit 10.2 contains the project's cash flow analysis. If all of the project's component cash flows (e.g., reimbursement rates, volume, operating costs) were known with certainty, the project's projected profitability would be known with certainty, and hence the project would be risk free.

However, in virtually all project analyses, future cash flows, and hence profitability, are uncertain, and in many cases highly uncertain, so risk is present. For example, forecasting patient volume for the open MRI system is not easy. If the forecasts are too high, and hence the actual (realized) volume is lower than that assumed in exhibit 10.1, then the realized NPV of the project would be less than the forecasted $82,493.

The nature of the component cash flow distributions and their correlations with one another determine the nature of the project's profitability distribution and hence the project's risk. In the following sections, two quantitative techniques for assessing project risk are discussed: sensitivity analysis and scenario analysis. Then, we explore a qualitative approach to risk assessment.

CRITICAL CONCEPT
Financial Risk

Capital investments are risky because a project's cash flows are not known with certainty when the project is being analyzed. For example, the estimate for the number of scans conducted by Bayside's new open MRI is based on historical volumes for the old system plus estimates of new volume created by the easier-to-use new system. If purchased and put into operation, the actual (realized) number of scans will likely be higher or lower than the initial estimate. The same reasoning applies to the average net reimbursement estimate, labor cost estimate, and the like. The bottom line is that the net cash flows in exhibit 10.2 are merely estimates of what is expected to happen financially rather than a sure bet. Because of the uncertainty in the cash flow forecasts, the $82,493 NPV (as well as the IRR) is also uncertain. After the project is terminated, and hence looking back on realized results, the actual NPV of the project could be much less than expected. In fact, the project could end up being a big loser. It is this fact that makes projects risky.

CRITICAL CONCEPT
Sensitivity Analysis

Sensitivity analysis is the process of assessing how changes in one variable affect another variable. In capital investment decisions, sensitivity analysis is used to determine how much a project's profitability—say, as measured by NPV—is affected when the value of an input cash flow component, such as volume, changes. Many of the component cash flow estimates are uncertain, so the realized values for these flows may be quite different from those used in the initial analysis. The greater the sensitivity of the project's profitability to changes in the component cash flow estimates, the greater the likelihood that the project's actual profitability will be far less than expected. Sensitivity analysis is most useful in identifying cash flow components that are critical to the analysis—that is, those components that, when changed, have the greatest impact on profitability.

Sensitivity Analysis

Historically, sensitivity analysis has been classified as a risk assessment tool, although it has many limitations in this regard. However, it does have significant value in project analyses, so we discuss it in some detail here (see "Critical Concept: Sensitivity Analysis").

Many of the input variables that determine a project's cash flows are subject to uncertainty. Let's face it, some of the inputs—say, volume—may be nothing more than educated guesses. If the realized (actual) value of such a variable is different from its expected value, the project's realized profitability will differ from that expected.

Sensitivity analysis shows how much a project's profitability (NPV or IRR) will change in response to a given change in a single component cash flow (input variable), with other inputs held constant. In other words, sensitivity analysis tells us how sensitive a project's profitability is to changes in selected input variable values.

To illustrate sensitivity analysis, assume that Bayside's managers believe that all of the open MRI project's component cash flows (except for weekly volume and salvage value) are known with relative certainty. (For ease of illustration, we are limiting the sensitivity analysis to two variables.) The expected (most likely, or best guess) values for these variables (volume = 20; salvage value = $750,000) were used in exhibit 10.2 to obtain the **base case** NPV of $82,493.

Base case
In a capital investment analysis, the situation that is expected (most likely) to occur.

Sensitivity analysis is designed to provide managers with the answers to questions such as what happens to profitability if volume is more or less than the expected level and what will result if salvage value is more or less than expected.

In a typical sensitivity analysis, each uncertain component cash flow is changed by a fixed percentage amount above and below its expected value, while all other component cash flows are held constant at their expected values. Thus, all input variables, except one, are held at their base case values. The resulting NPVs (or IRRs) are recorded and plotted. Exhibit 10.3 contains the NPV sensitivity analysis for the open MRI project, assuming only two uncertain variables: volume and salvage value.

Note that the NPV is a constant $82,493 when no change occurs in either of the component cash flow values, because a 0 percent change recreates the base case. Managers can examine values in exhibit 10.3 to get a feel for which component cash flow has the greatest impact on the MRI project's NPV—the larger the NPV change for a given percentage input

Exhibit 10.3
Open MRI Project Sensitivity Analysis

	Net Present Value	
Change from Base Case Level	**Volume**	**Salvage Value**
−30%	($814,053)	($ 57,215)
−20	(515,193)	(10,646)
−10	216,350	35,923
0	82,493	82,493
+10	381,335	129,062
+20	680,178	175,631
+30	979,020	222,200

change, the greater the impact. Such an examination shows that the MRI project's NPV is more affected by changes in volume than by changes in salvage value. This result should be somewhat intuitive because salvage value is a single cash flow in the analysis, occurring only at year 5, whereas volume influences the net cash flow in each year of operation.

Often, the results of sensitivity analyses are shown in graphical form. For example, the sensitivity analysis presented in tabular form in exhibit 10.3 is graphed in exhibit 10.4. Here, the slopes of the lines show how sensitive the open MRI project's NPV is to changes in each of the two uncertain component inputs—the steeper the slope, the more sensitive NPV is to a change in the variable.

Exhibit 10.4 vividly illustrates that the open MRI project's NPV is very sensitive to the volume forecast but only mildly sensitive to the salvage value forecast. A sensitivity plot showing a negative slope indicates that increases in the value of that input variable decrease the project's NPV.

If two projects are being compared, the one with the steeper sensitivity lines would be regarded as riskier because a relatively small error in estimating a component cash flow—for example, volume—would produce a large error in the project's forecasted NPV. If information were available on the sensitivity of NPV to input changes for Bayside's average project, we could make similar judgments regarding the riskiness of the open MRI project relative to the hospital's average project.

Although sensitivity analysis typically is considered to be a risk assessment tool, it does have severe limitations in this role. For example, suppose Bayside had a contract with an HMO that guaranteed a minimum MRI usage at a fixed reimbursement rate. In that situation, the project probably would have very little risk, in spite of the fact that the sensitivity analysis showed NPV to be highly sensitive to forecasted volume.

EXHIBIT 10.4
Open MRI Project Sensitivity Analysis Graphs

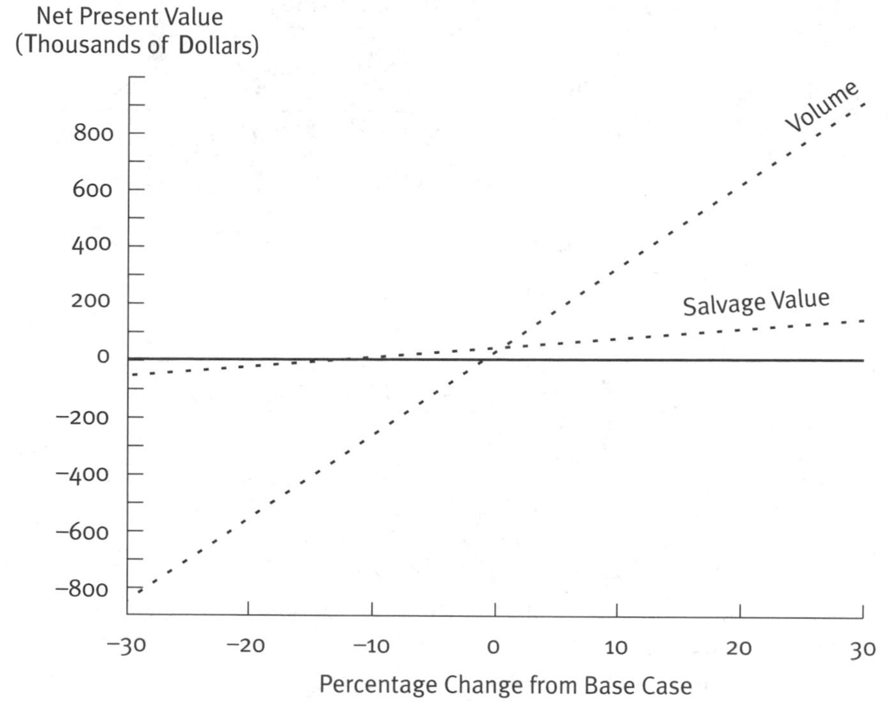

In general, a project's risk depends on both the sensitivity of its profitability to changes in key input variables and the ranges of likely values of these variables. Because sensitivity analysis considers only the first factor, it can give misleading results. Furthermore, sensitivity analysis does not consider any interactions among the uncertain cash flow components; it considers each component independently of the others.

In spite of the shortcomings of sensitivity analysis as a risk assessment tool, it does present managers with valuable information. First, it provides breakeven information for the project's uncertain variables. For example, exhibits 10.3 and 10.4 show that just a few percent decrease in expected volume makes the project unprofitable (a negative NPV), whereas the project remains profitable even if salvage value falls by more than 10 percent. Although somewhat rough, this breakeven information is clearly of value to Bayside's managers.

Second, and perhaps more important, sensitivity analysis identifies those cash flow components that are most critical to the analysis. By most critical, we mean those components that have the largest impact on profitability when their realized values differ from their forecasted values. For the open MRI project, volume is clearly the most critical input variable of the two being examined, so Bayside's managers should ensure that the volume estimate is the best possible.

A small overestimate in volume could make the project seem financially attractive when evaluated, yet the actual results could easily be disappointing. Bayside's managers have a limited amount of time to spend on analyzing the open MRI project, so they should expend their resources as productively as possible by focusing on those cash flow components that make the most difference (have the largest impact on profitability).

In addition, sensitivity analysis can be useful after a project has been initiated. For example, assume Bayside's open MRI project was accepted and the first year's postaudit indicates that the project is not meeting financial expectations. Bayside's managers must take actions to improve the project's financial results.

What actions should they take? Sensitivity analysis identifies the variables that have the greatest impact on profitability. Thus, managers can try to influence those variables that have the greatest potential for improving financial performance, such as volume, rather than those variables that have little impact on profitability.

Scenario Analysis

Scenario analysis is a project risk analysis technique that considers the sensitivity of NPV to changes in uncertain cash flow components, the likely range of component values, and the interactions among components (see "Critical Concept: Scenario Analysis").

To conduct a scenario analysis, managers start with the base case and then pick a bad set of circumstances (e.g., low volume, low salvage value, high labor costs) and a good set

CRITICAL CONCEPT
Scenario Analysis

Scenario analysis is a risk assessment technique that overcomes the problems associated with sensitivity analysis. In essence, scenario analysis examines the impact of several (often three) economic scenarios on a project's profitability. For example, assume a group practice is considering the purchase of an electrocardiogram (EKG) machine. The most likely (base case) estimate for volume is 200 procedures in the first year at an average reimbursement of $40 per procedure. These values result in a base case estimate of $8,000 in annual revenue. In a scenario analysis, the best-case estimate may be 250 procedures at $45 and the worst case may be 150 procedures at $35. Thus, the revenue estimate is 250 × $45 = $11,250 for the best case and 150 × $35 = $5,250 for the worst case. By combining these revenue values with the best- and worst-case estimates for the other uncertain component cash flows, we obtain the net cash flows for all three scenarios. Once the net cash flows are forecasted, the profitability (NPV and IRR) of each scenario can be estimated. The difference between the most likely (base) case and worst-case NPV (or IRR) gives managers a feel for the riskiness of the project—the greater the difference in these values, the higher the risk.

(e.g., high volume, high salvage value, low labor costs). Next, managers use the component cash flow values from the bad and good circumstances (scenarios) to forecast profitability under assumptions other than those used in the base case.

To illustrate scenario analysis, again consider Bayside's open MRI project. Assume that Bayside's managers regard a drop in weekly volume below 15 scans as unlikely and consider a volume above 25 to be improbable. On the other hand, salvage value could be as low as $500,000 or as high as $1 million. The most likely values for these cash flow components are 20 scans per week for volume and $750,000 for salvage value. Thus, a volume of 15 and a $500,000 salvage value define the lower bound (worst-case scenario), while a volume of 25 and a salvage value of $1 million define the upper bound (best-case scenario).

Bayside can now use the worst-, most likely, and best-case values for these cash flow components to obtain the NPV that corresponds to each scenario. Bayside's managers use a spreadsheet model to conduct the analysis, and exhibit 10.5 summarizes the results. The most likely (base) case results in a positive NPV; the worst case produces a negative NPV; and the best case results in a large, positive NPV.

Typically, the scenario analysis would be interpreted by Bayside's financial staff as described in "Optional Discussion: Applying Statistical Concepts to Scenario Analysis." However, scenario analysis can also be interpreted in a less mathematical way. The difference between the most likely NPV ($82,493) and the worst-case NPV (–$819,844) is $902,337. The larger this difference, the greater the chance that the project will have a return far below that expected, and hence the greater the risk.

Note that the potential loss of almost $820,000 represents an estimate of the worst possible financial consequences of the MRI project. Bayside is a large hospital in sound financial condition, so it can absorb such a loss in value without much impact. Thus, the project does not represent a significant financial threat to the hospital.

Conversely, if the project were being analyzed by a small clinic in poor financial condition, such a loss might mean financial ruin, and its managers might be unwilling to undertake the project, regardless of its profitability under the base case and best-case scenarios. Note that, if the numerical analysis is identical at Bayside and the clinic, the risk of the project—the spread between the most likely and worst-case NPVs—has not changed. What has changed is the ability of the organization to bear that risk. Large businesses in excellent financial condition can afford to take on more capital investment risk than can smaller businesses in poor financial condition.

EXHIBIT 10.5
Open MRI Project Scenario Analysis

Scenario	Volume	Salvage Value	NPV
Worst case	15	$ 500,000	($819,844)
Most likely case	20	750,000	82,493
Best case	25	1,000,000	984,829

OPTIONAL DISCUSSION

Applying Statistical Concepts to Scenario Analysis

The statistical concepts of *expected value* and *standard deviation* can be applied to the data in exhibit 10.5 to determine the expected NPV and standard deviation of NPV. To do so, an estimate is needed of the probabilities of occurrence of the three scenarios. Suppose that Bayside's managers estimate the following probabilities: a 20 percent chance of the worst case, a 60 percent chance of the most likely (base) case, and a 20 percent chance of the best case. (Of course, it is difficult to estimate scenario probabilities with any confidence.)

Using these probabilities, the expected NPV can be found as follows:

$$\begin{aligned}\text{Expected NPV} &= [0.20 \times (-\$819{,}844)] + (0.60 \times \$82{,}493) + (0.20 \times \$984{,}829)\\ &= \$82{,}493.\end{aligned}$$

Note that the expected NPV in the scenario analysis is the same as the base case NPV, $82,493. The consistency of results occurs because, when coupled with the scenario probabilities, the values of the uncertain variables used in the scenario analysis—15, 20, and 25 scans for volume, and $500,000, $750,000, and $1,000,000 for salvage value—produce the same most likely values used in the base case analysis in exhibit 10.2.

Using the distribution of NPVs, we can calculate the standard deviation:

$$\begin{aligned}\sigma_{NPV} &= [0.20 \times (-\$819{,}844 - \$82{,}493)^2 + 0.60 \times (\$82{,}493 - \$82{,}493)^2\\ &\quad + 0.20 \times (\$984{,}829 - \$82{,}493)^2]^{1/2}\\ &= \$570{,}688.2\end{aligned}$$

The standard deviation of NPV measures the open MRI project's stand-alone risk. Bayside's managers can compare the standard deviation of NPV of this project to the uncertainty inherent in Bayside's aggregate cash flows, or average project.

Often, the coefficient of variation (CV) is used to measure the stand-alone risk of a project,

$$\text{CV} = \sigma_{NPV} \div \text{Expected NPV} = \$570{,}688 \div \$82{,}493 = 6.9,$$

for the open MRI project. The CV measures the risk per unit of return and hence is a better measure of comparative risk than is the standard deviation, especially when projects have widely differing NPVs.

Bayside's average project has a CV in the range of 8.0 to 10.0, so the statistical risk analysis indicates that the open MRI project has below-average risk relative to the hospital's average project.

While scenario analysis provides useful information about a project's risk, it is limited in two ways. First, it considers only a few possible outcomes, whereas, in reality, an almost infinite number of possibilities exist.

Second, scenario analysis implies a definite relationship among the uncertain variables. That is, the scenario analysis assumes that the worst value for volume (15 scans per week) would occur at the same time as the worst value for salvage value ($500,000) because the worst-case scenario is defined by combining the worst possible value of each uncertain variable. Although this relationship (all worst values occurring together) may hold in some situations, it may not hold in others. For example, if volume is low, maybe the open MRI will have less wear and tear and hence be worth more after five years of use. The worst value for volume, then, should be coupled with the best salvage value. Conversely, poor volume may be symptomatic of poor medical effectiveness of the open MRI and hence lead to limited demand for used equipment and a low salvage value. Scenario analysis tends to create extreme profitability values for the worst and best cases because it automatically combines all the worst and best input values, even if these values actually have only a remote chance of occurring together (see "For Your Consideration: How Many Scenarios in a Scenario Analysis?").

Qualitative Risk Assessment

In some situations, perhaps in many, conducting a quantitative risk assessment is difficult because predicting the values needed in a scenario analysis is hard to do. In such situations, rather than ignore project risk, some healthcare businesses use a **qualitative risk assessment** approach. For example, Bayside uses the following questions to assess project risk subjectively:

Qualitative risk assessment
A process for assessing project risk that focuses on qualitative factors as opposed to a statistical analysis of profit variability.

- *Market share.* Does the project require additional market share or represent a new service initiative?
- *Scope of expertise.* Is the project outside the scope of current management expertise?
- *Recruitment.* Does the project require difficult-to-recruit technical specialists?
- *Competition.* Will the project position us counter to a strong competitor?
- *Technology.* Does the project require the use of new, unproven technology?

To assess project risk, each "yes" answer is assigned one point. If the overall score is zero or one point, the project is judged to have low risk. If it has two or three points, it is judged to have average risk, while a score of four or five points indicates high risk.

When Bayside's managers applied the qualitative risk assessment tool to the open MRI project, they assigned "no" as the answer to all questions except one: Will the project position us counter to a strong competitor? This question was answered "yes," under the assumption that a competing outpatient imaging center would also purchase an open MRI. Thus, with a total of one point, the project was judged to have low risk when assessed qualitatively.

FOR YOUR CONSIDERATION
How Many Scenarios in a Scenario Analysis?

In the scenario analysis of Bayside's open MRI project, we used three scenarios. However, three is not a magic bullet—the more scenarios used, the more information obtained from the analysis. Furthermore, more scenarios lessen the problem associated with extreme values because the very best and very worst scenarios can be assigned low probabilities (which are probably realistic) without causing the risk inherent in the project to be understated.

While more scenarios add realism and provide more information for decision makers, a greater number of scenarios increases forecasting difficulty and makes the analysis more time consuming. Furthermore, the greater the number of scenarios, the more difficult it is to interpret the results. Thus, the entire process is easier if three scenarios are used rather than, say, nine.

What do you think? Are three scenarios sufficient, or should more be used? How many scenarios are too many? Is it better to have an odd number of scenarios than an even number? Is there an optimal number of scenarios?

Although such a subjective approach initially appears to have little theoretical foundation, a closer examination reveals that each question in the list is tied to cash flow uncertainty. Thus, the greater the number of "yes" answers, the greater the cash flow uncertainty and hence the greater the risk of the project. Even when a quantitative risk assessment is feasible, a separate qualitative assessment is a good idea. The value of using the qualitative risk assessment approach in conjunction with a quantitative risk assessment is that it forces managers to think about project risk in alternative frameworks. If the quantitative and qualitative assessments do not agree, then clearly the project's risk assessment requires more consideration.

SELF-TEST QUESTIONS

1. Define the concept of financial risk.
2. What makes one project riskier than another?
3. Briefly describe sensitivity analysis. Is sensitivity analysis a good risk assessment tool? If not, what is its value in the capital budgeting process?
4. Briefly describe scenario analysis. What are its strengths and weaknesses?
5. Describe qualitative risk assessment. Why does it work?
6. Assume a quantitative risk assessment has been conducted on a project. Is a qualitative risk assessment necessary?

10.5 INCORPORATING RISK INTO THE DECISION PROCESS

It may be possible to reach the general conclusion that one project is more or less risky than another or to compare the riskiness of a project with the business as a whole. However, it is difficult to develop a really good measure of project risk—one that tells managers that project A is, say, twice as risky as project B. This lack of confidence in measuring project risk adds to the difficulties in incorporating differential risk into the capital investment decision. Still, it is not enough to merely measure project risk—differential risk must be incorporated into the capital investment decision process.

The Risk-Adjusted Discount Rate Method

Risk-adjusted discount rate (RADR)
A risk adjustment method that changes the discount (opportunity cost) rate to reflect the unique riskiness of the project being analyzed.

The method used most often to incorporate risk into the capital investment decision process is the **risk-adjusted discount rate (RADR)** method. Here, the project's most likely (base case) cash flows are discounted using an opportunity cost rate based on the project's risk assessment.

The starting point for the risk adjustment is the corporate cost of capital, which is covered in detail in chapter 8. Remember that this rate reflects the organization's aggregate risk—that is, the riskiness of the business's average project. In project risk analysis, a project's risk is assessed relative to the firm's average project. The corporate cost of capital is then adjusted to reflect any differential risk, resulting in a project cost of capital (see "Critical Concept: Project Cost of Capital").

In general, above-average-risk projects are assigned a project cost of capital that is higher than the corporate cost of capital, average-risk projects are evaluated at the corporate cost of capital, and below-average-risk projects are assigned a discount rate that is less than the corporate cost of capital.

CRITICAL CONCEPT
Project Cost of Capital

The project cost of capital is the discount rate that reflects the unique riskiness of the project being analyzed. Usually, the project cost of capital is estimated by adding or subtracting a specified number of percentage points from the corporate cost of capital. If the project is assessed to be riskier than average, the project cost of capital is greater than the corporate cost of capital. If the project is less risky, the project cost of capital is less than the corporate cost of capital.

Although widely used, the RADR method does have some disadvantages. First, there is no theoretical basis for the size of the adjustment, so the amount remains a matter of judgment. Second, the RADR method combines both time value and risk incorporation into a single discount rate applied to all cash flows. By lumping together risk and time value, the premium applied to above-average-risk projects is compounded over time; just as interest compounds over time, so does the risk premium. Thus, use of the RADR method implies that risk increases with time, which imposes a greater burden on long-term than on short-term projects. The end result is that, all else the same, short-term projects tend to look better financially than long-term projects. In general, this outcome is not a problem, as long-term projects typically are riskier than short-term projects because of the difficulties in forecasting cash flows well into the future.

Making the Final Decision on the Open MRI Project

The business's corporate cost of capital provides the basis for estimating the project cost of capital (discount rate). However, there is no good way of specifying exactly how much the corporate cost of capital should be adjusted to account for differential project risk. Given the present state of the art, risk adjustments are necessarily subjective and somewhat arbitrary (see "Healthcare in Practice: Risk Analysis in Healthcare Organizations").

HEALTHCARE IN PRACTICE
Risk Analysis in Healthcare Organizations

Several surveys have been conducted over the last 20 years to assess how businesses, including health services organizations, assess and incorporate risk into their capital investment decision processes.

Most organizations consider a variety of factors when assessing project risk, including market characteristics, uncertainty of cash flow estimates, and strategic fit. When examining cash flow uncertainty, most attention is paid to the estimates for cost, volume, and reimbursement.

Although observers generally agree that the discount rate used in capital investment analyses should be adjusted for project risk, they do not agree on the method used. Practically speaking, many organizations set a range of discount rates (for example, one used a range of 10.5 to 21.5 percent) and then apply these rates to projects on the basis of relative risk. Higher-risk projects are assigned higher rates, and vice versa.

Still, the entire capital investment process brings out many concerns. For example, one chief financial officer stated: "I do not believe in NPV. You can make any project look good or bad by selecting the right discount rate. Or you can spend all of your time arguing about which discount rate is correct." Although this statement has merit, we should not denigrate the entire process because of the difficulties involved. Clearly, some projects are suitable for a quantitative risk analysis, as described in this chapter, and other projects are not. One key to developing good analyses is to be able to make such distinctions.

Note: This Healthcare in Practice is based on information in K. L. Reiter, D. G. Smith, J. R. C. Wheeler, and H. L. Rivenson, 2000, "Capital Investment Strategies in Health Care Systems," *Journal of Health Care Finance* (Summer): 31–41.

Bayside's standard procedure is to add 4 percentage points to its 10 percent corporate cost of capital when evaluating higher-risk projects and to subtract 2 percentage points when evaluating lower-risk projects. Because Bayside's open MRI project was judged to have below-average risk, the project cost of capital is reduced to 10% – 2% = 8%. Thus, the final NPV estimate, which incorporates the risk analysis, is $243,969. Because the NPV is larger than before ($82,493), the risk analysis makes the open MRI project even more attractive financially than indicated in chapter 9, which excluded risk analysis.

On the other hand, what if the project had been judged to have above-average risk? In this situation, the project cost of capital would be 10% + 4% = 14%, and the project's expected (base case) net cash flows shown in exhibit 10.2 would be discounted at that project cost of capital. The resultant NPV is –$200,017, so the project becomes unprofitable if the analysis were to judge the project as having above-average risk. Bayside's managers might still decide to go ahead with the open MRI project for other reasons, but at least they would know that its expected profitability is not sufficient to make up for its riskiness.

Self-Test Questions

1. Explain the risk-adjusted discount rate (RADR) method for incorporating risk in the capital investment decision process.
2. What assumptions about time and risk are inherent in the RADR method?
3. What is the difference between the corporate cost of capital and a project cost of capital?
4. Is the risk adjustment objective or subjective?

10.6 AN OVERVIEW OF THE CAPITAL INVESTMENT DECISION PROCESS

For capital planning purposes, health services managers need to forecast the total number of projects that will be undertaken and the dollar amount of capital needed to fund these projects. The list of projects to be undertaken is called the **capital budget**.

Capital budget
A plan (budget) that outlines a business's expected future expenditures on new capital assets, such as land, buildings, and equipment.

While every healthcare provider estimates its optimal capital budget in its unique way, some procedures are common to all firms. This process is illustrated by the procedures followed by the Dallas Medical Group:

- *Estimate the corporate cost of capital.* The practice manager estimates the group's corporate cost of capital. As discussed in chapter 8, this estimate depends on market conditions, the business's inherent risk, and its optimal capital structure.

- *Assign project costs of capital.* Each project is assigned a project cost of capital that reflects its risk relative to the overall business.
- *Calculate NPVs.* The project costs of capital are used to discount each project's base case net cash flows. From a purely financial standpoint, all projects with positive NPVs are acceptable, while those with negative NPVs should be rejected.
- *Consider the relevant subjective factors.* Subjective factors are considered, and these factors may result in a capital budget that differs from a budget based solely on financial considerations. For example, could the project significantly increase the group's liability exposure? Conversely, does the project have any strategic or social value or other attributes that could affect its acceptability? Typically, if the project involves new services and is large (in capital requirements) compared to the group's average project, then the additional subjective factors will be important to the final decision.

Ultimately, capital budgeting decisions require an analysis of a mix of objective and subjective factors, such as risk, profitability, medical staff and patient needs, and social value. To help incorporate nonfinancial factors, many organizations use a project scoring approach similar to the one we discussed in chapter 9. The process is not precise, and often managers are tempted to ignore one or more important factors because such factors are so nebulous and difficult to measure. Despite the imprecision and subjectivity, a project's risk, as well as its other attributes, should be assessed and incorporated into the capital investment decision process.

? Self-Test Questions

1. **Describe a typical capital investment decision process.**
2. **Are decisions made solely on the basis of quantitative factors? Explain your answer.**

10.7 CAPITAL RATIONING

Standard capital investment decision processes assume that businesses can raise virtually unlimited amounts of capital to meet investment needs. Presumably, as long as a business is investing the funds in profitable (positive NPV) projects, it should be able to raise the debt and equity financing needed to fund all worthwhile projects.

This picture of the capital financing and capital investment process is probably appropriate for most large investor-owned businesses. However, not-for-profit businesses do not have unlimited access to capital. Their equity capital is limited primarily to retentions and contributions, and their debt capital is limited to the amount supported by the equity capital base. In addition, small businesses typically do not have unlimited supplies of capital. Thus, many businesses face periods in which the capital needed for investment in new projects exceeds the amount available. This situation is called **capital rationing**.

Capital rationing
The condition of having more acceptable projects than funds (capital) needed to undertake those projects.

If capital rationing exists, from a purely financial perspective it is best to accept the set of projects that maximizes aggregate NPV and still meets the capital constraint. This approach could be called "getting the most bang for the buck" because it picks projects that have the most positive impact on the organization's financial condition. Of course, priority may be assigned to some low or even negative NPV projects because of mission considerations, which is fine as long as these projects are offset by the selection of profitable projects to sustain the business's financial strength.

Self-Test Questions

1. What is capital rationing?
2. From a financial perspective, how are projects chosen when capital rationing exists?

Theme Wrap-Up: Estimating a Project's Cash Flows and Assessing Risk

At the beginning of chapter 9, we introduced a proposal by Palm Coast Radiology Associates that Bayside Memorial Hospital purchase a new, $2.5 million open MRI system. Although the medical benefits of the new system are clear, there were concerns expressed about the financial implications of the purchase.

To begin, Bayside's managers conducted a base case analysis assuming that the project had average risk. Among the results was an NPV of $82,493. Then, they performed a project risk analysis, first using sensitivity analysis to identify the key cash flow components. (For ease of illustration, we only examined two components of sensitivity analysis: volume and salvage value.) After conducting scenario and qualitative analyses, the managers concluded that the project had below-average risk. Thus, the 10 percent corporate cost of capital was adjusted downward to obtain an 8 percent project cost of capital, resulting in a final NPV estimate of $243,969.

After all factors (including recommendations from the physicians of Palm Coast Radiology Associates) were considered, and after the estimation and analysis processes were explained to Dr. Fisher, Bayside decided to go ahead with the open MRI project. Bayside's new MRI system went into service one full year before the competition (the outpatient imaging center) brought its own system to the marketplace.

Today, the open MRI system has proved to be a financial (and patient satisfaction) success and is still going strong. Clearly, Bayside's managers made the right decision.

Key Concepts

This chapter discusses project cash flow estimation and risk analysis. Here are the key concepts:

- The most critical and most difficult step in analyzing a capital investment proposal is estimating the incremental cash flows for the project.
- In determining incremental cash flows, *opportunity costs* (cash flows forgone by using an asset) must be considered, but *sunk costs* (cash outlays that cannot be recouped) are not included. Furthermore, any impact of the project on the firm's other projects must be included in the analysis.
- A project may have some strategic value that is not accounted for in the estimated cash flows. At a minimum, strategic value should be noted and considered qualitatively in the analysis.
- The effects of inflation must be considered in project analyses. The best procedure is to build inflation effects directly into the component cash flow estimates.
- Project risk is associated with the chance of earning a smaller return than expected. The greater the probability of a subpar return, the higher the risk. Two techniques are commonly used to assess a project's risk: (1) sensitivity analysis and (2) scenario analysis.
- *Sensitivity analysis* shows how much a project's profitability (for example, as measured by NPV) changes in response to a given change in an input variable, such as volume, with other variables held constant. Although its use in risk assessment is limited, sensitivity analysis is a valuable tool for identifying a project's critical component cash flows.
- *Scenario analysis* typically defines a project's best, most likely, and worst cases and then uses these data to assess risk.
- In many situations, conducting a quantitative project risk assessment is impractical. In these cases, many healthcare businesses use a qualitative approach to risk assessment.
- Projects generally are classified as *high risk*, *average risk*, or *low risk* relative to the business's average project. Higher-risk projects are evaluated at a project cost of capital that is greater than the firm's corporate cost of capital. Average-risk projects

are evaluated at the firm's corporate cost of capital, while lower-risk projects are evaluated at a rate less than the corporate cost of capital.

- The *capital budget* is the list of all projects expected to be undertaken during the next planning period.
- *Capital rationing* occurs when a business does not have access to sufficient capital to fund all profitable projects. Under these conditions, the best financial outcome results from accepting the set of projects that has the highest aggregate NPV.
- Ultimately, capital budgeting decisions require an analysis of a mix of objective and subjective factors such as risk, profitability, medical staff and patient needs, and service to the community. The process is not precise, but good managers do their best to ensure that none of the relevant factors is ignored.

This chapter concludes our discussion of financing and capital investment decisions. In chapter 11, we address how businesses report financial results.

End-of-Chapter Questions

10.1 Briefly define the following cash flow estimation concepts:
- a. Incremental cash flow
- b. Sunk cost
- c. Opportunity cost
- d. Strategic value
- e. Inflation effects

10.2 Define *financial risk*. Why is risk analysis so important to capital investment decisions?

10.3 a. Briefly describe sensitivity analysis.
b. What are its strengths and weaknesses?

10.4 a. Briefly describe scenario analysis.
b. What are its strengths and weaknesses?

10.5 Describe the qualitative approach to risk assessment. Why does this approach, which does not rely on numerical data, work?

10.6 How is project risk incorporated into the capital investment decision?

10.7 What is the difference between the corporate cost of capital and a project cost of capital?

10.8 What is meant by the term *capital rationing*? From a purely financial standpoint, what is the best capital budget under capital rationing?

10.9 Santa Roberta Clinic has estimated its corporate cost of capital to be 11 percent. What are reasonable values for the project costs of capital for lower-risk, average-risk, and higher-risk projects?

End-of-Chapter Problems

10.1 Great Lakes Clinic has been asked to provide exclusive healthcare services for next year's World Exposition. Although flattered by the request, the clinic's managers want to conduct a financial analysis of the project. An up-front cost of $160,000 is needed to get the clinic ready. Then, a net cash inflow of $1 million is expected from operations in each of the two years of the exposition. However, the clinic has to pay the organizers of the exposition a fee for the marketing value of the opportunity. This fee, which must be paid at the end of the second year, is $2 million.

a. What are the net cash flows associated with the project?

b. What is the project's internal rate of return (IRR)?

c. Assuming a project cost of capital of 10 percent, what is the project's net present value (NPV)?

10.2 California Imaging Center, a not-for-profit business, is evaluating the purchase of new diagnostic equipment. The equipment, which costs $600,000, has an expected life of five years and an estimated salvage value of $200,000 at that time. The equipment is expected to be used 15 times a day for 250 days a year for each year of the project's life. On average, each procedure is expected to generate $80 in cash collections during the first year of use. Thus, net revenues for year 1 are estimated at 15 × 250 × $80 = $300,000.

Labor and maintenance costs are expected to be $100,000 during the first year of operation, while utilities will cost another $10,000 and cash overhead will increase by $5,000 in year 1. The cost for expendable supplies is expected to average $5 per procedure during the first year. All costs and revenues are expected to increase at a 5 percent inflation rate after the first year. The center's corporate cost of capital is 10 percent.

a. Estimate the project's net cash flows over its five-year estimated life. (Hint: Use the following format as a guide.)

	Year					
	0	1	2	3	4	5
Equipment cost						
Net revenues						
Less: Labor/maintenance costs						
Utilities costs						
Supplies						
Incremental overhead						
Operating income						
Equipment salvage value						
Net cash flow						

b. What are the project's NPV and IRR? (Assume for now that the project has average risk.)
c. Assume that the project is assessed to have high risk and that California Imaging Center adds or subtracts 3 percentage points to adjust for project risk. Now, what is the project's NPV? Does the risk assessment change how the project's IRR is interpreted?

10.3 You have been asked to evaluate the proposed acquisition of a new clinical laboratory test system. The system's price is $50,000, and it will cost another $10,000 for transportation and installation. The system is expected to be sold after three years because the laboratory is being moved at that time. The best estimate of the system's salvage value after three years is $20,000. The system will have no impact on volume or reimbursement (and hence revenues), but it is expected to save $20,000 per year in operating costs. The not-for-profit business's corporate cost of capital is 10 percent, and the standard risk adjustment is 4 percentage points.
a. What is the project's net investment outlay at time 0?
b. What are the project's operating cash flows in years 1, 2, and 3?
c. What is the terminal cash flow at the end of year 3?
d. If the project has average risk, is it expected to be profitable?
e. What if the project is judged to have lower-than-average risk? Higher-than-average risk?

10.4 The staff of Jefferson Medical Services has estimated the following net cash flows for a food services operation that it may open in its outpatient clinic:

Year	Expected Net Cash Flow
0	($100,000)
1	30,000
2	30,000
3	30,000
4	30,000
5	30,000
5 (salvage value)	20,000

The time 0 cash flow is the net investment outlay, while the final amount is the terminal cash flow. (The clinic is expected to move to a new building in five years.) All other flows represent net operating cash flows. Jefferson's corporate cost of capital is 10 percent.
a. What is the project's IRR?
b. Assuming the project has average risk, what is its NPV?

c. Now, assume that the operating cash flows in years 1 through 5 could be as low as $20,000 or as high as $40,000. Furthermore, the salvage value cash flow at the end of year 5 could be as low as $0 or as high as $30,000. What are the worst-case and best-case IRRs? The worst-case and best-case NPVs?

10.5 The managers of United Medtronics are evaluating the following four projects for the coming budget period. The firm's corporate cost of capital is 14 percent.

Project	Cost	IRR (%)
A	$15,000	17
B	15,000	16
C	12,000	15
D	20,000	13

a. What is the firm's capital budget?
b. Now, suppose Medtronics's managers want to consider differential risk in the capital budgeting process. Project A has average risk, B has below-average risk, C has above-average risk, and D has average risk. What is the firm's optimal capital budget when differential risk is considered? (Hint: The firm's managers lower the IRR of high-risk projects by 3 percentage points and raise the IRR of low-risk projects by the same amount.)

10.6 This optional problem requires knowledge of statistics.

Heywood Home Healthcare is evaluating a project with the following net cash flows and probabilities:

	Time 0	Year 1	Year 2	Year 3	Year 4	Year 5
Prob = 0.2	($100,000)	20,000	20,000	20,000	20,000	30,000
Prob = 0.6	($100,000)	30,000	30,000	30,000	30,000	40,000
Prob = 0.2	($100,000)	40,000	40,000	40,000	40,000	50,000

The year 5 values include salvage value. Heywood's corporate cost of capital is 10 percent.

a. What is the project's most likely (base case) NPV, assuming average risk?
b. What are the project's most likely, worst-case, and best-case NPVs?
c. What is the project's expected NPV on the basis of the scenario analysis?
d. What is the project's standard deviation of NPV?
e. Assume that Heywood's managers judge the project to have lower-than-average risk. Furthermore, the company's policy is to adjust the corporate cost of capital up or down by 3 percentage points to account for differential risk. Is the project financially attractive?

PART IV

REPORTING RESULTS

In part IV, our focus is on how organizations report overall financial results and how those results are analyzed to assess financial condition. Clearly, information on financial results and condition are of vital interest to managers, investors, employees, and a whole host of parties that have a financial interest in the organization (stakeholders).

An organization's financial status is reported by its financial statements—the three most important are the income statement, the balance sheet, and the statement of cash flows. Our coverage of financial statements is spread over two chapters. Chapter 11 provides an introduction to financial statements as a whole and to the income statement (which reports profitability) specifically, while chapter 12 covers the balance sheet (which reports a business's assets and the way those assets are financed) and the statement of cash flows (which concerns the cash flowing into and out of a business). Together, chapters 11 and 12 offer a comprehensive treatment of the format and content of a business's financial statements.

Financial statements contain a great deal of information about an organization's financial condition, but much of this information is masked by the vast amount of data reported. Chapter 13 illustrates several techniques applied to financial statement data that facilitate judgments about an organization's financial condition.

CHAPTER 11

REPORTING PROFITS

THEME SET-UP: INTERPRETING AN INCOME STATEMENT

Five years ago, Lori Gibbs, a nurse practitioner, opened Park Ridge Homecare, an investor-owned home health agency located in a suburb of Chicago. After working for almost 15 years at a gerontology group practice, she felt ready to embark on a new career that would combine her nursing knowledge with a desire to run her own business.

In the beginning, the business provided basic healthcare services—such as wound and dressing care, catheter care, IV (intravenous) therapy, and colostomy care—to patients who are homebound. To support these services, the business sold medical supplies and equipment such as bandages, IV solutions, wheelchairs, and walkers. After the first year, the business expanded to offer additional services, including physical, occupational, and speech therapy.

The first several years of the business were hectic. In fact, Lori devoted most of her time to the work, often putting in 12 or more hours per day. Much of her effort involved identifying sources of financing, and she realized that running a start-up business was no piece of cake. Her time off was limited to emergencies and a few days here and there. However, all of her work eventually paid off—the business prospered, and she was able to hire an administrator to handle day-to-day operations.

Now, Lori is considering opening a second location in Barrington, a relatively affluent suburb about 20 miles northwest of Park Ridge. The success of Park Ridge Homecare makes her feel confident that she can start a second business. She wants to use the financial resources of the Park Ridge business to open the Barrington site.

Lori faces a question: What is the current financial condition of Park Ridge Homecare, and can it be used to support the opening of a second location? By the end of the chapter, you will learn how Park Ridge Homecare reports its profitability and get a feel for how financial statements are used to assess financial condition. By the end of part IV, you will be able to conduct a basic assessment of your own organization's financial condition on the basis of the data reported in its financial statements.

Note that the data we present for Park Ridge and selected sector measures are purely fictitious and should not be used for other purposes. For simplicity of presentation, the thousands (000s) in the calculations shown in the book have been omitted.

Learning Objectives

After studying this chapter, you will be able to do the following:

- Explain why financial statements are important to managers and to outside parties.
- Discuss the basic concepts behind the creation of financial statements.
- Describe the components of the income statement (revenues, expenses, profitability) and the relationships among these components.
- Differentiate among operating income, net income, and cash flow.

11.1 INTRODUCTION

When you think about a healthcare business, what do you visualize? Most people see buildings, equipment, and people. What we often do not readily consider are the costs involved—for example, salaries, medical supplies, and interest on debt financing. To be successful, these costs must be covered by revenues from patients and third-party payers (private and public insurance). The bottom line is that a large number of economic (financial) events support the physical elements (facilities and people) of the business.

In this chapter, we begin our discussion of how an organization reports its financial status.

Financial accounting
The field of accounting that focuses on the measurement and communication of the economic events and status of an entire organization.

11.2 FINANCIAL ACCOUNTING

Financial accounting involves identifying, measuring, recording, and communicating the economic events and status of an organization. This information is summarized and presented in a set of financial statements, the three most important of which are the income statement, the balance sheet, and the statement of cash flows (see "Critical Concept: Financial Statements"). Because these statements communicate financial information, financial accounting is often called *the language of business*.

Stakeholder
A party that has an interest—typically financial—in an organization. For example, owners (in for-profit businesses), managers, patients, and suppliers are some stakeholders of healthcare businesses.

Most people consider only the actual statements, such as the income statement shown in exhibit 11.1 (p. 325), when looking for financial data. However, the notes that follow the statements typically are extensive and contain a wealth of information that supplements the statements. These notes, sometimes referred to as *footnotes*, provide details that are left out of the primary documents. The note system ensures that important information is provided to financial statement users without clogging up the actual statements with excessive detail.

The predominant users of financial statements are **stakeholders**—parties who have a financial interest in the organization and hence are concerned with its economic welfare. In a not-for-profit organization, such as a community hospital, stakeholders include managers, staff physicians, employees, suppliers, creditors, government agencies, patients, and even the community at large. Investor-owned organizations, such as a private medical practice, have essentially the same set of stakeholders, plus the owners.

> **CRITICAL CONCEPT**
> Financial Statements
>
> Financial statements are reports that summarize the financial status of an organization. The three most important financial statements are the income statement, the balance sheet, and the statement of cash flows, which together provide information about the profitability, cash flows, assets, and liabilities of a business. Along with the notes section, financial statements provide information that is useful to a wide range of users, including investors and managers.

Although financial statements were developed primarily to meet the information needs of outside parties, the owners and managers of an organization, including its board of directors (trustees), also are important users of these statements. After all, managers are charged with ensuring that the organization has the financial strength to accomplish its mission. Managers are involved not only in creating financial statements but also in assessing current financial condition and formulating plans to ensure that the organization will be able to support its mission in the future.

Annual report
A report issued annually by a business that contains descriptive information about operations over the past year and several years of historical financial statements.

Financial statements usually are distributed to the public as part of a business's **annual report**. Many large businesses, both for-profit and not-for-profit, make their annual reports available on their websites. In addition, for-profit corporations with publicly traded stock must submit financial information, including financial statements, to the Securities and Exchange Commission (SEC), which in turn makes the information available to the public. (Obtain financial statement and other related data on not-for-profit organizations at www.guidestar.org.)

SELF-TEST QUESTIONS

1. What is the purpose of a business's financial statements?
2. Who are the primary users of financial statements?

11.3 HISTORICAL FOUNDATION

It is too easy to think of financial statements as mere pieces of paper with numbers. However, if you know how and why financial statements were developed and used, you can better understand what happens in a business and why financial statements play an important role.

Thousands of years ago, individuals or families were self-contained in the sense that they gathered their own food, made their own clothes, and built their own shelters. When specialization began, some individuals became good at hunting, others at making arrowheads, others at making clothing, and so on. With specialization came trade, initially by bartering one type of goods for another.

At first, each producer worked alone, and trade was strictly local. Over time, some people set up production shops that employed workers, simple forms of money were developed, and trade expanded beyond the local area. As these simple economies expanded, more formal monetary systems developed and a primitive form of banking began, with wealthy merchants lending profits from past dealings to enterprising shop owners and traders who needed money to expand their operations.

When the first loans were made, lenders could physically inspect borrowers' assets and judge the likelihood of repayment. Eventually, though, lending became much more complex. Industrial borrowers were developing large factories, merchants were acquiring fleets of ships and wagons, and loans were being made to finance business activities at distant locations. At that point, lenders could no longer easily inspect the assets that backed their loans, and they needed a practical way of summarizing the value of those assets.

In addition, certain loans were made on the basis of a share of the profits of the business, so a uniform, widely accepted method for expressing income was necessary. In addition, owners required reports to see how effectively their own enterprises were being operated, and governments needed information for use in assessing taxes. For all these reasons, a need arose for financial statements, for accountants to prepare the statements, and for auditors to verify the accuracy of the accountants' work.

The economic systems of industrialized countries have grown enormously since the early days, and financial statements have become much more complex. However, the original reasons for these statements still apply: Bankers and other investors need the information to make intelligent investment decisions, managers rely on it to operate their organizations efficiently, and taxing authorities use it to assess taxes in an equitable manner.

Although many challenges can arise when translating physical assets and economic events into accounting numbers, healthcare businesses must do so when they construct financial statements. To illustrate the translation challenge, the numbers used to reflect a business's assets and liabilities generally reflect historical costs and prices. However, land, buildings, and equipment may have current values that are much higher or lower than their historical costs. Similarly, costs that are reported may be understated or overstated, and some costs, such as depreciation, do not even represent current cash expenses. When examining a set of financial statements, you should keep in mind the physical reality that underlies the numbers and recognize that many challenges can arise in the translation process. The presentation of financial accounting data necessarily requires businesses to make estimates and assumptions.

? SELF-TEST QUESTIONS

1. What are the historical foundations of financial statements?
2. Do any challenges arise when translating physical assets and economic events into monetary units? Give one or two illustrations to support your answer.

11.4 FINANCIAL STATEMENT REGULATION AND STANDARDS

As a consequence of the Great Depression of the 1930s, which caused many businesses to fail with subsequent large losses to investors, the federal government began regulating the form and content of financial information reported by businesses. This regulation is

Securities and Exchange Commission (SEC)
The government agency that regulates the sale of securities and the content and format of financial statements.

Generally accepted accounting principles (GAAP)
The set of guidelines, which have evolved over time, that prescribes the content and format of financial statements.

External audit
An examination of a business's financial statements by an outside party to ensure that the statements follow GAAP and are a fair representation of the economic status of the business.

based on the theory that financial information constructed and presented according to standardized rules allows investors and other stakeholders to make well-informed decisions.

During this era, the **Securities and Exchange Commission (SEC)**, an independent regulatory agency of the US government, was given the authority to establish and enforce the form and content of financial statements for large, shareholder-owned corporations. In addition, not-for-profit corporations must file financial statements with state authorities that conform to SEC standards. Most small for-profit businesses that are not technically bound by SEC-established guidelines still follow these standards to ensure uniformity of presentation of financial data. The end result is that most businesses create SEC-conforming financial statements.

Rather than directly manage the process, the SEC relies on other organizations, such as the Financial Accounting Standards Board (FASB) and the American Institute of Certified Public Accountants, to develop and implement the rules and regulations. Over time, the regulating organizations developed guidelines called **generally accepted accounting principles (GAAP)**. GAAP can be thought of as a set of objectives, conventions, and principles that have evolved through the years (and are still evolving) to guide the preparation and presentation of financial statements. In essence, GAAP set the rules for preparing financial statements.

For large organizations, the final step in the financial statement preparation process is the **external audit**, which is performed by an independent (outside) accounting firm. The purpose of this audit is to verify the quality of the organization's financial statements. The results of the external audit are reported in a letter (opinion) attached to the financial statements saying whether the statements are judged to be a fair presentation of the business's financial status as specified by GAAP.

The preparation of financial statements is as much art as it is science. Furthermore, the GAAP in force today represent years of negotiation, compromise, and interpretation, and the organizations involved are continually reviewing and revising the standards to ensure that they stay relevant as business operations and financing sources evolve over time (see "For Your Consideration: International Financial Reporting Standards").

? Self-Test Questions

1. Why are widely accepted principles important for measuring and recording economic events?
2. What does GAAP stand for, and what are their primary purpose?
3. What is the purpose of the auditor's opinion?

FOR YOUR CONSIDERATION
International Financial Reporting Standards

As the globalization of business continues, the International Accounting Standards Board has developed a common set of accounting standards in hopes that it would be accepted worldwide.

These standards, called *international financial reporting standards (IFRS)*, were intended to be applicable to for-profit businesses in more than 150 countries, including the United States. However, despite years of effort, the FASB and the International Accounting Standards Board have not yet reached convergence of IFRS with US GAAP (a process that was intended to resolve differences between US and international standards). As a result, domestic public companies must continue to prepare reports in accordance with US GAAP.

What do you think? Should financial accounting standards applicable to for-profit businesses apply worldwide as opposed to country by country? What is the rationale behind your opinion? Should the United States continue to pursue convergence of the standards?

11.5 REPORTING METHODS

Two methods can be used to prepare financial statements: cash accounting and accrual accounting (see "Critical Concept: Cash Accounting Versus Accrual Accounting"). Although each method has its own set of advantages and disadvantages, GAAP require the accrual method, so it dominates the preparation of financial statements. Still, many small businesses use the cash method, and knowledge of the cash method will help you understand the accrual method, so we discuss both.

Cash Accounting

Under cash accounting, economic events are recognized when a cash transaction occurs. For example, suppose Sunnyvale Clinic, a large multispecialty group practice, provided services to a patient in December 2016. At that time, the clinic billed the insurer, Blue Cross Blue Shield of Florida, $700, which represents the full amount that the insurer is obligated to pay. However, Sunnyvale did not receive payment from the insurer until February 2017.

If it used cash accounting, the $700 payment obligation on the part of the insurer would not appear in Sunnyvale's 2016 financial statements. The books would be closed

CRITICAL CONCEPT
Cash Accounting Versus Accrual Accounting

Financial transactions can be reported in two ways. Under cash accounting, economic events are defined by the transfer of cash. Thus, revenues are reported when the payments for services are actually received and costs are reported when the payments are made. Under accrual accounting, economic events are defined by the creation of payment obligations. Revenues are reported when the service is rendered (payment obligation is created), and costs are reported when the obligation to pay is created. Cash accounting is simpler and closely mimics the data needed for income tax filing, but accrual accounting creates statements that better represent the financial status of the business. Because GAAP require accrual accounting, most businesses, including for-profit and not-for-profit, use this method. However, many small businesses, which do not have to provide financial statements to the public, use cash accounting.

on December 31, and the $700 payment expected from Blue Cross Blue Shield of Florida would be nowhere in sight. Rather, the revenue would not be recognized (included in the financial statements) until the cash was actually received in February 2017. The core argument in favor of cash accounting is that the most important financial event is the receipt of cash, not the provision of the service and the resulting obligation to pay.

Similarly, Sunnyvale's costs of providing services would be reported when the cash is physically paid out: Inventory costs would be recognized as supplies are purchased, labor costs would be recognized when employees are paid, new equipment purchases would be recognized when the invoices are paid, and so on. To put it simply, cash accounting records the actual flow of money into and out of a business.

Cash accounting provides two advantages:

- It is simple and easy to understand. No complex rules are required for the preparation of financial statements.
- It is closely aligned to accounting for income tax purposes, and hence cash accounting statements are easy to translate into tax filing data.

Because of these advantages, some medical practices—typically smaller ones—use cash accounting. However, cash accounting has one big disadvantage: It does not present information on a business's revenue or cost obligations, which clearly affect financial condition.

Accrual Accounting

Under **accrual accounting**, the economic event that creates the financial transaction, rather than the transaction itself, is the basis for reporting. When applied to revenues, the accrual concept implies that revenue earned does not necessarily correspond to the receipt of cash. Why? Earned revenue is recognized in financial statements when a service has been provided that creates an expectation of payment, rather than when the payment is actually received.

Accrual accounting
A method of accounting that uses economic events, not cash transactions, as the basis for reporting.

For healthcare providers, the payment obligation typically falls on the patient, a third-party payer, or both. If the obligation is satisfied immediately, such as when a patient makes full payment at the time the service is rendered, the revenue is in the form of cash. Thus, the revenue is reported at that time, whether cash accounting or accrual accounting is used. However, in most situations, the bulk of the payment for services is not received until later—perhaps several months after the service is provided. In this situation, the revenue reported from the service does not indicate an immediate cash payment.

Consider the Sunnyvale example presented in the last section. Although the services were provided in December 2016, the clinic did not receive its $700 payment until February 2017. Sunnyvale's accounting (fiscal) year ended on December 31, so the clinic's books were closed after the revenue obligation was created but before the cash was received. However, because Sunnyvale uses accrual accounting, it reported this $700 of revenue on its 2016 financial statements even though no cash was collected. Under cash accounting, the $700 in revenues would not be reported until 2017, when the cash was actually received. (Note that when accrual accounting is used, the fact that the $700 in reported income was not actually received in 2016 will be disclosed elsewhere in the financial statements.)

The accrual accounting concept also applies to expenses. To illustrate, assume that Sunnyvale had payroll obligations of $50,000 for employees' work during the last week of 2016 that would not be paid until the first payday in 2017. Because the employees actually performed the work, the obligation to pay the salaries was created in 2016. Thus, the $50,000 expense would be reported on the 2016 financial statements even though no cash payment will be made until 2017. (The fact that the cash has not actually been paid out will also be disclosed elsewhere in the financial statements.)

As we discuss the specific financial statements in detail, remember the difference between cash accounting and accrual accounting. This knowledge will make it much easier for you to understand and interpret the statements.

? Self-Test Questions

1. Briefly explain the difference between cash accounting and accrual accounting.
2. Why do GAAP favor accrual accounting over cash accounting?

> **CRITICAL CONCEPT**
> Income Statement (Statement of Operations)
>
> The income statement (statement of operations or statement of revenues and expenses) reports the results of operations of a business over some period—often one year. The three major sections are revenues, expenses, and profitability (the difference between revenues and expenses). Many healthcare businesses create income statements that report two different types of profitability: (1) profits that stem solely from patient service activities (operating income) and (2) profits from all activities (net income). Other businesses report only net income. Because the income statement itself only summarizes the financial results of business operations, a great deal of explanatory and supplementary information is contained in the notes to the financial statements.

11.6 INCOME STATEMENT BASICS

In this section, we begin our discussion on the content and interpretation of a business's financial statements. The financial statements of large organizations can be long and complex, and significant leeway is afforded companies regarding the format used, even in healthcare organizations. Thus, to keep our discussion manageable, we provide simplified illustrations of the key issues.

The most frequently asked, and perhaps the most important, question about an organization's financial status is whether it is making money. The income statement summarizes the operations of an organization with a focus on its revenues, expenses, and profitability. Thus, the income statement is also called the *statement of operations* or *statement of revenues and expenses* (see "Critical Concept: Income Statement [Statement of Operations]").

While the income statements of all businesses report results using the same three major sections, the format and details can differ based on the specific industry in which the organization operates, or based on the organization's ownership. To illustrate these differences, we present income statements for two organizations: Park Ridge Homecare, an investor-owned home health agency, and Good Samaritan Medical Center, a not-for-profit hospital. First, consider the income statements of Park Ridge Homecare in exhibit 11.1. Most financial statements contain two or three years of data, with the most recent year presented first. The idea is that newer data are more important than older data, so the statements are listed in descending order of age.

The title tells us that these are annual income statements, ending on December 31, for the years 2016 and 2015. Whereas the balance sheet, which is covered in chapter 12, reports a business's financial position at a single point in time, the income statement contains operational results over a specified period. Because these income statements are part of Park Ridge Homecare's annual report, the period is one year. (Most businesses also prepare quarterly income statements, and many prepare monthly statements.) Also, note that the dollar amounts reported are listed in thousands of dollars, so the $3,996 reported as net service revenues for 2016 is actually $3,996,000.

The core components of the income statement are straightforward: revenues, expenses, and profitability. In this illustration, there are three profitability measures—one based solely on service revenues and costs, called gross profit; one based on only operating revenues and

Exhibit 11.1
Park Ridge Homecare: Statements of Income for Years Ended December 31, 2016 and 2015 (in Thousands)

	2016	2015
Net service revenues	$3,996	$2,666
Cost of service revenues	2,937	1,944
Gross profit	$1,059	$ 722
General and administrative expenses	909	649
Depreciation	21	15
Total operating expenses	$ 930	$ 664
Operating income	$ 129	$ 58
Interest income	89	86
Interest expense	16	19
Total interest income, net	$ 73	$ 67
Income before income taxes	$ 202	$ 125
Income tax expense	39	26
Net income	$ 163	$ 99

expenses, called operating income; and the third, based on total revenues and expenses, called *net income* (by for-profits) and *excess of revenues over expenses* (by not-for-profits).

Note that profitability, as measured by gross profit, operating income, or net income, may be positive or negative. When expenses exceed revenues, the result is an operating loss or net loss. In general, the greater the profitability of a business, the better the business's financial position. Although gross profit, operating income, and net income are important measures of Park Ridge's profitability, several other measures may also be used. (Chapter 13 discusses these.)

The income statement, then, summarizes the ability of an organization to generate profits. Basically, it lists the organization's income (revenues), the costs that must be incurred to produce the income (expenses), and the differences between the two (profitability). The following section discusses the major components of the income statement in detail and compares and contrasts Park Ridge Homecare's income statement with that of Good Samaritan Medical Center (shown in exhibit 11.2).

Before we close this section, be aware that the notes to the income statement usually run many pages, while the statement itself typically takes up only a single page. The explanatory and supplemental information contained in the notes is as important to read and understand as is the actual income statement.

? SELF-TEST QUESTIONS

1. What is the primary purpose of the income statement?
2. In regard to time, how do the income statement and balance sheet differ?
3. What are the major components of the income statement?
4. Are the notes to the financial statements important?

11.7 REVENUES

As discussed previously, revenues represent both the cash received to date and the unpaid obligations of payers for services provided during the period. For healthcare businesses, revenues result mostly from the provision of patient services, although some revenues result from nonoperating (financial) activities, such as interest earned on investments or contributions (for not-for-profit providers).

Revenues can be shown on the income statement in several ways. In fact, companies have more latitude in the construction of the income statement than of the balance sheet, so the income statements of different healthcare providers tend to vary somewhat in presentation. Park Ridge Homecare breaks its revenues into two sections: operating revenues, which appear at the top of the statement, and nonoperating (interest) revenues, which appear near the bottom. The income statement of Good Samaritan Medical Center, shown in exhibit 11.2, reports revenues similarly; however, the hospital reports several types of revenue that Park Ridge Homecare does not have. In addition, the complexity of the services provided by a hospital creates some differences, as discussed in the following text.

Patient service revenue
The amount of revenue collected or expected to be collected as a direct result of providing patient services without considering potential bad debt losses.

Park Ridge Homecare reported net service revenues of $3,996,000 for 2016. This line contains revenues from providing homecare services directly to consumers on an hourly basis. Other than a small amount of interest income, this money is the only source of revenue for Park Ridge.

Good Samaritan Medical Center also reported **patient service revenue** of $150,118,000 for 2016, along with several additional sources of income. The key term here is *patient service*. These are revenues that stem exclusively from the provision of patient services, as opposed to revenues from other sources, such as cafeteria sales, parking garage fees, charitable contributions, or interest earned on securities investments.

Chargemaster
A provider's official list of charges (prices) for goods and services rendered.

Determining patient services revenue for a hospital is more complicated than determining the revenue received from sales in many other organizations. Good Samaritan Medical Center, like all hospitals, has a **chargemaster** that contains the charge code and gross price for each service (or product) that it provides. However, the chargemaster price rarely represents the amount the provider expects to be paid for a particular service (see "Historical Perspective: Gross Revenues Versus Net Revenues").

EXHIBIT 11.2
Good Samaritan Medical Center: Statements of Operations for Years Ended December 31, 2016 and 2015 (in Thousands)

	2016	2015
Operating revenues		
Patient service revenue	$ 150,118	$123,565
Less: Provision for bad debts	2,000	1,800
Net patient service revenue	$ 148,118	$ 121,765
Premium revenue	18,782	16,455
Other revenue	3,079	2,704
Net operating revenues	$169,979	$140,924
Expenses		
Salaries and benefits	$126,223	$102,334
Supplies	20,568	18,673
Insurance	4,518	3,710
Lease	3,189	2,603
Depreciation	6,405	5,798
Interest	5,329	3,476
Total expenses	$166,232	$136,594
Operating income	$ 3,747	$ 4,330
Nonoperating income		
Contributions	$ 243	$ 198
Investment income	3,870	3,678
Total nonoperating income	$ 4,113	$ 3,876
Excess of revenues over expenses (net income)	$ 7,860	$ 8,206

HISTORICAL PERSPECTIVE
Gross Revenues Versus Net Revenues

Until 1996, large healthcare providers such as hospitals reported both gross patient service revenue (based on chargemaster prices) and deductions from revenue (for contractual discounts and charity care) in the revenue section of the income statement. This made the revenue reporting for healthcare providers different from businesses in virtually every other sector.

(continued)

HISTORICAL PERSPECTIVE
Gross Revenues Versus Net Revenues *(continued)*

For example, airlines have a set of full fares, such as $1,500 for a round-trip coach ticket from New York to Chicago. Most travelers in coach do not pay this fare, however. Rather, they pay restricted excursion fares that could be as low as $200. When an airline prepares its income statement, it does not list revenues at full fares and then subtract an allowance for discount fares. Only those revenues that it actually expects to receive are shown on the income statement. For reporting consistency across industries, healthcare providers eventually were forced to report revenues the same way as other companies—net of all discounts and charity care.

Under the old guidance, a healthcare provider's charity care was reported directly on the income statement as a deduction to gross patient service revenue. Thus, if $500 worth of charity services were provided to an indigent patient, the income statement would include this $500 in gross patient service revenue but deduct the $500 as charity care, resulting in $0 net patient service revenue for those services. This accounting treatment allowed providers, particularly those with not-for-profit status, to highlight the amount of charity care provided.

Today, a broad description of the organization's charity care policy, along with an estimate of the value of such care provided, typically is contained in the notes to the financial statements and is reported to the Internal Revenue Service on Form 990 (Return of Organization Exempt from Income Tax).

For example, the chargemaster price for a session with an MRI (magnetic resonance imaging) machine might be $3,500, but the contract with a particular payer might specify a reimbursement amount of only $1,300, which reflects a discount of $2,200. Discounts are accounted for before the revenue is recorded on a hospital's income statement, so the patient service revenue amounts shown on the income statement are net of discounts. For this MRI, the amount of patient service revenue reported on Good Samaritan's income statement would be $1,300, rather than the $3,500 chargemaster "price."

In addition to services provided to paying patients, some services have been provided by the hospital as **charity care** to indigent patients who do not have the ability to pay for those services. Good Samaritan has no expectation of ever collecting for these services, so, like discounts, charges for charity care services are not reflected in the $150,118,000 patient service revenue reported for 2016.

Charity (indigent) care Care provided to patients who do not have the capacity to pay.

Although Good Samaritan Medical Center reports a total of $150,118,000 for patient services provided in 2016, past experience indicates that it will not collect every dollar that it reported, though payers are assumed to have the ability to pay. Of the reported patient service revenue, Good Samaritan expects that, for one reason or another, $2,000,000 will never be collected. This amount is reported as a provision for bad debts that is subtracted from patient service revenue on the income statement. Thus, the business has already collected, or expects to collect, a total of $150,118,000 – $2,000,000 = $148,118,000 for patient services provided in 2016. This amount is reported as net patient service revenue, where *net* implies that patient service revenues have been adjusted for expected **bad debt losses**. Does the absence of a provision for bad debts on the income statement of Park Ridge imply that it has no uncollectible accounts? The answer is no. Park Ridge also has some revenues that will ultimately become uncollectible; however, the amount is small enough that it need not be reported as a separate line on the income statement. Service revenues are simply reported net of uncollectible amounts.

Bad debt losses
Revenue that is expected, but never collected, from patients (or third-party payers) who have the capacity to pay.

With bad debt losses running at about $2,000,000 ÷ $150,118,000 = 0.013 = 1.3% of patient service revenue, Good Samaritan Medical Center is not losing a high percentage to deadbeat payers. Still, margins are thin on healthcare services, so Good Samaritan should review its collection procedures to ensure that they are effective. (As discussed in chapter 7, one of the goals of receivables management is to reduce the amount of bad debt losses.)

Note the fine distinction between charity care and bad debt losses. Charity care represents services that are provided to patients who do not have the capacity to pay. Bad debt losses result from the failure to collect for services provided to patients or third-party payers who do have the ability to pay.

Beginning in 2018 (for public entities) and 2019 (for nonpublic entities), the classification and reporting of bad debt losses will change under GAAP. A new revenue recognition standard will require that hospitals and other healthcare providers consider both explicit and implicit price concessions when reporting net revenue. As discussed in earlier paragraphs, under existing GAAP, discounts and allowances and charity care are subtracted from revenue before it is reported on the income statement. These deductions are defined as explicit price concessions in the new revenue recognition standard and will be treated the same way under the new standard. However, many of the bad debt losses that are currently reported as revenue deductions under existing GAAP will be defined as implicit price concessions under the new standard and will be treated differently. For example, a patient may owe the hospital a copayment of $800 for services provided. Historical experience with similar patients, or a credit assessment performed on the specific patient, may suggest that the patient will not pay the $800. Under current GAAP, the $800 copayment is classified as a bad debt loss and is recorded as a revenue deduction on the income statement. However, under the new revenue recognition standard, the $800 would be considered an implicit price concession and would be treated similarly to charity care and discounts and allowances. In other words, the $800 would be deducted from patient service revenue before it is reported on the income statement. Only unanticipated nonpayments, such as might be associated with a patient bankruptcy, will be considered bad debt losses, and these will be recorded as an operating expense rather than a revenue deduction. The net result is an expected decline in the total amount of bad debt losses that appear as such on the income statements of healthcare providers.

new rule

Even though Good Samaritan ultimately expects to receive all of its reported net patient service revenue not yet collected, the hospital did not actually receive $148,118,000 in cash payments in 2016; some of the revenue for services provided toward the end of the year has not been received. As discussed in chapter 12, the yet-to-be-collected portion of the net patient service revenue appears on the balance sheet (exhibit 12.2) as net patient accounts receivable. The same is true for net service revenues for Park Ridge (exhibit 12.1). In addition, some of the revenue reported for services provided toward the end of 2015 (hence reported for 2015) was not collected until 2016. The point is that the actual cash revenues collected for 2016 will likely differ from the amounts reported on the income statement because both organizations use the accrual method of accounting.

Premium revenue
Revenue arising from capitated patients as opposed to fee-for-service patients.

The service revenue discussed so far reflects contracts in which the healthcare provider is paid on a fee-for-service basis. If a provider has a significant amount of revenue stemming from capitation contracts, it is often reported separately in the operating revenue section as **premium revenue**. Good Samaritan reported premium revenue of $18,782,000 for 2016.

Other revenue
Revenue that is related to patient services but not directly tied to the provision of clinical services. One common example for hospitals is cafeteria revenue.

Finally, most large healthcare organizations, such as Good Samaritan, receive some revenue related to patient service operations that does not result directly from treating patients. This revenue, which stems from such activities as cafeteria services and parking garages, is reported in the operating revenue section as **other revenue**. In 2016, Good Samaritan reported $3,079,000 of such revenue.

A description of the policies regarding revenue recognition often appear in the notes to the financial statements. To illustrate, Good Samaritan's financial statement notes include the following information:

- *Patient service revenue.* Patient service revenue represents the estimated realizable revenue amounts from patients, third-party payers, and others for services rendered. Approximately 58 percent of net patient service revenue in 2016 and 37 percent in 2015 was derived from federal and state reimbursement programs.

- *Charity care.* Good Samaritan Medical Center has a policy of providing charity care to patients who are unable to pay. Such patients are identified through financial information obtained from the patient and subsequent analysis. Because Good Samaritan Medical Center does not expect payment from these patients, estimated charges for charity care are not included in revenue. Charity care represented approximately 6 percent of revenues in 2016 and 5 percent of revenues in 2015.

- *Provision for bad debts.* The provision for bad debts is based on management's assessment of historical and expected net collections, considering business and economic conditions, trends in governmental healthcare coverage, and other collection indicators. Throughout the year, management reviews this amount and makes any modifications necessary either to recognize collections or to write off those amounts that are deemed uncollectible.

? Self-Test Questions

1. What categories of revenue may be reported on the income statement?
2. Briefly, what is the difference between patient service revenue based on chargemaster prices and reported patient service revenue? Between patient service revenue and net patient service revenue? Between net patient service revenue and other operating revenue?
3. Describe how the following types of revenue are reported on the income statement: (a) discounts from charges, (b) charity care, and (c) bad debt losses.

11.8 EXPENSES

To produce revenues (and nonoperating income listed separately on the income statement), businesses must incur expenses. Depending on the nature and complexity of the organization, the number and nature of expense items reported on the income statement can vary widely. For example, some businesses (such as Park Ridge Homecare) may report only a few categories of expenses. As shown in exhibit 11.1, Park Ridge Homecare reports its expenses in three categories: cost of service revenues, general and administrative expenses, and depreciation. This format allows readers to differentiate between the costs of providing direct care services and the costs required to operate the administrative functions of the organization. However, it does not provide a lot of detail as to the breakdown of expenses by type (e.g., wages and benefits, insurance, supplies). To find this detail, readers must look to the footnotes.

In contrast, Good Samaritan Medical Center takes a middle-of-the-road approach to the number of expense categories. Most readers of financial statements would prefer more detail than less because they can glean more insight if an organization reports revenues and expenses both by service breakdown (e.g., inpatient vs. outpatient) and by type (e.g., salaries vs. supplies).

Both Park Ridge and Good Samaritan are typical of most healthcare providers, in that the dominant portion of their cost structures (more than 70 percent) is related to labor. Good Samaritan reported salaries and benefits of $126,223,000 for 2016. The details of how these costs are broken down by service or contract, or the relationship of these expenses to volume, are typically not included in the income statement. However, some organizations provide additional details on expenses in the notes to the financial statements.

The expense item titled "supplies" represents the cost of supplies (primarily medical) used in providing patient services. Good Samaritan does not order and pay for supplies when a particular patient visit requires them. Rather, the business's managers estimate the usage of individual supply items, order them ahead of time, and then maintain a medical supplies inventory. (As discussed in chapter 12, the amount of supplies on hand is reported as inventory on the balance sheet.)

The income statement expense listing for supplies represents the cost of the items actually consumed in providing patient services. Thus, the expense reported for supplies does not reflect the actual cash spent on inventory purchases. In theory, Good Samaritan could have several years' worth of inventories at the beginning of 2016 but may have used some of these items without replenishing the stocks—hence it might not have actually spent one dime of cash on supplies during that year.

Good Samaritan uses commercial insurance to protect against many risks, including property risks, such as fire and damaging weather, and liability risks, such as managerial malfeasance and professional (medical) liability. The cost of this protection is reported on the income statement as insurance expense.

Good Samaritan owns all of its land and buildings but leases (rents) much of its diagnostic equipment. The total amount of lease payments—$3,189,000 for 2016—is reported as lease expense on the income statement. There are many reasons that health services organizations lease rather than purchase equipment, including protection against technological obsolescence. Chapter 15, which is available online, contains more information on leases and how they are analyzed (visit ache.org/books/FinanceFundamentals3).

The next expense category, depreciation, warrants closer examination. For virtually all businesses, long-lived assets such as buildings and equipment are necessary to providing goods and services. When these assets were initially purchased, Good Samaritan did not report their purchase price as an expense on the income statement, but they were listed on the balance sheet as property and equipment owned by the business.

The logic of not reporting the cost of such assets when purchased is that it would be improper to allocate the acquisition costs of long-lived assets to a single accounting period because these assets are used to produce revenues for many years. A more pragmatic reason for not reporting long-lived asset costs when they occur is that such outlays would have a severe impact on reported profitability in years when large amounts are purchased. Thus, reported profitability would fluctuate widely from year to year depending on the amount of such assets acquired.

To match the cost of long-lived assets to the revenues produced by such assets, accountants use the concept of depreciation expense, which amortizes (spreads out) the cost of a long-lived asset over many years (see "Critical Concept: Depreciation Expense"). Most people use the terms *cost* and *expense* interchangeably, but to accountants, the terms can have different meanings. Depreciation expense is a good example: The cost is the actual cash outlay for a long-lived asset, while the expense is the allocation of that cost over time.

The calculation of depreciation expense is somewhat arbitrary, so the amount of depreciation expense applied to a long-lived asset in any year generally is not closely related to the actual usage of the asset or its loss in market value. To illustrate, assume that Good

CRITICAL CONCEPT
Depreciation Expense

Depreciation expense stems from the purchase of long-lived assets such as buildings and equipment. Because such assets create revenues over many years, it makes little sense to list their entire cost in the year of purchase as an expense. To match the cost of a long-lived asset with the revenues that it is expected to produce more closely, the cost is spread over the asset's expected useful life. For example, assume an X-ray machine that costs $100,000 is purchased at the end of 2017 and is expected to have a five-year useful life and a salvage value of $25,000. For income statement purposes, the $100,000 cost, less the $25,000 salvage value estimate, would be spread over five years, so $75,000 ÷ 5 = $15,000 would be expensed in each of the next five years (from 2018 through 2022). The $15,000 amortized (spread over many years) cost of the X-ray machine when expensed (listed) on the income statement is called depreciation expense.

Samaritan owns a piece of diagnostic equipment that it uses infrequently. In 2015, the equipment was used 100 times, while in 2016 it was used only 75 times. Still, the depreciation expense associated with this equipment was the same ($1,725) in both years. In addition, Good Samaritan owns another piece of equipment that could be sold today for about the same price as the business paid for it four years ago, yet each year the hospital reports a depreciation expense for that equipment, which implies loss of value.

Depreciation expense, like all other financial statement entries, is calculated in accordance with GAAP. The calculation typically uses the **straight-line method**—that is, the depreciation expense is obtained by dividing the cost of the asset (less its estimated **salvage value**) by the number of years of its estimated useful life. The result is the asset's annual depreciation expense, which is the charge reflected in each year's income statement over the estimated life of the asset and, as discussed in chapter 12, accumulated over time on the balance sheet.

Straight-line method
A method for calculating the depreciation expense of a long-lived asset that assumes the loss of value is constant over time (follows a straight line).

Salvage value
The estimated value of a long-lived asset at the end of its useful life.

The term *straight-line* stems from the fact that the depreciation expense is constant in each year, and hence the implied value of the asset declines evenly (like a straight line) over time. How is the useful life of a long-lived asset determined? Accountants use tables that list the useful lives of various classes of assets. For example, certain medical equipment has a five-year useful life, while office furniture has a 20-year life.

Both the income statements of Park Ridge and Good Samaritan report interest expense. Park Ridge had an obligation to pay its lenders $16,000 in interest expense for debt capital supplied during 2016, while Good Samaritan had a similar obligation of $5,329,000.

Not all of the interest expense reported was paid in 2016, because Park Ridge and Good Samaritan typically pay interest monthly or semiannually, and hence some portion of the interest owed on 2016 borrowings will not be paid until 2017. Note, Park Ridge reports interest expense as a nonoperating expense, while Good Samaritan classifies interest as an operating expense. The difference reflects the leeway afforded to healthcare providers in determining the format of their income statements.

The amount of interest expense reported by an organization is influenced primarily by its capital structure, which reflects the amount of debt that it uses. In addition, interest expense is affected by the borrower's creditworthiness, its mix of long-term and short-term debt, and the general level of interest rates. (These factors are covered in chapter 8.)

The final expense line on the income statement of Park Ridge Homecare reports income tax expense. Park Ridge has an obligation to pay state and local taxing authorities $39,000 on income earned in 2016. No income tax expense is reported on Good Samaritan's income statement because it is a not-for-profit entity that is tax-exempt (except for payroll taxes).

In closing our discussion of expenses, note that many income statements contain a catchall expense category labeled "other." Listed here are general and administrative expenses that are too small to list separately, including items such as marketing expenses and external auditor's fees. Although organizations cannot possibly report every expense item separately, it is frustrating for readers of financial statements to come across a large, unexplained expense item. Thus, income statements that include the "other" category often add a note that provides additional detail.

? Self-Test Questions

1. What is an expense?
2. Briefly, what are some of the commonly reported expense categories?
3. What is the logic behind depreciation expense, and how is it calculated?

11.9 OPERATING INCOME

Although the reporting of revenues and expenses is clearly important, the most important information on the income statement is profitability. As shown in exhibits 11.1 and 11.2, different profit measures can be reported on the income statement. (Not all healthcare organizations report all measures; some report only the final measure, net income.)

The first profitability measure reported by Park Ridge Homecare is gross profit, calculated in exhibit 11.1 as net service revenues minus cost of service revenues. This measure reflects the amount of profit earned from providing direct patient services, excluding administrative costs. The next measure, reported by both Park Ridge and Good Samaritan, is operating income (see "Critical Concept: Operating Income"). In exhibit 11.1, operating income is calculated as gross profit minus total operating expenses, and in exhibit 11.2 as net operating revenues minus total expenses. The precise calculation is tied to the format of the income statement, but the general idea of operating income is to focus on revenues and expenses that are related to operations (the provision of patient services).

> **CRITICAL CONCEPT**
> **Operating Income**
>
> Operating income measures the profitability of a healthcare organization's core activities—the provision of patient services and those activities that are directly related. It eliminates any income resulting from sources unrelated to patient services, such as contributions and securities investments. Many analysts consider operating income to be the most important income statement measure of a healthcare business's profitability. After all, if an organization cannot make a profit on its core business, its financial sustainability is in doubt.

Operating income measures the profitability of core operations (patient services and related endeavors). Many healthcare providers, especially large ones, have significant revenues that stem from activities unrelated to patient services, so it is useful to report the inherent profitability of the core business separately from the overall profitability of the enterprise.

For example, Good Samaritan reported $3,747,000 of operating income in 2016, which means that the provision of healthcare services and directly related activities generated a profit of $3,747,000. Operating income is an important measure of a healthcare business's profitability because it focuses on the core activities of the business (see "For Your Consideration: Will the Real Operating Income Please Stand Up?"). Some healthcare businesses report a positive net income (net income is discussed in section 11.11) but a negative operating income (an operating loss). This situation is worrisome, because a business is on shaky financial ground if its core operations are losing money, especially if they do so year after year.

Note that the operating income reported on the income statement represents an estimate of the long-run operating profitability of the business. It has some shortcomings—for one, it does not represent cash flow—that are similar to the shortcomings related to net income discussed later. Still, measuring the profitability of a business is critical to understanding its financial status, and measuring operating income gives managers and other interested parties a feel for the profitability of a health services organization's core operations.

Self-Test Questions

1. What is operating income?
2. Why is operating income such an important measure of profitability?

FOR YOUR CONSIDERATION
Will the Real Operating Income Please Stand Up?

Who would think it would be hard to measure operating income? After all, the basic definition is straightforward: operating revenues minus operating expenses. Still, different analysts can look at the same set of revenue and expense data and calculate different values for operating income.

The problem with calculating operating income lies primarily in the definition of what constitutes a provider's operations (core activities). Defining operations can be approached in at least three ways: (1) by including patient care activities only; (2) by including patient care and directly related activities, such as cafeteria and parking garage operations; and (3) by including patient care, directly related activities, and government appropriations. Each definition results in a different value for operating income. In general, as the definition of core operations expands, the value calculated for operating income increases.

What do you think? Consider the hospital field. What activities should be considered part of core operations? Should hospitals be required by GAAP to report multiple measures of operating income, each using a different definition of core activities?

11.10 NONOPERATING INCOME

Nonoperating income The income of a healthcare provider that is unrelated to the provision of patient services. The two most obvious examples are income from securities investments and income from charitable contributions (for not-for-profit businesses).

The next section of the income statement lists **nonoperating income**. As mentioned earlier, reporting the revenues of operating and nonoperating activities separately is useful. The revenues from Good Samaritan Medical Center's operating activities, for example, are reported in the revenue section of exhibit 11.2. However, the income (revenues) generated from activities unrelated to the provision of healthcare services is reported separately in a lower section on the income statement.

The first category of nonoperating income listed for Good Samaritan is contributions. Many not-for-profit organizations, especially those with large, well-endowed foundations, rely heavily on charitable contributions—as well as earnings on securities investments—as a revenue source. Those charitable contributions that can be used immediately (spent now) are reported as nonoperating income. However, contributions that create a permanent endowment fund, and hence are not available for immediate use, are not reported on the income statement.

The second category of nonoperating income is investment income, which stems from two primary sources:

1. Healthcare businesses usually have funds available that exceed the minimum necessary to meet current cash expenses. Because cash earns no interest, these

"excess" funds usually are invested in short-term, interest-earning securities, such as Treasury bills or money market mutual funds. Sometimes these invested funds can be quite large—say, when a business is building up cash to make a tax payment or to start a large construction project. In addition, prudent businesses keep a reserve of funds on hand to meet unexpected emergencies. The interest earned on such funds is listed as investment income.

2. Not-for-profit businesses may have a large amount of endowment fund contributions. When these contributions are received, they are not reported as income because the funds are not available to be spent. However, the income from securities purchased with endowment funds is available to the healthcare organization, and hence this income is reported as nonoperating (investment) income.

In total, Good Samaritan reported $4,113,000 of nonoperating income for 2016, consisting of $243,000 in spendable contributions and $3,870,000 earned on the investment of excess cash and endowments. Nonoperating income is not central to the core business, which is providing healthcare services. Overreliance on nonoperating income to create profitability could mask operational inefficiencies that, if not corrected, could lead to future financial problems.

Note that the costs associated with creating nonoperating income are not separately reported. Thus, the expenses associated with soliciting contributions or investing excess cash and endowments are mixed in with the operating expenses listed in the expense section of the income statement. Thus, the amounts reported for nonoperating income really represent revenues because no costs have been deducted. Some organizations may report nonoperating income net of associated expenses, while others may report both nonoperating income and expenses in a single nonoperating section of the income statement.

Finally, note that the income statements of some providers do not contain a separate section titled "nonoperating income." Rather, nonoperating income is included in the revenue section that heads the income statement. In this situation, total revenues reported in the top section include both operating and nonoperating revenues.

? Self-Test Questions

1. What is nonoperating income?
2. Why is nonoperating income reported separately from revenues? Is this always the case?
3. Is nonoperating income truly income, or is it actually a type of revenue?

> **CRITICAL CONCEPT**
> Net Income
>
> Net income measures the total profitability of a business, including both operating and nonoperating income. Although operating income is an important profitability measure because it focuses on a healthcare business's core operations, the financial condition of the business ultimately depends on overall profitability, which is reported as net income. Healthcare providers can lose money on core operations yet still be above water financially if operating losses are covered by nonoperating income. However, this situation is not desirable in the long run.

11.11 NET INCOME

The final profitability measure reported by Park Ridge Homecare is net income, which on exhibit 11.1 is equal to Income before income taxes − Income tax expense. Park Ridge reported net income of $163,000 for 2016, so $202,000 − $39,000 = $163,000. In exhibit 11.2, Good Samaritan reported net income of $7,860,000, calculated as Operating income + Total nonoperating income, or $3,747,000 + $4,113,000. (Not-for-profit organizations, such as Good Samaritan, use the term *excess of revenues over expenses* in place of *net income*, but for purposes of this discussion, we call this measure net income. See "Critical Concept: Net Income.")

Because of its location on the income statement and its importance, net income is referred to as the bottom line. In spite of the fact that Good Samaritan is a not-for-profit organization, it still must make a profit. If the business is to offer new services in the future, it must earn a profit today to produce the funds needed to purchase new assets. Furthermore, because of inflation, Good Samaritan could not even replace its existing assets as they wear out or become obsolete without the funds generated by positive profitability. Thus, turning a profit is essential for the long-term viability of all businesses, including not-for-profits.

What happens to a business's net income? For the most part, it is reinvested in the business. Not-for-profit corporations must reinvest all earnings in the business. An investor-owned corporation, on the other hand, may return a portion or all of its net income to owners in the form of dividend payments. The profits reinvested in an investor-owned business, therefore, equal Net income – Dividends. (Some for-profit businesses distribute profits to owners in the form of bonuses, which often occurs in medical practices. However, when such distributions are made, they become an expense item that reduces net income rather than a distribution of net income. The result is the same—profits are distributed to owners—but the reporting mechanism is different.)

Note that both operating income and net income measure profitability as defined by GAAP. In establishing GAAP, accountants have created guidelines that attempt to measure the economic income of a business, which is a difficult task because economic gains and losses often are not tied to easily identifiable events.

Furthermore, some of the income statement items (e.g., provision for bad debt losses) are estimates and others (e.g., depreciation expense) do not represent actual cash revenues or costs. Because of accrual accounting and other factors, the fact that Park Ridge reported net income of $163,000 for 2016 does not mean that the business experienced a net cash inflow of that amount. This point is discussed in greater detail in the next section (see also "Healthcare in Practice: Sources of Hospital Profitability").

Self-Test Questions

1. Why is net income called the bottom line?
2. What is the difference between net income and operating income?

HEALTHCARE IN PRACTICE
Sources of Hospital Profitability

Ask the average healthcare manager this question: "Do hospitals make money?" Most would answer, "Yes, but not very much." Follow up with this question: "How do hospitals make money?" The answers here might differ somewhat, but in general, most responses would be, "By providing patient services." Following are the results of one study on the components of hospital profitability.

Hospital revenues, and hence profits, come from many sources. In general, the revenue sources can be broken down into three major categories:

- *Patient service revenue*. The most obvious source of revenue stems from the provision of patient services. Hospitals generally provide both inpatient and outpatient services, including emergency, ancillary, and other patient services. The monies received from patients and insurers for these services constitute the largest source of hospital revenue. About 94 percent of total hospital revenues are generated by patient services.
- *Other operating revenue*. The second source of revenue comes from activities that are related to hospital operations but do not stem directly from the provision of patient services. Examples here include cafeteria sales and parking garage revenues. Other operating revenue constitutes 1.5 percent of hospital total revenues.
- *Nonoperating revenue*. The third source of revenue stems from activities that are totally unrelated to operations. The primary sources in this category are earnings

(continued)

HEALTHCARE IN PRACTICE
Sources of Hospital Profitability *(continued)*

on financial investments and unrestricted contributions. Nonoperating revenue accounts for about 4.5 percent of total revenues.

What is the contribution of each revenue source to overall profitability? Patient service revenue contributes about 27 percent, or less than one-third, of total before-tax profitability. Other operating revenue contributes 33 percent, while nonoperating revenue contributes 40 percent. Thus, the largest contributor, on average, to a hospital's total profitability is nonoperating revenue, while other operating revenue contributes somewhat more to profitability than does patient service revenue. Combined, non–patient service revenue accounts for 73 percent of the total profitability of an average hospital.

The largest contributor, by far, to other operating revenue is cafeteria (noninpatient food) services. Other significant sources are gift shop revenue and parking revenue. The largest source of nonoperating revenue is investment income, followed by revenue from physician office rentals and unrestricted contributions.

Although the specific contribution of patient service versus non–patient service revenue varies by ownership, non–patient service revenue clearly contributes substantially to hospital profitability. In fact, in many periods, not-for-profit hospitals would be barely profitable without the contribution of non–patient service revenue. Furthermore, for-profit hospitals, when income taxes are considered, would have their total profits cut by slightly more than half were it not for the contribution of non–patient service revenue.

These results confirm the conventional wisdom that holds that the profit earned on patient services is very thin or, for many hospitals, even negative. Thus, without non–patient service revenue, most hospitals would be facing a difficult financial future.

Note: This Healthcare in Practice is based on information in N. L. McKay and L. C. Gapenski, 2009, "Nonpatient Revenues in Hospitals," *Health Care Management Review* (July–September): 234–41.

11.12 NET INCOME VERSUS CASH FLOW

As stated previously, the income statement reports total profitability as net income, which is determined in accordance with GAAP. Although net income is an important measure of profitability, an organization's financial condition, at least in the short run, depends more on the actual cash that flows into and out of the business than it does on reported profitability. Thus, occasionally a business will go bankrupt despite a historically positive net income. More commonly, many businesses that have reported negative net incomes (net losses) for several years have survived with little or no financial damage.

How can these things happen? The problem is that the income statement is like a mixture of apples and oranges. Consider exhibit 11.1. Park Ridge Homecare reported total revenues (including interest income) of $4,085,000 for 2016. Yet, this amount of cash is not actually equal to what was collected during the year, because some of these revenues will not be collected until 2017. Furthermore, some revenues reported for 2015 were actually collected in 2016, but these do not appear at all on the 2016 income statement. Thus, because of accrual accounting, reported revenue is not the same as cash revenue.

The same logic applies to expenses. Few of the values reported as expenses on the income statement are the same as the actual cash outflows. To make matters even more complex, not one cent of depreciation expense was paid out as cash. Depreciation expense is an accounting reflection of the cost of long-lived assets, but Park Ridge did not actually pay out $21,000 in cash to someone called the "collector of depreciation." The actual cash outlays associated with reported depreciation expense occurred in past years when the long-lived assets were purchased.

Can net income be converted to net cash flow—the actual amount of cash generated during the year? As a rough estimate, net cash flow can be thought of as net income plus **noncash expenses**. Thus, the net cash flow generated by Park Ridge in 2016 is not merely the $163,000 reported net income, but this amount plus the $21,000 shown for depreciation, for a total of $184,000. Depreciation expense must be added back to net income to estimate net cash flow because initially it was subtracted from revenues to obtain net income, though there was no associated cash outlay.

Noncash expenses
Expenses that are listed on the income statement that do not represent actual cash outlays. The most prominent noncash expense is depreciation.

Here is another way of looking at cash flow versus accounting income: If Park Ridge showed zero net income for 2016, it would still be generating cash of $21,000 because that amount was listed as an expense item but not actually paid out in cash. The idea behind the income statement treatment of depreciation is that Park Ridge would be able to set aside the depreciation amount, which is above and beyond its actual operating expenses, this year and in future years.

Eventually, the accumulated total of depreciation cash flow would be used by Park Ridge to replace its existing assets as they wear out or become obsolete. Thus, the incorporation of depreciation expense into the cost, and ultimately the price structure, of services provided is designed to ensure the ability of a business to replace its buildings and equipment as needed, assuming that they could be purchased at their historical cost. To be more realistic, businesses must plan to generate net income, in addition to the accumulated depreciation funds, sufficient to replace existing assets in the future at inflated costs or to expand (grow) the business.

Understand that because of accrual accounting, the $184,000 net cash flow calculated here is only an estimate of actual cash flow for 2016, because virtually no item of revenues and expenses listed on the income statement equals its cash flow counterpart. The greater the difference between the reported values and cash values, the less reliable is the net cash flow estimate. The value of knowing the precise amount of cash generated or lost has not gone unnoticed by accountants. In chapter 12, you will learn about the statement of cash flows, which can be thought of as an income statement that has been recast to focus on cash flow.

SELF-TEST QUESTIONS

1. Why is there a difference between net income and cash flow?
2. How can income statement data be used to estimate cash flow?
3. Why do not-for-profit businesses need to make a profit?

11.13 INCOME STATEMENTS OF INVESTOR-OWNED FIRMS

What do the income statements of investor-owned firms look like? They are generally similar to those of not-for-profit businesses, except for those transactions, such as tax payments, that are applicable only to one form of ownership. Because the transactions of all healthcare organizations in the same core business are similar, ownership plays only a minor role in the presentation of financial statement data. For the most part, the differences involve labeling (e.g., net income vs. excess of revenues over expenses). In reality, more differences exist in financial statements because of lines of business (e.g., hospitals vs. home care agencies) than because of ownership.

SELF-TEST QUESTION

1. Are there appreciable differences in the income statements of not-for-profit and investor-owned businesses?

11.14 A LOOK AHEAD: FINANCIAL CONDITION ANALYSIS

Chapter 13 details the techniques used to analyze financial statements to gain insights into a business's financial condition. At this point, however, it is worthwhile to introduce

ratio analysis, one method used in financial condition analysis. In ratio analysis, values found on the financial statements are combined to form ratios that have economic meaning and hence help managers and investors interpret the numbers.

To illustrate, **total profit margin**, usually just called total margin, is defined as net income divided by total (all) revenues. For Park Ridge Homecare, net income for 2016 was \$163,000, while total (all) revenues were \$3,996,000 + \$89,000 = \$4,085,000, so the total margin was \$163,000 ÷ \$4,085,000 = 0.040 = 4.0%. Thus, each dollar of revenues produced 4.0 cents of total profit (net income). By implication, the production of each dollar of revenues required 96.0 cents of expenses.

The total margin is a measure of expense control; for a given amount of revenues, the higher the net income—and hence total margin—the lower the expenses. If the total margin for other home health businesses were known, judgments about how well Park Ridge is doing in the area of expense control, relative to its peers, could be made.

Note that the **operating margin** for 2016 was Operating income ÷ Operating revenues = \$129,000 ÷ \$3,996,000 = 0.032 = 3.2%. (On Park Ridge's income statement, operating revenues are labeled as net service revenues.) Thus, in 2016, roughly 80 percent (3.2% ÷ 4.0%) of the overall profitability of the business was generated by the provision of healthcare services (operations), while 20 percent stemmed from nonoperating sources (interest income).

Park Ridge's total margin for 2015 was \$99,000 ÷ \$2,752,000 = 0.036 = 3.6%, so the total margin increased from 2015 to 2016. In effect, Park Ridge's revenues increased faster than its expenses, which resulted in increasing profitability as measured by total margin. Managers should identify the conditions that contributed to the increase in profitability and attempt to continue this positive trend into 2017.

A complete discussion of ratio analysis can be found in chapter 13. The discussion here, along with a brief return in chapter 12, is intended to give you a preview of how financial statement data can be used to make judgments about a business's financial condition.

Ratio analysis
The process of creating and analyzing ratios from the data contained in a business's financial statements and elsewhere to help assess financial condition.

Total (profit) margin
Net income divided by all (both operating and nonoperating) revenues. It measures the amount of total profit per dollar of total revenues.

Operating margin
Operating income divided by operating revenues. It measures the amount of profit per dollar of operating revenues and hence focuses on the profitability of a business's core activities.

? Self-Test Questions

1. Explain how ratio analysis can be used to help interpret income statement data.
2. What is the total margin, and what does it measure?
3. How does the total margin differ from the operating margin?

Theme Wrap-Up: Interpreting an Income Statement

As Lori considers opening another home health care business, she wonders if she can use the financial resources of her existing facility, Park Ridge Homecare, as a springboard to support the second location. After reviewing two years' worth of Park Ridge's income statements, Lori has learned a fair amount about the revenues, expenses, and profitability of the business (and so have you).

The business significantly increased its revenues from 2015 to 2016, but, at the same time, its cost of providing services (expenses) also increased. The net result was a more than doubling of operating income from $58,000 in 2015 to $129,000 in 2016. The largest revenue source was services, while the largest expense was the cost of providing those services (primarily salaries and benefits of employees).

Because Park Ridge also had nonoperating income in 2015 and 2016, its net income (excess of revenues over expenses) was greater than its operating income. In total, the business generated $163,000 + $99,000 = $262,000 in net income over the two-year period. The business's estimated cash flow was even greater, because a noncash charge (depreciation) was subtracted as an expense even though no cash transaction occurred. Thus, operating and nonoperating revenues provided the business with cash flow that it could use in the future to improve or expand its services.

Although Lori now has a clearer picture of Park Ridge's profit status, she still does not have sufficient information to make a sound judgment about its ability to support a second location financially. For example, how much cash does Park Ridge Homecare have on hand? Does the business have any savings available to help finance a new location? Where is the business's cash coming from, and what is it used for?

To learn the answers to these questions, Lori needs to examine Park Ridge's two other financial statements: the balance sheet and statement of cash flows. These statements are the focus of chapter 12.

Key Concepts

This chapter lays out the basics of financial reporting and the income statement. Here are the key concepts:

- The field of *financial accounting* involves identifying, measuring, recording, and communicating the economic events and status of an organization.
- The financial status of an organization is reported by a set of financial statements. The three most important statements are the *income statement*, the *balance sheet*, and the *statement of cash flows*.

- The predominant users of financial statement information are the business's *stakeholders*—parties (primarily managers and investors) who have a direct financial interest in the business.
- *Generally accepted accounting principles (GAAP)* establish the standards for financial measurement and reporting. Although these principles are sanctioned by the Securities and Exchange Commission, they are developed by other organizations.
- Under *cash accounting*, economic events are recognized when the financial (cash) transaction occurs. Under *accrual accounting*, economic events are recognized when the obligation to make payment occurs. GAAP require that businesses use accrual accounting because it provides a better picture of a business's true financial status.
- The *income statement* reports on an organization's operations over a period of time. Its basic structure consists of revenues, expenses, and profitability.
- *Revenues* are monies collected or expected to be collected by the business. Revenues are broken down into categories—often, *net patient service revenue* and *other operating revenue*.
- *Expenses* are the economic costs associated with generating revenues.
- *Operating income* is the dollar amount of profit earned from patient services and other sources directly related to patient services.
- *Nonoperating income* represents income (revenue) from sources unrelated to patient services, such as contributions and earnings on securities investments.
- *Net income*, or *excess of revenues over expenses* for not-for-profits, is the dollar amount of total profit earned from both patient service operations and nonoperating sources.
- Because the income statement is constructed using accrual accounting, net income does not represent the actual amount of cash that has been earned or lost during the reporting period. To estimate cash flow, noncash expenses (primarily depreciation) must be added back to net income.
- The income statements of investor-owned and not-for-profit businesses tend to look alike. However, the income statements of healthcare organizations in different lines of business can vary in format. The good news is that all income statements have essentially the same economic content.
- *Ratio analysis*, which combines values that are found in the financial statements, helps managers and investors interpret the data with the goal of making judgments about the financial condition of the business.

In chapter 12, our discussion continues with the remaining two statements: the balance sheet and the statement of cash flows.

End-of-Chapter Questions

11.1 a. What is a stakeholder?

b. What stakeholders are most interested in the financial condition of a healthcare business?

11.2 a. What are generally accepted accounting principles (GAAP)?

b. What is the purpose of GAAP?

c. What organizations are involved in establishing GAAP?

11.3 Explain the difference between cash accounting and accrual accounting.

11.4 Briefly describe the format of the income statement.

11.5 a. What is the difference between gross (chargemaster) revenue and net patient service revenue? (Hint: Think about discounts, bad debts, and charity care.)

b. What is the difference between net patient service revenue and other operating revenue?

c. What is the difference between charity care, or financial assistance, and bad debt losses? How is each handled on the income statement?

11.6 a. What is meant by the term *expense*?

b. What is depreciation expense, and what is its purpose?

c. What are some other categories of expenses?

11.7 a. What is operating income?

b. What is net income, and how does it differ from operating income?

c. Why is net income called the bottom line?

d. What is the difference between net income and cash flow?

e. Is financial condition more closely related to net income or to cash flow?

END-OF-CHAPTER PROBLEMS

11.1 Entries for the Warren Clinic 2016 income statement are listed in the following exhibit in alphabetical order. Reorder the data to reflect income statement format.

Depreciation expense	$ 90,000
General/administrative expenses	70,000
Interest expense	20,000
Net income	30,000
Nonoperating income	40,000
Other operating revenue	10,000
Patient service revenue	440,000
Provision for bad debts	40,000
Purchased clinic services	90,000
Salaries and benefits	150,000

11.2 Consider the following income statement:

BestCare Health Insurer Statement of Operations Year Ended June 30, 2016 (in Thousands)

Revenue:	
Healthcare premiums	$26,682
Fees and other revenue	1,689
Net investment income	242
Total revenues	$28,613
Benefits and expenses:	
Healthcare costs	$15,154
Operating expenses:	
Selling expenses	3,963
General and administrative expenses	7,893
Interest expense	385
Total benefits and expenses	$27,395
Net income	$ 1,218

a. Compare and contrast this income statement with the ones presented in exhibits 11.1 and 11.2.

b. What is BestCare's total margin? How can it be interpreted?

11.3 Consider this income statement:

Green Valley Nursing Home Inc. Statement of Income, Year Ended December 31, 2016

Revenue	
Resident services revenue	$3,163,258
Provision for bad debts	(110,000)
Other revenue	106,146
Total revenues	$3,159,404
Expenses	
Salaries and benefits	$ 1,515,438
Medical supplies and drugs	966,781
Insurance and other	296,357
Depreciation	85,000
Interest	206,780
Total expenses	$3,070,356
Operating income	$ 89,048
Income tax expense	31,167
Net income	$ 57,881

a. How does this income statement differ from the ones presented in exhibits 11.1 and 11.2 and problem 11.2?
b. Why does Green Valley show an income tax expense?
c. What is Green Valley's total profit margin? How does this value compare with the values for Park Ridge Homecare and BestCare Health Insurer?
d. The before-tax profit margin for Green Valley is operating income divided by total revenues. Calculate Green Valley's before-tax profit margin. Why might this be a better measure of expense control when comparing an investor-owned business with a not-for-profit business?

11.4 Great Forks Hospital reported net income for 2016 of $2.4 million on total revenues of $30 million. Depreciation expense totaled $1 million.

a. What were total expenses for 2016?
b. What were total cash expenses for 2016? (Hint: Assume that all expenses, except depreciation, were cash expenses.)
c. What was the hospital's 2016 estimated cash flow?

11.5 Brandywine Clinic, a not-for-profit business, had revenues of $12 million in 2016. Expenses other than depreciation totaled 75 percent of revenues, and depreciation expense was $1.5 million. All revenues were collected in cash during the year, and all expenses other than depreciation were paid in cash.

a. Construct Brandywine's 2016 income statement.
b. What were Brandywine's net income, total profit margin, and cash flow?
c. Now, suppose the company changed its depreciation calculation procedures (still within GAAP) such that its depreciation expense doubled. How would this change affect Brandywine's net income, total profit margin, and cash flow?
d. Suppose the change had halved, rather than doubled, the firm's depreciation expense. Now, what would be the impact on net income, total profit margin, and cash flow?
e. Explain the reason for the similarities or differences in your answers to parts b, c, and d.

11.6 Assume that Harkers Healthcare, a for-profit corporation, also experiences the situation reported in problem 11.5. However, Harkers must pay taxes at a rate of 40 percent of pretax income. Assuming that the same revenues and expenses reported for financial accounting purposes would be reported for tax purposes, redo problem 11.5 for Harkers. Compare your answers to problem 11.5 and interpret and explain the results.

CHAPTER 12

REPORTING ASSETS, FINANCING, AND CASH FLOWS

Theme Set-Up: Understanding the Balance Sheet and the Statement of Cash Flows

Lori Gibbs, founder of Park Ridge Homecare, is considering opening a second location of her home health care business. Rather than start from scratch, she wants to use the resources of the existing organization as a financial springboard. Her task is to assess the financial condition of the current business to determine whether it can support the opening of a new enterprise.

So far, Lori knows these facts: Over the past two years, Park Ridge generated $262,000 in net income (earnings). Its estimated cash flow was even greater, because a noncash charge (depreciation) was subtracted as an expense on the income statement, though no cash transaction occurred. However, she does not know if these earnings have already been spent or are still available to help fund the new business. To find out more about these earnings, plus other information relevant to Park Ridge's financial condition, Lori set out to study two other financial statements: the balance sheet and the statement of cash flows.

By the end of the chapter, you will see how a business reports assets, financing, and cash flows.

Learning Objectives

After studying this chapter, you will be able to do the following:

- Explain the purpose of the balance sheet.
- Describe the organization and contents of the balance sheet, including the basic accounting equation.
- State the purpose of the statement of cash flows.
- Detail the contents of the statement of cash flows and the way it differs from the income statement.
- Discuss the interrelationships among the income statement, balance sheet, and statement of cash flows.

12.1 INTRODUCTION

As discussed in chapter 11, the income statement contains information about an organization's revenues, expenses, and profitability. However, it does not provide data related to what assets a business owns or how those assets are financed. Those specifics are contained in the balance sheet, the second financial statement we discuss.

In addition to the balance sheet, investors and managers recognize that financial condition, especially in the short run, is related more to the actual flow of cash into and out of a business than to economic income as reported on the income statement. The statement of cash flows focuses on this important determinant of financial condition.

Understanding the composition of each financial statement (income statement, balance sheet, statement of cash flows) is essential, but it is similarly critical to be aware of how these statements fit together. Thus, throughout this chapter, we emphasize the interrelationships among the statements.

12.2 BALANCE SHEET BASICS

Whereas the income statement reports the results of operations over a period of time, the balance sheet presents a snapshot of a business's assets and financing at a given point in time (see "Critical Concept: Balance Sheet"). The balance sheet changes every day as a business increases or decreases its assets or changes the composition of its financing. Note that the balance sheet, unlike the income statement, reflects a business's financial position as of a given date, so the data typically become invalid one day later, even when both dates are in the same accounting period.

> **CRITICAL CONCEPT**
> Balance Sheet
>
> The balance sheet is one of the three primary financial statements. Unlike the income statement, which reports the results of operations over a period (often a year), the balance sheet reports the financial position of a business at a single point in time. Specifically, the balance sheet lists the assets (resources) of a business and the claims against those assets (obligations), or how the assets are financed. The balance sheet has three basic sections: total assets, total liabilities, and equity. Perhaps the most important feature of this financial statement is that it must balance. That is, Total assets = Total liabilities + Equity.

Healthcare providers with seasonal demand, such as a walk-in clinic in Fort Lauderdale, Florida, have especially large changes in their balance sheets during the year. For such businesses, a balance sheet constructed in February can look quite different from one prepared in August. Moreover, businesses that are growing rapidly will have significant changes in their balance sheets over relatively short periods.

The balance sheet lists, as of the end of the reporting period, the resources of an organization and the claims against those resources. In other words, the balance sheet reports the assets of an organization and how those assets are financed. The balance sheet has the following basic structure:

ASSETS	
Current (short-term) assets	
Long-term assets	
Total assets	
LIABILITIES AND EQUITY	
Current (short-term) liabilities	
Long-term liabilities	
Equity	
Total liabilities and equity	

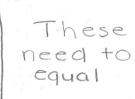

These need to equal

The upper section (assets) lists all the resources (in dollar terms) owned by the organization. In general, assets are broken down into categories that distinguish short-lived assets from long-lived assets. The lower section (liabilities and equity) lists the claims (again in dollar terms) against these resources. By claims, we mean that if the business closes and the assets are sold, the funds obtained would have to be distributed to the claimants listed in the lower section.

In essence, the lower section reports the sources of financing (capital) used to acquire the assets listed in the upper section. The sources of capital are divided into two broad categories: liabilities (financial obligations fixed by contract) and equity (a residual claim that depends on asset values and the amount of liabilities). As with assets, liabilities are listed by maturity (short-term vs. long-term).

Perhaps the most important characteristic of the balance sheet is that it must balance—that is, the total of the upper section must equal the total of the bottom section. This relationship, called the **basic accounting equation**, can be expressed in equation form:

Basic accounting equation
The relationship between balance sheet accounts that requires the balance sheet to balance. That is, total assets must equal total liabilities plus equity.

$$\text{Total assets} = \text{Total liabilities} + \text{Equity}.$$

Because liability claims are paid before equity claims if a healthcare organization is liquidated, liabilities are shown before equity, both on the balance sheet and in the basic accounting equation.

Note that the basic accounting equation can be rearranged:

$$\text{Equity} = \text{Total assets} - \text{Total liabilities}.$$

This format reinforces the concepts that equity represents an ownership (residual) claim against the total assets of the business and that equity can be negative.

To illustrate, suppose a for-profit business has \$100,000 in total assets, financed by \$50,000 in debt financing (total liabilities) and \$50,000 in ownership (equity) financing. If a business writes down (decreases) the value of some of its assets because they become obsolete, its liabilities are unaffected because it still owes these amounts to creditors and others. If total assets are written down so much that their value drops below that of total liabilities, then the equity reported on the balance sheet becomes a negative amount.

In our example, if total assets are now considered to be worth only $40,000 (as compared to $100,000 initially) but the business still owes its lenders $50,000, the only way for the basic accounting equation to hold is to have a negative equity value (in this example, –$10,000). Negative equity, which can also result from a long period of losses (negative net income), is relatively rare and reflects an ominous financial situation.

Exhibit 12.1 contains Park Ridge Homecare's balance sheets, which follows the basic structure discussed earlier. The title of the balance sheet reinforces the fact that the data are presented for the entire business. The balance sheet will not provide much information, if any, about the subparts of an organization, such as departments or service lines. Rather, the balance sheet will provide an overview of the economic position of the organization as a whole.

The timing of the balance sheet is apparent in the title. The data are reported for 2016 and 2015 as of December 31. Whereas Park Ridge's income statement indicates the data were for the years ended on December 31, the balance sheet merely indicates a closing date. This minor difference in terminology reinforces the fact that the income statement reports operational results over a period of time, while the balance sheet reports financial position at a single point in time. Finally, the amounts reported on Park Ridge's balance sheet, just as on its income statement, are expressed in thousands of dollars.

The format of the balance sheet emphasizes the basic accounting equation. For example, as of December 31, 2016, Park Ridge Homecare had a total of $1,220,000 in assets financed by a total of $1,220,000 of liabilities and equity. In addition to this obvious confirmation that the balance sheet balances, this statement indicates that the total assets of Park Ridge were valued, according to generally accepted accounting principles (GAAP), at $1,220,000.

The lower section of the balance sheet reflects the manner in which Park Ridge raised the capital needed to acquire its $1,220,000 in assets. Liabilities and equity represent claims against the assets of the business by various classes of creditors, other parties with fixed claims, and owners. Creditors and other claimants have first priority in claims for $742,000, while the owners (which, in the case of Park Ridge, means Lori Gibbs and any partners who have invested in the business) follow with a residual claim of $478,000.

If, for some reason, Park Ridge went out of business on December 31, 2016, and its assets were sold for exactly $1,220,000, liability holders would receive $742,000 of the proceeds, and the remaining $478,000 would go back to the owners. (In the case of liquidation of a not-for-profit organization, any proceeds from the sale or liquidation of the business must be used for charitable purposes.)

If the assets were worth less than $1,220,000 (but more than $742,000), the liability holders would still get their $742,000, but the amount remaining to be returned to the owners would be reduced. Conversely, sale of the assets for more than $1,220,000 would create a greater amount for the owners.

For comparison, exhibit 12.2 presents the balance sheets of Good Samaritan Medical Center. Despite the differences in lines of business and ownership, the two organizations' balance

EXHIBIT 12.1
Park Ridge Homecare: Balance Sheets as of December 31, 2016 and 2015 (in Thousands)

	2016	2015
ASSETS		
Current assets		
Cash and cash equivalents	$ 113	$ 67
Short-term investments	147	137
Accounts receivable, net	727	476
Inventories	27	22
Total current assets	$1,014	$702
Investments	$ 125	$100
Property and equipment		
Medical and office equipment	$ 56	$ 54
Vehicles	70	47
Total	$ 126	$ 101
Less: Accumulated depreciation	(45)	(24)
Net property and equipment	$ 81	$ 77
Total Assets	$1,220	$879
LIABILITIES AND EQUITY		
Current liabilities		
Notes payable	$ 13	$ 13
Accounts payable	40	21
Accrued expenses	535	363
Total current liabilities	$ 588	$397
Long-term debt	154	167
Total liabilities	$ 742	$564
Equity	$ 478	$315
Total liabilities and equity	$1,220	$879

EXHIBIT 12.2
Good Samaritan Medical Center: Balance Sheets as of December 31, 2016 and 2015 (in Thousands)

	2016	2015
ASSETS		
Current assets		
Cash and cash equivalents	$ 12,102	$ 6,486
Short-term investments	10,000	5,000
Net patient accounts receivable	28,509	25,927
Inventories	3,695	2,302
Total current assets	$ 54,306	$ 39,715
Long-term investments	54,059	31,837
Net property and equipment	52,450	49,549
Total assets	$160,815	$121,101
LIABILITIES AND NET ASSETS		
Current liabilities		
Notes payable	$ 4,334	$ 3,345
Accounts payable	5,022	6,933
Accrued expenses	6,069	5,037
Total current liabilities	$ 15,425	$ 15,315
Long-term debt	85,322	53,578
Total liabilities	$100,747	$68,893
Net assets		
Unrestricted	$ 54,068	$46,208
Temporarily restricted	1,000	1,000
Permanently restricted	5,000	5,000
Total net assets	$ 60,068	$52,208
Total liabilities and net assets	$160,815	$121,101

sheets look quite similar. The primary difference is in the labeling and reporting of equity (equity is called *net assets* in a not-for-profit), a topic that will be discussed further in the sections that follow.

In the following sections, we discuss the structure and individual balance sheet accounts in more detail.

? SELF-TEST QUESTIONS

1. What is the purpose of the balance sheet?
2. What are the three major sections of the balance sheet?
3. What is the basic accounting equation, and what information does it provide?

12.3 ASSETS

Assets either possess or create economic benefit for the organization (see "Critical Concept: Assets"). Exhibit 12.1 contains three major categories of assets: current assets, long-term investments, and property and equipment. The following sections describe each asset category in detail.

Current assets
Cash and other assets that are expected to be converted into cash within one accounting period (often a year). Examples of noncash current assets include cash equivalents, short-term investments, receivables, and inventories.

CURRENT ASSETS

Current assets include cash and other assets that are expected to be converted into cash within one accounting period, which in this example is one year. For Park Ridge Homecare, current assets totaled $1,014,000 at the end of 2016.

Suppose that the short-term investments were converted into cash as they matured; the receivables were collected; and the inventories were used, billed to patients, and collected—all at the values stated on the balance sheet. With all else the same, Park Ridge would have $1,014,000 in cash at the end of 2017. Of course, all else will not be the same, so Park Ridge's 2017 reported cash balance will undoubtedly be different from that amount. Still, this little exercise reinforces the concept behind the current asset category: the assumption that these assets will be converted into cash during the next accounting period.

The conversion of current assets into cash is expected to provide some or all of the funds needed to pay off the $588,000 in current liabilities outstanding at the end of 2016 as they become due in 2017. At the end of 2016, Park Ridge had $1,014,000 – $588,000 = $426,000 more in current assets than in current liabilities. In general, the greater this difference, the better, because more funds are expected to be converted into cash during the next year than will be required to pay the bills that are expected to become due.

! CRITICAL CONCEPT
Assets

The assets of a business represent items of value owned by the business. Some items are tangible (can be touched and felt), such as buildings, equipment, cash, and supplies inventories. Also included in tangible assets are those that are financial in nature, such as securities investments and monies owed to the business for services rendered (accounts receivable). Intangible assets include such items as the value of a trademark (think Coca-Cola) or the value created by research and development efforts. Businesses list assets on the balance sheet in order of liquidity, or the speed at which they are converted to cash. Thus, cash itself is listed first, and long-lived physical assets (property and equipment) are listed last.

CRITICAL CONCEPT
Cash and Cash Equivalents

Cash and cash equivalents make up the first current asset account listed on a business's balance sheet. Cash is actual (petty) cash plus the amount of money held in commercial checking accounts, so cash is immediately (more or less) available for disbursement. Cash equivalents are those securities investments that have a maturity of 90 days or less, such as money market funds. Such funds can be quickly converted into cash at known prices. The cash and cash equivalents account is the most liquid of a business's balance sheet accounts; that is, it consists of either cash or securities that can be turned quickly into cash at a known price.

Among Park Ridge's current assets, there is $113,000 in cash and cash equivalents (see "Critical Concept: Cash and Cash Equivalents"), an account that represents actual cash in hand plus money held in commercial checking accounts plus securities investments with a maturity of three months or less (such as money market mutual funds). There is also $147,000 of **short-term investments** (sometimes called *marketable securities*), which represent investments in highly liquid, low-risk securities, such as US Treasury bills, that have maturities greater than three months but not greater than one year. Note that cash equivalents and short-term investments are similar in nature; they differ only slightly in maturity.

Organizations hold cash equivalents and short-term investments because cash and funds held in commercial checking accounts earn no interest. Thus, businesses should hold only enough cash and checking account balances to pay their recurring operating expenses; any funds on hand in excess of immediate needs should be invested in safe, short-term, easily sellable, interest-bearing securities.

Short-term investments
Securities that are held in lieu of cash. Typically very safe, short-term securities with maturities greater than 90 days but less than one year, such as Treasury bills.

In addition to holding excess cash, short-term investments are built up periodically to meet projected nonoperating cash outlays, such as tax payments, investments in property and equipment, and legal judgments. Even though short-term investments pay relatively low interest, any return is better than none, so such investments are preferable to cash and checking account holdings.

Accounts receivable represents money owed to Park Ridge for services that have already been provided. As discussed in chapters 3 and 7, third-party payers make most payments for healthcare services, and these payments often take weeks or months to be billed, processed, and ultimately paid. The accounts receivable balance of $727,000 represents monies owed to the business for services rendered in 2016 that have not yet been received. Note that the $727,000 amount is net of allowances for uncollectible accounts. In other words, the amount listed represents the actual amount expected to be collected. Thus, the presentation on the balance sheet is consistent with the chapter 11 discussion concerning the net patient service revenue of Good Samaritan, in which only the amount actually expected to be collected is reported.

Accounts receivable
A current asset created when a service is performed but payment has not yet been received. The receivable is eliminated when the payment is collected.

The $727,000 net receivable amount listed on the balance sheet stems from the income statement's 2016 net service revenues of $3,996,000 (see exhibit 11.1 in chapter 11). The fact that $727,000 of the net service revenues remains to be collected suggests that the difference between $3,996,000 and $727,000, which totals $3,269,000, was collected during

2016. (The total is actually greater than $3,269,000 because some revenues reported for 2015 were collected in 2016.) Where is this collected cash? It could be anywhere. Most of it went right out the door to pay operating expenses, primarily for salaries and benefits. Some of the collected cash may have been spent on new equipment or on inventories that have not yet been used, and hence may be sitting in one of the asset accounts on the balance sheet.

If the business were to close its doors on the last day of 2016, its accounts receivable balance of $727,000 would fall to zero when the entire amount was eventually collected (except for any errors in the uncollectible accounts forecast). However, if Park Ridge continues as an ongoing enterprise, the receivables balance really never falls to zero because, while Park Ridge's collections are lowering it, new services are constantly being provided that create new billings—and hence new receivables—that are added to this balance.

The final current asset in exhibit 12.1, inventories, primarily reflects Park Ridge's investment in medical supplies, including drugs. The value of supplies on hand at the end of 2016 was $27,000. As with the cash account, it is not in a business's best interest to hold excessive inventories. A certain level of supplies is necessary to meet immediate expected needs and to maintain a safety stock to guard against unexpected surges in usage. Any inventories held that are above this level create unnecessary costs. Thus, many healthcare organizations limit their investment in inventories through aggressive inventory management techniques, as discussed in chapter 7.

It should be obvious that the primary purpose of the current asset accounts is to support the operations of the organization. However, current assets do not generate high returns. For example, cash earns no return, and short-term investments generally earn relatively low returns. The receivables account does not earn interest income, nor does it generate new service revenues, and inventories are essentially dollar amounts invested in items sitting on shelves, which earn no return until patients are billed for their use. Because of the low (or zero) return earned on current assets, businesses try to minimize the amounts in these accounts but ensure that the levels on hand are sufficient to keep operations running smoothly.

> ***Financial asset***
> A security such as a stock or bond that gives the holder a claim against the issuing business's cash flows.

The importance of converting inventories, accounts receivable, and cash into securities investments as quickly as possible, and hence turning zero-return assets into some-return assets, cannot be overemphasized. Under most reimbursement methods, providers must first build the current assets necessary to provide the services; then actually do the work; and then later (often 50 days or more) get paid. This demonstrates the importance of revenue cycle management, as discussed in chapter 7.

> ***Real asset***
> Property and equipment, such as land, buildings, and machines, used to create a business's cash flows.

Long-Term Investments

The second major asset category is investments. Because these investments are not listed under current assets, they represent the money Park Ridge has invested in various forms of long-term securities (those with maturities that exceed one year). Note that this account represents investments in long-term **financial assets**, as opposed to investments in **real assets**, which are listed next on the balance sheet as property and equipment. The $125,000 reported at the end of 2016 represents the amount that the business has invested in stocks, bonds, and other securities that have a longer maturity than its short-term investments and that, Park Ridge hopes, will provide a higher return.

The income earned on near cash, short-term investments, and long-term investments is reported on Park Ridge's income statement as interest income. As discussed in chapter 11, Park Ridge reported interest income of $89,000 for 2016. Some of this money came from returns on its long-term investments, and some from payers that were required to pay interest penalties on late reimbursements. A note will often reveal the details of the types of security investments held by the organization and the sources of interest or investment income.

Not-for-profit organizations often carry large amounts of long-term securities investments, as shown in exhibit 12.2. Eventually, the funds that Good Samaritan Medical Center has invested in long-term securities investments will be used to purchase buildings and equipment and other real assets that provide new or improved services to its patients.

Accumulated depreciation
The total amount of depreciation expensed over time against the fixed assets listed on the balance sheet.

In contrast, well-established investor-owned businesses usually do not build up such large reserves. Any cash flow above the amount needed for near-term reinvestment in the business would likely be returned to owners, primarily as dividends. When additional capital is needed for property and equipment purchases, an investor-owned business simply accesses the capital (debt and equity) markets for additional financing.

CRITICAL CONCEPT
Property and Equipment (Fixed Assets)

The property and equipment account on the balance sheet lists a business's land; buildings; and equipment, including vehicles, office furniture, and computers. Such physical assets have lives greater than one year and are fundamentally different from short-term assets, which are converted into cash in a relatively short time. The categories of assets that are listed as property and equipment often are called *fixed assets* because they are left in place to produce income, as opposed to, say, inventories, which are consumed to produce income. Fixed assets are listed on the balance sheet at historical cost minus the cumulative amount of depreciation taken on the listed assets. The result—net property and equipment—is the book value of a business's fixed assets.

Property and Equipment (Fixed Assets)

The third asset category is property and equipment, often called fixed assets. Fixed assets, compared to current assets, and even compared to long-term securities investments, are highly illiquid (cannot easily be bought and sold) and are used over relatively long periods (see "Critical Concept: Property and Equipment [Fixed Assets]"). Whereas the levels of current assets rise and fall spontaneously with the organization's level of operations, fixed assets (land, buildings, equipment) are normally maintained at a level sufficient to handle peak patient demand (see "For Your Consideration: Should Governments Report Like Businesses?").

Fixed assets are listed at historical cost (the purchase price) minus accumulated depreciation as of the date of the balance sheet. **Accumulated depreciation** represents the total dollars of

FOR YOUR CONSIDERATION
Should Governments Report Like Businesses?

Historically, states and cities used cash accounting methods to report the cost of infrastructure assets such as roads, bridges, and water and sewer facilities. Thus, the cost of an infrastructure investment was reported as an expense on the income statement when it occurred, but the value of the physical asset did not appear on the balance sheet. In other words, the value of all infrastructure assets was off the books.

The theory behind this treatment is that infrastructure assets are, for the most part, immovable and of value only to the governmental unit (and its residents). Because infrastructure assets cannot be sold, there is no financial value to be reported on the balance sheet. In actuality, of course, physical infrastructure assets such as roads and bridges generally continue to have value, or usefulness, long after governmental units have incurred the cost of construction. And, just as business assets depreciate in value, the value of infrastructure assets declines over time.

Thus, in 2001, the Government Accounting Standards Board mandated that states and cities treat infrastructure assets just as businesses do—record them on the balance sheet at initial cost and depreciate this value over time. The idea is that the new treatment will (1) improve financial reporting, (2) enhance awareness of fiscal issues facing governmental units, and (3) emphasize the importance of maintaining infrastructure assets.

What do you think? Should governmental entities have been required to report financial status in the same way as businesses? Has the change in how infrastructure assets are treated caused states and cities to act differently?

depreciation that have been expensed on the income statement against the historical cost of the organization's fixed assets. (Depreciation expense, which is an income statement item, was discussed in chapter 11.)

Numerically, the amounts of depreciation expense reported on the income statement each year are accumulated over time to create the accumulated depreciation account on the balance sheet. Then, the accumulated depreciation amount is subtracted from the historical cost to obtain net fixed assets (net property and equipment), which is the balance sheet (GAAP) value of a business's property and equipment.

Park Ridge lists two categories of property and equipment: medical and office equipment (with a cost of $56,000) and vehicles (with a cost of $70,000), for a total acquisition cost of $126,000. However, the accumulated depreciation amount on these assets was $45,000, so the net property and equipment balance was $126,000 – $45,000 = $81,000 at the end of 2016. (The accumulated depreciation amount is shown as a negative number because it is subtracted on the balance sheet.) Example

Gross fixed assets
The historical cost of a business's property and equipment.

Note that the historical cost of these assets, often referred to as **gross fixed assets**, was $126,000. Some of the fixed assets were purchased in 2016 and some earlier, but the total acquisition cost of all the fixed assets used by Park Ridge on December 31, 2016, was $126,000. The accumulated depreciation on these assets through December 31, 2016, was $45,000, which accounts for that portion of the assets' value that was spent in producing income.

Net fixed assets
The current accounting (book) value of a business's property and equipment. Calculated as gross fixed assets minus accumulated depreciation.

The difference between the gross amount and the accumulated depreciation, $81,000, reflects the accounting estimate of the current value of the property and equipment, called **net fixed assets**. Note that the $81,000 amount represents a book value of the business's fixed assets, as opposed to a market value, which is the amount that could be realized if the assets were individually sold (see "Critical Concept: Book Value"). Often, a more detailed explanation of the fixed-asset accounts is found in the notes to the financial statements.

As mentioned earlier, depreciation expense is the connection between the balance sheet net property and equipment account and the income statement. The accumulated depreciation of $45,000 reported at the end of 2016 is $21,000 greater than the 2015 amount of $24,000. This increase in accumulated depreciation on the balance sheet reflects the $21,000 in depreciation expense reported on the 2016 income statement.

CRITICAL CONCEPT
Book Value

Book value is the value of a business's assets as reported on the balance sheet. Note that an asset's book value might be quite different from its current, or market, value. For example, an inventory item might be obsolete and worthless, but until disposed of, it typically would be carried on the balance sheet at cost. Alternately, because of inflation, a business's office building may be worth far more than the depreciated (net) value reported on the balance sheet.

Depreciation, though it rarely reflects the true change in value of a fixed asset over time, at least ensures an orderly recognition of value loss. On occasion, assets experience a sudden, unexpected loss of value. One example is when changing technology instantly makes a piece of diagnostic equipment obsolete and hence worthless. When this occurs, the asset that has experienced the decline in value is written down, which means that its value on the balance sheet is reduced (perhaps to zero, in which case the asset is written off) and the amount of the reduction is taken as an expense on the income statement.

SELF-TEST QUESTIONS

1. What are the three major categories of asset accounts?
2. What is the primary difference between current assets and the remainder of the assets listed on the balance sheet?
3. What is accumulated depreciation, and how does it tie into the income statement?

12.4 LIABILITIES

As shown in exhibit 12.1, liabilities and equity make up the lower section of the balance sheet. Together, they represent the capital that a business has raised to acquire the assets shown in the upper section of the balance sheet. Again, by definition, total liabilities and equity must equal total assets. Another way of looking at this concept is that every dollar of assets listed in the upper section of the balance sheet must be matched by a dollar of capital from the lower section.

Liabilities represent financing, provided by individuals and businesses that have claims against the organization, that is fixed by contract (see "Critical Concept: Liabilities"). For example, employees may have unpaid wages and salaries, tax authorities may have unpaid taxes, and vendors may have unpaid bills for supplies or equipment sold to the business. (Even not-for-profit organizations, which do not pay income taxes, typically must pay payroll and withholding taxes on their employees.)

> **CRITICAL CONCEPT**
> Liabilities
>
> Liabilities represent the payment obligations of a business. Thus, liabilities stem from many sources. Perhaps the most obvious liability is money owed to lenders for furnishing debt capital. Typically, borrowers must pay lenders interest and must, at some point, repay the principal amount. These debt obligations are listed as liabilities on the balance sheet. Other liabilities include monies owed to suppliers, employees, and tax authorities. The difference between liabilities and equity is that liabilities are contractual obligations that must be paid or severe consequences can result, including bankruptcy. Businesses, even for-profit ones, have no contractual obligations to make payments to their suppliers of equity capital.

However, the largest liability claims typically are by creditors (lenders) who supplied debt capital to the business, often in the form of bank loans or bonds (for large businesses). Most creditors' claims are against the total assets of the organization (unsecured), rather than tied to specific assets that were used as collateral for the loan (secured).

In the event of default (nonpayment of interest or principal) by the borrower, creditors have the right to force the business into bankruptcy, with liquidation as a possible consequence. If liquidation occurs, the law requires that any proceeds be used first to satisfy liability claims before any funds can be paid to owners or, in the case of not-for-profits, used for charitable purposes. Furthermore, the dollar value of each liability claim is fixed by the amount shown on the balance sheet, while the owners, including the community at large for not-for-profit organizations, have a claim to the residual proceeds of the liquidation rather than to a fixed amount.

As with assets, the balance sheet presentation of liabilities follows a logical format. Current liabilities, those that fall due (must be paid) within one accounting period (one year in this example), are listed first. Long-term debt, distinguished from short-term debt by having maturities greater than one accounting period, is listed second.

As shown in exhibit 12.1, Park Ridge Homecare had total liabilities at the end of 2016 of $742,000, which consisted of two parts: total current liabilities of $588,000 and total long-term debt of $154,000. The following sections describe each liability account in detail.

Current liability
A payment obligation (liability) of a business that is due in the next accounting period, often one year.

Current Liabilities

Current liabilities are liabilities that must be paid within one accounting period (one year in this example). Many healthcare businesses use both short-term and long-term debt financing. Short-term debt, with a maturity of one year or less, usually takes the form of a bank loan and generally is used to finance temporary (seasonal) asset needs. When listed on the balance sheet, short-term debt typically is called **notes payable**. We see that Park Ridge Homecare had $13,000 of short-term debt outstanding at the end of 2016.

Notes payable
The balance sheet name typically used for a business's short-term debt, often bank loans.

Accounts payable represent payment obligations to vendors (suppliers) that have been incurred as of the balance sheet date but have not yet been paid. Often, suppliers offer their customers credit terms, which allow payment some time after the purchase is made—say, 30 days. By allowing Park Ridge to pay 30 days after it has received the supplies, the supplier is acting as a creditor. The balance sheet tells us that Park Ridge, at the end of 2016, owed its suppliers $40,000 for such credit, often called *trade credit.*

Accounts payable
Monies owed to vendors for purchased supplies. Payables arise when vendors offer trade credit (terms that allow the buyer to pay some time (say, 30 days) after the supplies have been purchased).

Wages and benefits due to employees, interest due on debt financing, taxes due to state and federal taxing authorities, accrued utilities expenses, and similar items are included on the balance sheet as **accrued expenses (accruals)**. We can use Park Ridge's employees to illustrate the logic behind accruals.

The staff earns wages and benefits on a daily basis as the work is performed. However, the business pays its workers every two weeks on the Thursday following the pay period that ended the previous Friday. Therefore, there is always an obligation to pay for work that has already been performed. Whenever the obligation to pay wages extends into the next accounting period, an accrual is created on the balance sheet. This obligation, as well as taxes due to government authorities and interest due to lenders, appears on Park Ridge's balance sheet as an accrual. At the end of 2016, the business owed $535,000 to its employees, creditors, and tax authorities.

Accrued expenses (accruals)
Monies owed to various parties, such as to employees, for services rendered. Also includes interest owed to lenders and tax obligations.

In total, at the end of 2016, current liability accounts provided $588,000 in financing for Park Ridge. In effect, these funds represent "loans" provided to the business by lenders, suppliers, employees, and taxing authorities that must be paid in 2017. In fact, most of these obligations must be paid in a much shorter time than one year; many are due just a few days or weeks into the year.

Long-Term Debt

Long-term debt
Debt financing that has a maturity greater than one accounting period.

The **long-term debt** section of exhibit 12.1 includes debt financing to the organization with maturities of more than one year. The long-term debt section lists any debt owed to banks and other creditors, such as bondholders, as well as obligations under certain types of lease arrangements. Usually, detailed information relative to the specific characteristics of the long-term debt is disclosed in the notes to the financial statements. For example, the notes to Park Ridge's financial statements indicate that the business's long-term debt consists of a bank loan with a 10 percent interest rate that matures in 2026.

At the end of 2016, Park Ridge had total liabilities—combined current liabilities and long-term debt—of $742,000. As discussed in the next section, Park Ridge reported $478,000 in equity, for total financing (which must equal total assets) of $1,220,000. Thus, based on the values recorded on the balance sheet (book values), Park Ridge uses more debt financing than equity financing.

SELF-TEST QUESTIONS

1. What are liabilities?
2. What are some of the accounts that would be classified as current liabilities?
3. Use an example to explain the logic behind accruals.
4. What is the difference between notes payable and long-term debt?

12.5 EQUITY (NET ASSETS)

On the balance sheet, the equity (ownership) claim on an organization's assets is called **net assets** when the organization has not-for-profit status. As the term *net* implies, net assets represent the dollar value of assets remaining when a business's liabilities are stripped out. However, as detailed in chapter 2, the healthcare field has a variety of ownership types, which results in the various names used in the equity section of the balance sheet. To keep terminology manageable, we use the word *equity* to specify nonliability (ownership) capital (see "Critical Concept: Equity").

Net assets
The term used to designate the equity on a not-for-profit organization's balance sheet.

To determine what amount belongs to the owners, whether explicitly recognized in for-profit businesses or implied in not-for-profit organizations, fixed claims (liabilities) are subtracted from the value of the business's assets. The remainder, the equity, represents the residual value of the organization's assets.

CRITICAL CONCEPT
Equity

Equity represents the value of a business that remains when the value of its liabilities is subtracted from asset value. Perhaps the best way to consider this concept is in terms of home ownership. Suppose you own a home that is worth $200,000 today. However, you have a mortgage on the home with a $150,000 balance. In this situation, the balance sheet for the home would look like the following statement:

(continued)

CRITICAL CONCEPT
Equity *(continued)*

ASSETS	
Home	$200,000
Total assets	$200,000
LIABILITIES AND EQUITY	
Mortgage	$ 150,000
Equity	50,000
Total liabilities and equity	$200,000

The $50,000 represents the value of the home to the owner. If you sold the home today for $200,000 and paid off the mortgage balance of $150,000, you could pocket $50,000. (Of course, you would have no place to sleep!)

A business's equity is similar. If a business sold off its assets and realized the exact amounts listed on the balance sheet and then used the proceeds to pay off its liabilities, the amount in the equity section would be left. If the business were for-profit, the owners would receive that amount. If the business were not-for-profit, the amount would belong to the community at large and would have to be used for some charitable purpose.

Note that this balance sheet was created using market values. That is, the $200,000 value of the home is an estimate of its price if sold today, as opposed to book values, which are created following accounting rules (GAAP).

Also, note what would happen if the value of your home dropped to $150,000. Your equity value would drop to $0; you would be wiped out. Even worse, what would happen if the value dropped to $125,000? To make the balance sheet balance, your equity balance would have to be –$25,000. Now you owe more on the home than it is worth, which is called being *underwater*.

Park Ridge Homecare's equity increased by $163,000 from 2015 to 2016, which is the same amount that it reported on the income statement as net income (excess of revenues over expenses in a not-for-profit) for 2016. This connection between the bottom line of the income statement and the equity section of the balance sheet is a mathematical necessity. In the case of not-for-profit businesses, there is simply nowhere else for those earnings to go. This scenario highlights a second connection (the first was depreciation) between the balance sheet and the income statement.

Park Ridge's balance sheet balances because the increase in equity of $163,000 was matched by a like increase in assets, along with asset increases that resulted from other financing. The asset increases might be in cash, receivables, fixed assets (property and equipment), or some other account.

The key point is that the equity account is not a store of cash. As Park Ridge earns profits that increase the equity account, these funds are invested in supplies, property and equipment, and other assets to provide future services that would likely generate even larger profits in the future. Park Ridge's total assets grew by $1,120,000 – $879,000 = $341,000 in 2016, which was supported by an increase in total liabilities of $742,000 – $564,000 = $178,000 and an increase in equity (net assets) of $163,000. Thus, the increase in the lower section of the balance sheet, $178,000 + $163,000 = $341,000, was the same as the increase in the upper section. After all, the balance sheet must balance.

Thus far, the discussion of the balance sheet has focused on Park Ridge Homecare, a for-profit organization. In general, the asset and liability sections of the balance sheet are much the same, regardless of ownership status (see "Healthcare in Practice: The Average Home Health Care Business"). The equity section tends to differ in presentation for different types of ownership because the forms of equity differ. That is the bad news. The good news is that the economic substance of the equity section remains the same.

HEALTHCARE IN PRACTICE
The Average Home Health Care Business

When financial statements are created for entire industries, as opposed to individual businesses, it is most useful to express the balance sheet accounts and income statement items in percentages rather than in dollars. That way, easy comparison can be made between a specific business (e.g., Park Ridge Homecare) and the sector in which it operates. Financial statements that are expressed in percentages rather than dollars are called common-size statements.

The average home health care business's common-size income statement looks like the following:

Total revenues	100.0%
Operating expenses	90.3
Operating profit	9.7%
All other expenses	2.9
Profit before taxes	6.8%

(continued)

HEALTHCARE IN PRACTICE
The Average Home Health Care Business *(continued)*

Note that this format does not match the format of Park Ridge Homecare's income statement given in exhibit 11.1. Unfortunately, sectorwide data, which come from many sources, typically are summarized using a more generic format than specified by GAAP. This is just a fact of life.

The bottom line for the sector is that the average home health care business makes 6.8 percent (6.8 cents) before taxes on every dollar of revenue. But let's not get too far ahead of ourselves; we analyze Park Ridge's financial condition in detail in chapter 13. However, remember from chapter 11 that Park Ridge had a total margin—defined as total profits divided by total revenues—of 4.0 percent. As compared to the average 6.8 percent profit before taxes for the national average, Park Ridge is not as profitable.

Here is what the average home health care business's balance sheet looks like:

ASSETS	
Current assets	
Cash and cash equivalents	22.6%
Receivables	31.1
Inventories	1.7
Other current assets	3.9
Total current assets	59.3%
Fixed assets	17.5
Other long-term assets	23.2
Total long-term assets	40.7%
Total assets	100.0%
LIABILITIES AND EQUITY	
Current liabilities	
Short-term debt	13.5%
Accounts payable	8.5
Other short-term expenses	18.7
Total current liabilities	40.7%
Long-term debt	23.3
Total liabilities	64.0%
Equity	36.0%
Total liabilities and equity	100.0%

HEALTHCARE IN PRACTICE
The Average Home Health Care Business *(continued)*

Note that Park Ridge had a debt ratio—defined as total debt (total liabilities) divided by total assets—of 60.8 percent in 2016. The average home health care business has a debt ratio of 64.0 percent (the total liabilities percentage reported in the balance sheet). Thus, Park Ridge has less debt (liability) financing than the national average.

We could go on to examine other elements of the sector's financial statements, and you are welcome to do so. However, we do not want to steal the thunder from the next chapter, so we will wait until then.

Note: This Healthcare in Practice is based on data in Risk Management Association (RMA), 2016, *Annual Statement Studies: 2015–2016*, Philadelphia: RMA.

SELF-TEST QUESTIONS

1. What is equity (net assets)?
2. What is the relationship between the equity account on the balance sheet and earnings (net income) reported on the income statement?

Restricted account
An account with funds restricted to specific uses by donors.

12.6 FUND ACCOUNTING

One unique feature of many not-for-profit balance sheets is that they classify certain asset and equity accounts as **restricted accounts**. When a not-for-profit organization receives contributions that donors have indicated must be used for a specific purpose, the organization must create multiple funds to account for its assets and equity. Each fund typically has assets, liabilities, and an equity balance.

Because the balance sheet of an organization that receives restricted contributions is separated into restricted and unrestricted funds, this form of accounting is called *fund accounting* (see "Critical Concept: Fund Accounting"). Only contributions to not-for-profit organizations are tax

CRITICAL CONCEPT
Fund Accounting

Fund accounting involves the separation of balance sheet accounts into separate funds by designated purpose. Thus, an investment account shown on the balance sheet might be labeled as restricted, meaning that the dollar amount of that account must be used for a specific purpose, which often is designated by donors. Another investment account might be labeled as unrestricted, meaning it is available for any use deemed appropriate by management. Fund accounting typically is used by not-for-profit businesses (and charities), although such businesses are encouraged to also create a set of more standard financial statements for public distribution.

deductible to the donor, and hence few contributions are made to investor-owned healthcare businesses. Thus, fund accounting is only applicable to not-for-profit organizations.

Restricted contributions impose legal and fiduciary responsibilities on healthcare organizations to carry out the written wishes of donors. Thus, numerous rules are associated with fund accounting—however, as they go well beyond the scope of this book, they will not be discussed here.

The good news is that GAAP encourage organizations that use fund accounting to present balance sheets to outside parties using consistent formats. Through the end of 2017, balance sheets of organizations that use fund accounting will have roughly the same look as shown in exhibit 12.2. Good Samaritan Medical Center reports its net assets in three categories depending on the nature of donor restrictions. Unrestricted net assets reflect contributions with no restrictions on their use (either because the donor did not impose a restriction or the organization used the contribution in accordance with the donor's wishes). Unrestricted net assets is also the equity account that is increased by the organization's earnings (net income) during the accounting period. Temporarily restricted net assets reflect contributions with restrictions on use or time. Finally, permanently restricted net assets reflect contributions that are intended to be maintained and invested by the organization for its long-term support.

Starting with annual financial statements issued for fiscal years beginning after December 15, 2017, the display of net assets on the balance sheets of not-for-profit organizations will be simplified to include only two categories: net assets with donor restrictions and net assets without donor restrictions. Organizations will continue to be required to report total net assets as well. The new accounting standard will also increase the information available to users in the footnotes. Specifically, organizations will be required to disclose how various designations, appropriations, and restrictions on assets affect the use of resources.

The reporting of fund accounting information gives financial statement users a picture of limitations that may exist on the way resources may be spent. However, with the exception of further breakdown into unrestricted and restricted accounts, balance sheets of organizations that use fund accounting have the same economic content as those prepared by businesses that do not use fund accounting.

Self-Test Questions

1. What is fund accounting?
2. What type of a healthcare organization is most likely to use fund accounting?
3. Is there a significant difference in the economic content of balance sheets created by investor-owned and not-for-profit healthcare organizations?

12.7 THE STATEMENT OF CASH FLOWS

The balance sheet and income statement are traditional financial statements that GAAP have required for many, many years. In contrast, the statement of cash flows has only been required for for-profit businesses since 1989 and for not-for-profit businesses since 1995. The statement of cash flows was created in response to demands by users for better information about a firm's cash inflows and outflows (see "Critical Concept: Statement of Cash Flows").

> **CRITICAL CONCEPT**
> Statement of Cash Flows
>
> The statement of cash flows can be thought of as an income statement that has been converted from accrual accounting to cash accounting. In essence, the statement of cash flows reports where a business gets its cash and what it does with that cash. The statement is organized into three major sections: The first section focuses on operating flows, the second on investment flows, and the third on financing flows. In addition, there is a short section that reconciles the net cash flow reported on the statement to the change in the cash reported on the balance sheet.

While the balance sheet reports the cash balance on hand at the end of the period, it does not provide details on why the cash account is greater or smaller than the previous year's value, nor does the income statement give detailed information on cash flows.

In addition to the problems of accrual accounting and noncash expenses discussed in chapter 11, some cash raised by a business may not even appear on the income statement. For example, Park Ridge Homecare may have raised cash during 2016 by taking on more debt or by selling some equipment. The income statement does not show these flows, yet they affect a firm's cash balance.

Finally, the cash coming into a business does not just sit in the cash account. Most of it goes to pay operating expenses or to purchase other assets, or for investor-owned firms, some may be paid out as dividends. Thus, the cash account does not increase by the full amount of cash generated, and it would be useful to know how the difference was spent. The statement of cash flows details where cash resources came from and how they were used.

Park Ridge's 2016 and 2015 statements of cash flows are presented in exhibit 12.3. To simplify the discussion, the content of the statements has been reduced, so they are somewhat shorter and easier to comprehend than most real-world statements. Nevertheless, an understanding of the composition and presentation of exhibit 12.3 will give you an appreciation for the value of the statement of cash flows. Also, note that an alternative format of this statement differs in how the operational cash flows are reported but not in overall structure.

The format of the statement of cash flows makes it easy to understand why Park Ridge's cash position increased by $46,000 during 2016. In other words, the statement tells us Park Ridge's sources of cash and how this cash was used.

EXHIBIT 12.3
Park Ridge Homecare: Statements of Cash Flows for Years Ended December 31, 2016 and 2015 (in Thousands)

	2016	2015
Cash flows from operating activities		
Cash received from services	$3,740	$2,542
Cash paid to employees and suppliers	(3,694)	(2,536)
Interest paid	(16)	(19)
Interest earned	89	86
Net cash from operations	$ 119	$ 73
Cash flows from investing activities		
Purchase of property and equipment	(25)	(19)
Securities purchases	(35)	(15)
Net cash from investing activities	($ 60)	($ 34)
Cash flows from financing activities		
Repayment of long-term debt	($ 13)	$ 0
Net cash from financing activities	($ 13)	$ 0
Net increase (decrease) in cash and equivalents	$ 46	$ 39
Cash and equivalents, beginning of year	$ 67	$ 28
Cash and equivalents, end of year	$ 113	$ 67

The statement is divided into three major sections: cash flows from operating activities, cash flows from investing activities, and cash flows from financing activities.

Cash Flows from Operating Activities

The first section focuses on the sources and uses of cash tied to operations. Of course, the most important source is cash received from the provision of patient services, so its value for 2016—$3,740,000—is listed first.

Note that this amount is not the same as that listed for net service revenues on the income statement. As you know, income statement revenues follow accrual accounting guidelines, but the statement of cash flows follows cash accounting guidelines. Thus, Park Ridge "booked" $3,996,000 in operating revenues in 2016, but the cash collected in that year was only $3,740,000.

The next item in the section is cash paid to employees and suppliers. As we just discussed, because of accrual accounting, the total cash outlay in 2016—($3,694,000)—does not exactly match the total of the cost of service revenues, general and administrative expenses, and income tax expense listed on the income statement. The statement of cash flows focuses on the actual movement of cash into and out of a business, while the income statement centers on the obligations that create those cash flows. Note that the cash paid to employees and suppliers is enclosed in parentheses in exhibit 12.3. On the statement of cash flows, all outflows are shown in parentheses to differentiate them from inflows.

The interest paid and interest earned items are listed here as operating activities, which shows some leeway in formatting. These flows could also be listed in the financing activities section rather than the operating activities section.

Totaling all the operating activities entries, Park Ridge reported $119,000 in net cash from operations for 2016. For a business, whether investor owned or not-for-profit, to be financially sustainable, it must generate a positive cash flow from operations. Thus, at least for 2016 and 2015, Park Ridge's operations are doing financially what they should be doing—generating cash.

Furthermore, the business's cash flow from operations increased 63 percent from 2015 to 2016. Much of this increase was the result of growth in volume, but other factors also played a role. Lori Gibbs, the founder of Park Ridge Homecare, should identify those factors that contributed to the increase and take appropriate action to ensure another increase in 2017. Unlike the situation reported by Park Ridge, a consistent negative net cash flow from operations sends a warning to managers and other stakeholders that the business may not be economically sustainable.

Cash Flows from Investing Activities

The investing activities section contains cash flows related to investments in both fixed assets (property and equipment) and securities used as alternatives to cash holdings. Note that this section does not contain cash flows related to the financing of the business; such flows are listed in the next section.

As evidenced by the 2015 to 2016 change in total (gross) property and equipment derived from the balance sheets, Park Ridge spent $126,000 – $101,000 = $25,000 to acquire additional fixed assets. Thus, roughly one-quarter of the business's operating cash flow was spent on new property and equipment. This fact should not be alarming, as long as the investments are prudent. (Chapters 9 and 10 contain a great deal of insight into what makes a prudent capital investment, at least from a financial perspective.)

The next line in the investing activities section lists $35,000 in securities purchases (an outflow) for 2016. The changes in balance sheet accounts from 2015 to 2016 indicate that Park Ridge invested $10,000 in short-term investments and $25,000 in long-term investments (which require a use of cash).

When both entries are considered, Park Ridge experienced a net cash outflow from investing activities of $60,000 in 2016.

Cash Flows from Financing Activities

This third section focuses on financing flows, that is, those flows that arise from the financing of a business's assets and operations. This section shows that $13,000 was spent in 2016 to repay long-term debt financing.

Net Increase (Decrease) in Cash and Reconciliation

After the three major sections, the next line in the statement of cash flows is the net increase (decrease) in cash and equivalents. This number is the sum of the totals from the three major sections. For Park Ridge in 2016, the net increase in cash and equivalents is $119,000 – $60,000 – $13,000 = $46,000.

Unlike the so-called bottom line of the income statement, the change in cash line has limited value in assessing an organization's financial condition because it can be manipulated by investing and financing activities. If an organization is losing cash on operations, but its managers want to report an increase in the cash account, in most cases they simply can borrow the funds necessary to show a net cash increase on the statement of cash flows. Thus, the net cash from operations line is a more important indicator of financial well-being than is the net increase (decrease) in cash line.

The net increase (decrease) in cash line is used to verify the correctness of the entries on the statement of cash flows. As shown in exhibit 12.3, the $46,000 increase in cash reported by Park Ridge for 2016 added to the $67,000 beginning-of-year cash balance totals $113,000. A check of the end-of-2016 cash balance shown on the exhibit 12.1 balance sheet confirms the amount calculated on the statement of cash flows.

In summary, the income statement focuses on accounting profitability, while the statement of cash flows follows the movement of cash—that is, where did the money come from, and how did the organization use it? The major concern for the income statement is economic profitability as defined by GAAP; for the statement of cash flows, it is cash viability (see "For Your Consideration: Which Financial Statement Is the Most Important?"). Is the organization generating, and will it continue to generate, sufficient cash to meet both short-term and long-term needs?

FOR YOUR CONSIDERATION
Which Financial Statement Is the Most Important?

Although all of the financial statements are important, many argue that either the balance sheet or the cash flow statement is most important. The most common argument in support of the balance sheet is that it gives the broadest picture of the company's financial position. A comparison of assets to debt lets you know how leveraged the business is and hence whether or not bankruptcy is a concern. Managers, creditors,

FOR YOUR CONSIDERATION
Which Financial Statement Is the Most Important? *(continued)*

and investors (both creditors and owners of for-profit businesses) all are concerned with a business's liabilities compared to its assets and equity. A strong equity position indicates long-term viability.

Others argue that the statement of cash flows is most important. They contend that no matter what is reported on the income statement or balance sheet, managers and investors are ultimately interested in how much cash the company is generating. In addition to serving as an indicator of financial health, the cash flow statement shows managers whether the business has cash to pay dividends or, for a not-for-profit business, to increase its mission capabilities. Managers, suppliers, employees, and other stakeholders all have a direct interest in whether the company is generating substantial cash flows and what it is doing with those flows.

What do you think? Is the balance sheet or statement of cash flows more important? What about the income statement? If you had to consider only one financial statement, which would it be?

SELF-TEST QUESTIONS

1. How does the statement of cash flows differ from the income statement?
2. Briefly explain the three major sections on the statement of cash flows.
3. In your view, what is the most important piece of information reported on the statement of cash flows?

12.8 A LOOK AHEAD: FINANCIAL STATEMENT ANALYSIS

Here, we continue our discussion of ratio analysis (started in chapter 11) using balance sheet data.

The **debt ratio** (or **debt-to-assets ratio**) is defined as total debt divided by total assets. Total debt can be defined several ways, depending on the use of the ratio, but for our purposes, assume that total debt includes all liabilities—that is, all nonequity capital. (One alternative would be to include only interest-bearing debt in our definition.) Using exhibit 12.1 balance sheet data, Park Ridge Homecare's debt ratio at the end of 2016 was Total debt (Total liabilities) ÷ Total assets = \$742,000 ÷ \$1,220,000 = 0.608 = 60.8%.

Debt ratio (debt-to-assets ratio)
A ratio that measures the proportion of debt (versus equity) financing. Often defined as total debt (liabilities) divided by total assets.

This ratio reveals that each dollar of assets was financed by about 61 cents of debt and, by inference, about 39 cents of equity.

Park Ridge's debt ratio at the end of 2015 was $564,000 ÷ $879,000 = 0.642 = 64.2%. Thus, the business decreased its proportional use of debt financing by roughly 3 percentage points from 2015 to 2016. That information is important to Park Ridge's managers and creditors. Also, note that judgments about Park Ridge's capital structure could not be made easily without constructing the debt ratio and other ratios; interpreting the dollar values directly is just too difficult.

Self-Test Questions

1. Explain how ratio analysis can be used to help interpret balance sheet data.
2. What is the debt ratio, and what does it measure?

Theme Wrap-Up: Understanding the Balance Sheet and the Statement of Cash Flows

After reviewing Park Ridge Homecare's balance sheet and statement of cash flows, what has Lori learned about Park Ridge's ability to start a second location (and what have you)?

The business has nearly $385,000 in cash and securities investments. Of course, some cash must be held to meet day-to-day operating expenses and as a reserve, and some of the securities investments may take time to liquidate and hence could not be used immediately to fund a new location. Still, some portion of the $385,000 could likely be used to help open a second facility.

According to the balance sheet, Park Ridge currently has $27,000 in inventories and $126,000 in gross fixed assets (vehicles and equipment), for a total gross investment of $153,000. Assuming that a start-up location would require about the same amount (or perhaps less, initially) of these assets, it appears that the proposed business could be partially or wholly funded from Park Ridge's current securities investments.

Finally, the statement of cash flows indicates that Park Ridge has generated $192,000 of operating cash flow over the last two years of operations. This fact means that a new location, if it achieves the same level of success as the existing business, would quickly generate a positive operating cash flow and hence would be more or less self-sustaining in a short time.

All in all, Lori's plan to use Park Ridge's resources to fund another location seems feasible. However, a complete financial statement analysis will yield the best possible picture of Park Ridge's financial condition and hence its ability to support the opening of a new business. We will perform that analysis in chapter 13.

Key Concepts

This chapter extends the discussion of financial statements to the balance sheet and the statement of cash flows. Here are the key concepts:

- The *balance sheet* provides a snapshot of the financial position of a business at a given point in time.
- The *basic accounting equation* specifies that assets must equal liabilities plus equity (total assets must equal total financing).
- *Assets* are the resources (in dollar terms) owned by the organization. Assets are listed by maturity (order of when the assets are expected to be converted into cash). Current assets are expected to be converted into cash during the next accounting period—often, one year.
- *Liabilities* represent a business's payment obligations to employees, suppliers, tax authorities, and lenders. Current liabilities—those obligations that fall due within one accounting period—are listed first. Long-term liabilities (typically, debt with maturities greater than one accounting period) are listed second.
- *Equity* constitutes the residual (ownership) claim against a business's assets. Depending on the form of organization and ownership, this claim may be called *net assets* or some other term.
- There are two primary interrelationships between the balance sheet and the income statement. First, the annual depreciation expense shown on the income statement accumulates on the balance sheet in the accumulated depreciation account. Second, all earnings from the income statement that are reinvested in the business accumulate on the balance sheet in the equity account.
- *Fund accounting* is used by organizations that have restricted contributions. This accounting method complicates internal accounting procedures and adds detail to the balance sheet. However, fund accounting does not alter the basic format of the balance sheet or its economic interpretation.
- The *statement of cash flows* shows where an organization gets its cash from and how the cash is used. It combines information found on both the income statement and the balance sheet.
- The statement of cash flows has three major sections: *cash flows from operating activities*, *cash flows from investing activities*, and *cash flows from financing activities*.
- The *bottom line* of the statement of cash flows is the net increase (decrease) in cash. Although this amount is useful in verifying the accuracy of the statement, its

economic content is not as meaningful as the statement's component amounts, particularly net cash from operations.

In chapter 13, we focus on using the information in all three financial statements to assess a business's financial condition.

End-of-Chapter Questions

12.1 a. What is the difference in timing between the income statement and the balance sheet?

b. Explain what is wrong with this statement: "The clinic's cash balance for 2016 was $150,000, while its net income on December 31, 2016, was $50,000."

12.2 a. What is the basic accounting equation?

b. What is its implication for the numbers on a balance sheet?

c. What does the basic accounting equation tell us about a business's equity?

12.3 a. What are assets?

b. What are the three major categories of assets?

12.4 a. What makes an asset a current asset?

b. Provide some examples of current assets.

12.5 a. On the balance sheet, what is the difference between long-term investments and property and equipment?

b. What is the difference between gross fixed assets (gross plant and equipment) and net fixed assets?

c. How does depreciation expense on the income statement relate to accumulated depreciation on the balance sheet?

12.6 a. What is the difference between liabilities and equity?

b. What makes a liability a current liability?

c. Give some examples of current liabilities.

d. What is the difference between notes payable and long-term debt?

12.7 What is the relationship between net income on the income statement and the equity section on a balance sheet?

12.8 What is fund accounting, and why is it important to some healthcare providers?

12.9 a. What is the statement of cash flows, and how does it differ from the income statement?

b. What are the three major sections of the statement of cash flows?

c. What is the most important line on the statement of cash flows?

END-OF-CHAPTER PROBLEMS

12.1 Middleton Clinic had total assets of $500,000 and an equity balance of $350,000 at the end of 2015. One year later, at the end of 2016, the clinic had $575,000 in assets and $380,000 in equity. What was the clinic's dollar growth in assets during 2016, and how was this growth financed?

12.2 San Mateo Healthcare had an equity balance of $1.38 million at the beginning of the year. At the end of the year, its equity balance was $1.98 million. Assume that San Mateo is a not-for-profit organization. What was its net income for the period?

12.3 Here is the financial statement information on four not-for-profit clinics:

	Pittman	Rose	Beckman	Jaffe
December 31, 2015:				
Assets	$ 80,000	$100,000	g	$150,000
Liabilities	50,000	d	$ 75,000	j
Equity	a	60,000	45,000	90,000
December 31, 2016:				
Assets	b	130,000	180,000	k
Liabilities	55,000	62,000	h	80,000
Equity	45,000	e	110,000	145,000
During 2016:				
Total revenues	c	400,000	i	500,000
Total expenses	330,000	f	360,000	l

Fill in the missing values labeled a through l.

12.4 The following are selected entries for Warren Clinic for December 31, 2016, in alphabetical order. Create Warren Clinic's balance sheet.

Accounts payable	$ 20,000
Accounts receivable, net	60,000
Cash	30,000
Equity	230,000
Long-term debt	120,000
Long-term investments	100,000
Net property and equipment	150,000
Other assets	40,000
Other long-term liabilities	10,000

12.5 Consider the following balance sheet.

BestCare Health Insurer Balance Sheet June 30, 2016 (in Thousands)

ASSETS	
Current assets	
Cash and cash equivalents	$2,737
Net premiums receivable	821
Other current assets	387
Total current assets	$3,945
Long-term investments	$4,424
Net property and equipment	$ 1,500
Total assets	$9,869
LIABILITIES AND EQUITY	
Healthcare costs payable	$ 2,145
Accrued expenses	929
Unearned premiums	382
Total current liabilities	$3,456
Long-term debt	$4,295
Total liabilities	$ 7,751
Equity	$ 2,118
Total liabilities and equity	$9,869

a. How does this balance sheet differ from the one presented in exhibit 12.1 for Park Ridge Homecare?
b. What is BestCare's debt ratio? How does it compare with Park Ridge Homecare's debt ratio?

12.6 Consider the following balance sheet.

Green Valley Nursing Home Inc.
Balance Sheet December 31, 2016

ASSETS	
Current assets	
Cash and cash equivalents	$ 105,737
Short-term securities	200,000
Net accounts receivable	215,600
Supplies	87,655
Total current assets	$ 608,992
Property and equipment	2,250,000
Less accumulated depreciation	356,000
Net property and equipment	$1,894,000
Total assets	$2,502,992
LIABILITIES AND SHAREHOLDERS' EQUITY	
Current liabilities	
Accounts payable	$ 72,250
Accrued expenses	192,900
Notes payable	100,000
Current portion of long-term debt	80,000
Total current liabilities	$ 445,150
Long-term debt	$1,700,000
Shareholders' equity	
Common stock, $10 par value	$ 100,000
Retained earnings	257,842
Total shareholders' equity	$ 357,842
Total liabilities and shareholders' equity	$2,502,992

a. How does this balance sheet differ from the ones presented in exhibits 12.1 and 12.2 and problem 12.5?

b. What is Green Valley's debt ratio? How does it compare with the debt ratios for Park Ridge Homecare and BestCare?

CHAPTER 13

ASSESSING FINANCIAL CONDITION

THEME SET-UP: TECHNIQUES FOR EVALUATING FINANCIAL STATEMENTS

Following Lori Gibbs's story, we have learned that over the past two years, Park Ridge Homecare generated $262,000 in net income (earnings) and currently has nearly $385,000 in cash and securities investments. In addition, the balance sheet indicates that the business has a total gross (predepreciation) investment in property, equipment, and inventories of $153,000.

Assuming the second location being considered would require about the same amount of start-up resources as needed by Park Ridge today, it appears that the organization's current securities investments could fund the new enterprise.

In addition, by examining the statement of cash flows, Lori found out that, over the last two years of operations, Park Ridge has generated $192,000 of operating cash flow. This is good news. It shows that if the new location achieves the same level of success as Park Ridge has, it would quickly generate a positive operating cash flow and hence could sustain itself.

Lori's intention to use Park Ridge's success as a financial springboard for the new location appears feasible. At this point, a complete financial statement analysis should be performed. Doing so would generate the clearest picture of Park Ridge's current financial condition.

That is our task in this chapter.

Learning Objectives

After studying this chapter, you will be able to do the following:

- Explain the purpose of financial statement analysis.
- Describe the primary techniques used in financial statement analysis.
- Conduct basic financial statement analyses to assess the financial condition of a business.
- Discuss the problems associated with financial statement analysis.

13.1 INTRODUCTION

In the last two chapters, we presented an overview of a business's financial statements. The purpose of these statements is to provide relevant information about the operations and financial status of an organization. Now, we turn our attention to assessing financial condition: Does the organization have the financial capacity to perform its mission?

Although the information contained in the financial statements is logically organized and presented, to gain a better understanding of a business's financial condition it is necessary to reformat the financial statement data. Furthermore, data found outside of the financial statements can be used to provide additional insights. By using various techniques applied to a variety of data, analysts can make the best possible judgments about a business's financial capabilities.

In this chapter, we explore several analytical techniques used in financial condition analysis and the problems inherent in such analyses. Along the way, you will discover that such analyses generate a great deal of data. A significant problem in assessing financial condition is separating the important factors from the unimportant and presenting the results in a simple format that is easy to understand and monitor.

13.2 FINANCIAL STATEMENT ANALYSIS

Often, initial judgments about financial condition are made on the basis of financial statement analysis, which focuses on the data contained in a business's financial statements (see "Critical Concept: Financial Statement Analysis"). Financial statement analysis is applied both to historical data, which reflect the results of past managerial decisions, and to forecasted data, which provide the road map for the business's future. Therefore, managers use financial statement analysis not only to assess current conditions but also to plan.

> **CRITICAL CONCEPT**
> Financial Statement Analysis
>
> Financial statement analysis involves using financial statement data to make judgments about a business's financial condition. Several techniques can be used in financial statement analysis, but the most important is ratio analysis. Because financial statement analysis does not provide much information about the underlying operational factors that contribute to financial condition, often it is supplemented by an analysis of operating data. The results of a financial statement analysis usually are presented as a list of financial (and operational) strengths and weaknesses.

Although financial statement analysis provides a wealth of information regarding financial condition, it often fails to provide insight into the operational causes of that condition. Thus, financial statement analysis typically is supplemented by an analysis of the business's operating data, such as occupancy rate, patient mix, length of stay, and productivity measures. (Some of these operational measures are discussed in chapter 7.)

By examining operational data in conjunction with financial data, managers can more easily identify factors that contributed to the assessed financial condition. Through such combined analyses, managers are better able to develop and implement strategies that ensure a sound financial condition in the future.

In this chapter, we continue to use Park Ridge Homecare, an investor-owned home health care business, as our illustration, but now we focus on financial statement analysis. However, all the techniques we present here can be applied to any healthcare organization, with only minor modification, regardless of setting.

? SELF-TEST QUESTIONS

1. What is financial statement analysis, and what is its purpose?
2. Why is financial statement analysis typically accompanied by an operational analysis?

13.3 INTERPRETING THE STATEMENT OF CASH FLOWS

We begin our financial statement analysis of Park Ridge Homecare by examining the statement of cash flows, presented first in exhibit 12.3 and repeated here in exhibit 13.1. We look at this statement first because it is constructed in a way that allows us to make judgments without having to reformat the data. (Consider this discussion to be a review of chapter 12 material—it never hurts to cover basic concepts a second time.)

The statement of cash flows answers the following questions:

- Are the business's core operations profitable?
- How much capital did the business raise? How was this capital used?
- What impact did operating and financing decisions have on the business's cash position?

The top section of the statement shows cash generated by and used in operations. For Park Ridge, operations in 2016 provided $119,000 in net cash flow, which is certainly a step in the right direction. A positive cash flow from operations indicates that the business's operations are inherently profitable on a cash flow basis. Furthermore, the substantial increase in operating cash flow from 2015 to 2016 shows an excellent trend.

The next section focuses on investments in fixed assets (property and equipment) and securities. Park Ridge spent $25,000 on capital expenditures in 2016, but is this amount large or small? To answer this question, note that the income statement (exhibit 11.1) reported a depreciation expense of $21,000 for 2016, so the business spent only slightly more on fixed assets in 2016 than the amount expensed for wear and tear. Furthermore, according to the balance sheet (exhibit 12.1), the bulk of the fixed-assets addition was a $23,000

EXHIBIT 13.1 Park Ridge Homecare: Statements of Cash Flows for Years Ended December 31, 2016 and 2015 (in Thousands)

	2016	2015
Cash flows from operating activities:		
Cash received from services	$3,740	$2,542
Cash paid to employees and suppliers	(3,694)	(2,536)
Interest paid	(16)	(19)
Interest earned	89	86
Net cash from operations	$ 119	$ 73
Cash flows from investing activities:		
Purchase of property and equipment	($ 25)	($ 19)
Securities purchases	(35)	(15)
Net cash from investing activities	($ 60)	($ 34)
Cash flows from financing activities:		
Repayment of long-term debt	($ 13)	$ 0
Net cash from financing activities	($ 13)	$ 0
Net increase (decrease) in cash and equivalents	$ 46	$ 39
Cash and equivalents, beginning of year	$ 67	$ 28
Cash and equivalents, end of year	$ 113	$ 67

increase in vehicles. Thus, Park Ridge likely added a vehicle to its fixed-assets base, which appears to be a sound capital investment for a growing home care business. In addition, the 2016 investment in fixed assets was only slightly larger than the 2015 amount, which confirms that no unusual activity occurred.

As indicated by account changes on the balance sheet, the $35,000 investment in securities for 2016 consisted of $10,000 in short-term investments and $25,000 in long-term investments. Considering both fixed assets and securities, investing activities used $60,000 in 2016, which constitutes about half of the cash flow from operations. However, more than half of the investment amount is in financial securities that, if necessary, could be sold and converted back into cash (assuming the long-term investments could be sold at a value equal to or greater than their purchase price). The fact that Park Ridge placed $10,000 of the $35,000 securities investment in short-term securities indicates that these funds are likely to be needed in the near term.

The third section highlights the fact that Park Ridge used cash to pay off $13,000 of previously incurred debt financing, resulting in a net cash outflow from financing of $13,000 in 2016 compared to $0 in 2015.

When the three major sections are totaled, the result is a $119,000 – $60,000 – $13,000 = $46,000 net increase in cash (net cash inflow) during 2016 and a cash increase of $39,000 in 2015. The bottom of exhibit 13.1 reconciles the net cash flow with the ending cash balance shown on the balance sheet. For 2016, Park Ridge began with $67,000, experienced a cash inflow of $46,000 during the year, and ended the year with $67,000 + $46,000 = $113,000 in its cash and cash equivalents account. Cash and cash equivalents is also presented on the balance sheets in exhibit 13.2, and we can verify the value reported.

EXHIBIT 13.2 Park Ridge Homecare: Balance Sheets as of December 31, 2016 and 2015 (in Thousands)

	2016	2015
ASSETS		
Current assets		
Cash and cash equivalents	$ 113	$ 67
Short-term investments	147	137
Accounts receivable, net	727	476
Inventories	27	22
Total current assets	$1,014	$702
Investments	$ 125	$100
Property and equipment		
Medical and office equipment	$ 56	$ 54
Vehicles	70	47
Total	$ 126	$ 101
Less: Accumulated depreciation	(45)	(24)
Net property and equipment	$ 81	$ 77
Total assets	$1,220	$879
LIABILITIES AND EQUITY		
Current liabilities		
Notes payable	$ 13	$ 13
Accounts payable	40	21
Accrued expenses	535	363
Total current liabilities	$ 588	$397
Long-term debt	154	167
Total liabilities	$ 742	$564
Equity	$ 478	$ 315
Total liabilities and equity	$1,220	$879

Park Ridge's statement of cash flows shows nothing unusual or alarming. It does reveal that the business's operations are inherently profitable, at least in 2015 and 2016. Had the statement shown an operating cash drain, Lori would have had something to worry about; if it continued, such a drain could bleed the business to death.

The statement of cash flows also provides easily interpreted information about Park Ridge's financing and fixed-asset investing activities for the year. In essence, the business's cash flow from operations was used primarily to purchase new fixed assets, to invest in securities, and to pay off long-term debt. Such uses of operating cash flow do not raise any red flags regarding the business's financial actions. In fact, the statement of cash flows indicates a business that is generating excess cash flow, which is a very positive sign.

Managers and investors must pay close attention to the statement of cash flows. Financial condition is driven by cash flows, and the statement gives a clear picture of the annual cash flows generated by the business. An examination of exhibit 13.1—or, better yet, a series of such exhibits going back the last five years (if the business is that old) and projecting five years into the future—would give managers and creditors an idea of whether the business's operations are self-sustaining.

? Self-Test Questions

1. What type of financial condition information is provided in the statement of cash flows?
2. Does the fact that its cash position has improved provide much insight into the business's financial condition?
3. What did Park Ridge's 2016 statement of cash flows tell us?

13.4 RATIO ANALYSIS

Now we can turn our attention to interpreting the income statement and balance sheet. Although both of these statements contain a wealth of information, they yield raw data that do not help managers in making meaningful judgments about the business's financial condition. For example, a hospital may have $5,248,760 in long-term debt and interest charges of $419,900. The true burden of this debt, and the hospital's ability to pay the interest and principal due, cannot be easily determined without additional analysis.

Ratio analysis combines data to create single numbers that have easily interpreted significance (for our purposes, numbers that measure various aspects of financial condition). An almost unlimited number of financial ratios can be constructed, and the choice of ratios depends in large part on the nature of the business being analyzed, the purpose of the analysis, and the availability of comparative data (see "Critical Concept: Ratio Analysis"). Generally, ratios are grouped into categories to make them easier to interpret.

In the paragraphs that follow, we use the data presented in exhibits 13.2 and 13.3 to calculate selected 2016 financial ratios for Park Ridge Homecare. Then, we compare the calculated ratios with average ratios for the home health sector. Note that in a real analysis, many more ratios would be calculated and analyzed. The specific ratios used in any analysis depend on the type of healthcare provider (in our case, a home health care business). Some ratios are meaningful for hospitals, some for long-term care facilities, some for group practices, and so on.

CRITICAL CONCEPT
Ratio Analysis

Ratio analysis is a technique that helps interpret the data contained in a business's financial statements as well as in other contexts. By combining values (sometimes from different statements or sources), analysts can gain a more complete view of the business's financial condition. The idea is to create single values (ratios) from the raw data that have economic meaning and can be easily interpreted. For example, a business with $100,000 in debt and $250,000 in assets has a debt ratio of $100,000 ÷ $250,000 = 0.040 = 40.0%, which tells us that it is financed with 40 percent debt and, by definition, 60 percent equity. Thus, this single value summarizes the business's financing situation (capital structure). Furthermore, it is easy to compare this value to industry averages or to other comparative values.

Profitability Ratios

Profitability is the net result of a large number of managerial policies and decisions. As such, profitability ratios provide a measure of the aggregate financial condition of a business. As you know, an organization must be profitable to meet mission goals.

Exhibit 13.3
Park Ridge Homecare: Statements of Income for Years Ended December 31, 2016 and 2015 (in Thousands)

	2016	2015
Net service revenues	$3,996	$2,666
Cost of service revenues	2,937	1,944
Gross profit	$1,059	$ 722
General and administrative expenses	909	649
Depreciation	21	15
Total operating expenses	$ 930	$ 664
Operating income	$ 129	$ 58
Interest income	89	86
Interest expense	16	19
Total interest income, net	$ 73	$ 67
Income before income taxes	$ 202	$ 125
Income tax expense	$ 39	$ 26
Net income (excess of revenues over expenses)	$ 163	$ 99

Margin Measures

Margin measures focus on how much money a business earns on its revenues. In other words, they reflect how much of its revenues are converted into earnings (profits). Because expenses are subtracted from revenues to create earnings, margin measures indicate the ability of an organization to control its expenses.

Total (profit) margin Net income divided by all (both operating and nonoperating) revenues. It measures the amount of total profit per dollar of total revenues.

The **total margin**, often called *profit margin*, is defined as net income (excess of revenues over expenses) divided by total revenues, including nonoperating revenues (nonoperating income):

Total margin = Net income ÷ Total revenues = \$163 ÷ (\$3,996 + 89) = \$163 ÷ \$4,085
= 0.04 = 4.0%.
Sector average = 5.9%.

Park Ridge's total margin of 4.0 percent shows that the business makes 4.0 cents on every dollar of total revenues, including both operating and nonoperating revenues. The total margin measures the ability of a business to control its expenses. With all else the same, the higher the total margin, the lower the expenses relative to revenues.

Park Ridge's total margin is below the home health sector average of 5.9 percent, indicating that the business's expenses are higher than they should be or that revenues are too low for the expense structure of the business. Thus, low margins suggest a problem with expenses, revenues, or both. Park Ridge's total margin may also be compared to national quartiles; suppose that for total margin, the upper quartile was 10.4 percent, meaning that 25 percent of the sector had total margins higher than 10.4 percent, while the lower quartile was 2.1 percent. Although Park Ridge's total margin was below average, it did not fall in the lower quartile (lower 25 percent) of all home health care businesses.

The industry average is not a magic number that all businesses should strive to achieve. In fact, some well-managed businesses are above the average, while other good firms are below it. However, if a business's ratios are far removed from the average for the industry, its managers should be concerned about why this difference occurs.

As mentioned, Park Ridge's relatively low total margin could mean that its revenues (reimbursements) are relatively low, its costs are relatively high, or a combination of the two. A thorough examination of relevant operational data, such as average cost per home visit and average reimbursement per visit, would help pinpoint the cause or causes of the low total margin.

When data are available, as in our example, another useful margin measure is the operating margin, defined as operating income divided by operating revenues:

Operating margin = Operating income ÷ Operating revenues = \$129 ÷ \$3,996
= 0.032 = 3.2%.
Sector average = 5.6%.

Park Ridge's operating margin of 3.2 percent shows that the business makes 3.2 cents on every dollar of operating revenues. (On Park Ridge's income statement [exhibit 13.3], operating revenues are listed as net service revenues.) Park Ridge's operating margin is below the sector average of 5.6 percent, suggesting that Park Ridge should take a close look at its costs of providing services and its general and administrative expenses. The advantage of the operating margin over the total margin is that it focuses on core business operations and hence removes the influence of nonoperating income, which often is transitory and unrelated to core operations. However, the format of some healthcare organizations' financial statements makes this ratio difficult to determine without additional information.

Return Measures

Return measures focus on how much a business earns on its asset or equity investment. The ratio of net income to total assets measures the **return on total assets**, often just called *return on assets (ROA)*:

Return on total assets (ROA)
Net income divided by the book value of total assets; measures the amount of profit per dollar of investment in total assets. ROA indicates the financial productivity of a business's total assets.

Return on assets = Net income ÷ Total assets = \$163 ÷ \$1,220 = 0.134 = 13.4%.
Sector average = 12.7%.

Park Ridge's 13.4 percent ROA, which means that each dollar of assets generated 13.4 cents in profit, is above the 12.7 percent average for the home health care sector.

ROA alerts managers to the productivity, in a financial sense, of a business's total assets. The higher the ROA, the greater the net income for each dollar invested in assets and hence the more productive the assets. ROA measures a business's ability to control expenses (as expressed by the total margin) and ability to use its assets to generate revenue.

Another return measure is return on equity (ROE), defined as the ratio of net income to total equity (net assets):

Return on equity = Net income ÷ Total equity = \$163 ÷ \$478 = 0.341 = 34.1%.
Sector average = 36.5%.

Park Ridge's 34.1 percent ROE is below the 36.5 percent sector average. The business was able to generate 34.1 cents of income for each dollar of equity investment, while the average home health care business produced 36.5 cents.

ROE is especially meaningful for investor-owned businesses because owners are concerned with how well the business's managers are using owner-supplied capital to generate returns, and ROE gives the answer to this question. In essence, ROE is the return that owners are earning on their investment in the business. For not-for-profit businesses, such as Good Samaritan Medical Center, ROE tells its board of trustees and managers how well, in financial terms, its community-supplied capital is being managed.

Note that Park Ridge's 2016 total margin, operating margin, and return on equity were below the sector average, yet its return on assets was above the sector average. As explained later in section 13.6, on DuPont analysis, this seeming inconsistency is a result of the business's smaller asset base.

Liquidity Ratios

Liquidity
The ability of a business to meet its cash obligations as they become due.

One of the first concerns of managers, and the major concern of a firm's short-term creditors, is the business's **liquidity**, which means its ability to meet its cash obligations as they become due.

Park Ridge had obligations totaling $588,000 (its current liabilities) at the end of 2016 that must be paid off during 2017. Will the business be able to make these payments? A full liquidity analysis requires the use of tools that are beyond the scope of this text. However, here are two measures that are quick and easy to use.

Current ratio
Total current assets divided by total current liabilities; measures the number of dollars of current assets available to pay each dollar of current liabilities.

The most basic liquidity measure is the **current ratio**, which is defined as total current assets divided by total current liabilities:

$$\text{Current ratio} = \text{Current assets} \div \text{Current liabilities} = \$1{,}014 \div \$588$$
$$= 1.7, \text{ or } 1.7 \text{ times.}$$
$$\text{Sector average} = 1.9.$$

The current ratio tells managers that the liquidation of Park Ridge's current assets at book value would provide $1.70 of cash for every $1 of current liabilities. If a business is getting into financial difficulty, it will begin paying its accounts payable more slowly and building up short-term bank loans (notes payable). If these current liabilities rise faster than current assets, the current ratio will fall, and this trend could indicate financial trouble. Because the current ratio is an indicator of the extent to which short-term obligations are covered by assets that are expected to be converted to cash in the near term, it is a commonly used measure of liquidity.

Park Ridge's current ratio is slightly below the average for the home health care sector. Because current assets should be converted to cash in the near future, these assets are highly likely to be liquidated at close to their stated values. With a current ratio of 1.7, the business could liquidate current assets at only 59 percent of book value and still pay off current creditors in full. (To obtain this value, divide 1 by the current ratio: 1 ÷ 1.7 = 0.59 = 59%.)

Days cash on hand (DCOH)
The number of days it would take to run out of cash if the business does not receive any additional revenues or financing.

The current ratio measures liquidity on the basis of balance sheet accounts, and hence it is a static measure of liquidity. However, the true measure of a business's liquidity is whether the business can meet its payments as they become due, so liquidity is more related to cash flows than to assets and liabilities.

The **days-cash-on-hand (DCOH)** ratio moves closer to those factors that truly determine liquidity:

$$\text{DCOH} = \frac{\text{Cash and cash equivalents} + \text{Short-term investments}}{(\text{Operating expenses} - \text{Depreciation}) \div 365}$$

$$= \frac{\$113 + \$147}{(\$2{,}937 + \$930 - \$21) \div 365} = \frac{\$260}{\$3{,}864 \div 365} = \frac{\$260}{\$10.54} = 24.7 \text{ days.}$$

Sector average = 22.6 days.

The denominator of the equation estimates average daily cash operating expenses by stripping out noncash expenses (depreciation) from reported total operating expenses and then dividing by 365 days per year. The numerator is the cash and securities that are available to make those cash payments. Because Park Ridge's DCOH is slightly higher than the sector average, its liquidity position as measured by DCOH is a little better than that of the average home health care business. Including nonoperating expenses (interest and taxes) in the denominator would only slightly reduce Park Ridge's DCOH, to 24.3 days.

For Park Ridge, the two measures of liquidity—current ratio and DCOH—give a picture of about-average liquidity. However, both of these measures are rough, so additional analysis is required to make a supportable judgment concerning Park Ridge's liquidity position. (The best measure of a business's liquidity is provided by a cash budget, which details the business's expected cash inflows and outflows. Cash budgeting is beyond the scope of this book.)

Debt Management (Capital Structure) Ratios

The degree to which a firm uses debt financing, or financial leverage, is an important measure of financial performance for several reasons. First, by raising funds through debt, owners of for-profits can maintain control of the firm with a limited investment. For not-for-profits, debt financing allows the organization to provide more services than it could if it were solely financed with contributed and earned capital.

Second, creditors look to equity capital to provide a margin of safety; if the owners (or community) have provided only a small proportion of total financing, the risks of the enterprise are borne mainly by its creditors.

Third, if a firm earns more on investments financed with borrowed funds than it pays in interest, its return on equity capital is increased when debt financing is used.

Two types of ratios are used to assess debt management:

1. *Capitalization ratios.* These ratios use balance sheet data to determine the extent to which borrowed funds have been used to finance assets.
2. *Coverage ratios.* Here, income statement data are used to determine the extent to which fixed financial charges are covered by reported profits or cash flow.

The two sets of ratios are complementary, so most financial statement analyses examine both types.

Capitalization Ratios

The ratio of total debt (total liabilities) to total assets (total liabilities and equity), generally called the debt ratio, is a capitalization ratio that measures the percentage of total capital provided by creditors and other capital suppliers that have fixed claims:

Debt ratio = Total liabilities ÷ Total assets = $742 ÷ $1,220 = 0.608, or 60.8%.
Sector average = 63.9%.

For our purposes, we define debt as all debt, including current liabilities and long-term debt—that is, everything but equity. However, as illustrated by the next ratio discussed, capitalization ratios have numerous variations, many of which use different definitions of what constitutes debt financing.

Creditors prefer low debt ratios (low leverage) because the lower the ratio, the greater the cushion against creditors' losses in the event of bankruptcy and liquidation. Conversely, owners of for-profit firms may seek high leverage either to increase returns or to prevent giving up some degree of control when they sell new stock. In not-for-profit organizations, managers may seek high leverage to offer more services. However, as discussed in chapter 8, the greater the amount of debt financing, the higher the interest rate on that debt and the greater the risk of bankruptcy.

Park Ridge's debt ratio is 60.8 percent. This result means that its creditors (and other fixed claimants) have supplied about 61 percent of the business's total financing. Put another way, each dollar of assets was financed with roughly 61 cents of debt and, consequently, 39 cents of equity. Because the average debt ratio for the home health care sector is more than 63 percent, Park Ridge uses a little less nonequity financing than does the average home health care business. The slightly lower-than-average debt ratio indicates that Park Ridge probably could borrow a limited amount of additional funds at a relatively reasonable rate.

Debt-to-capitalization ratio
Long-term debt divided by long-term capital (long-term debt plus equity); measures the proportion of long-term debt in a business's permanent (long-term) financing mix.

The **debt-to-capitalization ratio** is another capitalization ratio. It is defined as long-term debt divided by long-term capital (long-term debt plus equity), and it focuses on the proportion of debt used in a business's permanent (long-term) capital structure. This ratio is also called the *long-term-debt-to-capitalization ratio* or just *capitalization ratio*.

Debt-to-capitalization ratio = Long-term debt ÷ (Long-term debt + Equity)
= $154 ÷ ($154 + $478) = $154 ÷ $632 = 0.244, or 24.4%.
Sector average = 31.2%.

Many analysts believe that the debt-to-capitalization ratio best reflects the capital structure of a business. This belief is based on the fact that most businesses use as much free credit (current liabilities less short-term bank loans) as they can get. Furthermore, short-term interest-bearing debt typically is used only to fund temporary current asset needs. Thus, the so-called true capital structure of a business—the one that reflects its target structure—is best measured by the debt-to-capitalization ratio, which focuses on long-term (permanent) financing.

Park Ridge's debt-to-capitalization ratio is 24.4 percent, compared to the sector average of 31.2 percent. This low use of debt financing in the business's permanent capital mix confirms the conclusion we made earlier that the business has some unused debt capacity. That is, the business could easily obtain additional debt financing at relatively favorable rates.

Another common capitalization ratio is the *debt-to-equity ratio*, which is defined as Total liabilities ÷ Total equity. This ratio gives the number of dollars of debt financing per dollar of equity. The higher the ratio, the greater the use of financial leverage. In essence, the debt ratio and debt-to-equity ratio provide the same information, but in slightly different ways. Finally, the *assets-to-equity ratio* (called the equity multiplier), which is defined as Total assets ÷ Total equity, is used in DuPont analysis. (Section 13.6 discusses DuPont analysis.)

Coverage Ratios

The most basic coverage ratio is the **times interest earned (TIE) ratio**, which is defined as earnings before interest and taxes (EBIT) divided by interest charges. EBIT is used in the numerator because it represents the amount of income that is available to pay interest expense. For a not-for-profit business, which does not pay taxes, EBIT = Net income + Interest expense.

Times interest earned (TIE) ratio
Earnings before interest and taxes divided by interest charges; measures the number of times that a business's interest expense is covered by the earnings available to pay that expense. This ratio provides insight into how much earnings could fall before the business has trouble meeting its interest payments.

$$\text{TIE ratio} = \text{EBIT} \div \text{Interest expense} = (\$163 + \$16 + \$39) \div \$16$$
$$= \$218 \div \$16 = 13.6 \text{ times.}$$
$$\text{Sector average} = 10.4.$$

The TIE ratio measures the number of dollars of accounting income (as opposed to cash flow) available to pay each dollar of interest expense. In essence, it is an indicator of the extent to which income can decline before it is less than annual interest costs—the higher the ratio, the greater the safety margin. Failure to pay interest might trigger legal action by creditors, which could result in the firm's bankruptcy.

Park Ridge's interest is covered 13.6 times, so it has $13.60 of accounting income to pay each dollar of interest expense. Because the sector average TIE ratio is 10.4 times, the business is covering its interest charges by a decent margin of safety. Thus, the TIE ratio reinforces the previous conclusions based on capitalization ratios—namely, Park Ridge could potentially expand its use of debt financing.

Coverage ratios often are better measures of a firm's debt use than capitalization ratios are because coverage ratios discriminate between low–interest rate debt and high–interest rate debt. For example, a large group practice might have $10 million of 4 percent debt on its balance sheet, while another might have $10 million of 8 percent debt. If both practices have the same income and assets, both would have the same debt ratio. However, the group that pays 4 percent interest would have lower interest charges and hence would be in better financial condition than the group that pays 8 percent. This difference in financial condition is captured by the TIE ratio.

Although the TIE ratio is easy to calculate, it has two major deficiencies:

1. The TIE ratio ignores lease payments, which, like debt payments, are contractual obligations. Also, many debt contracts require that principal payments be made over the life of the loan, rather than only at maturity. Thus, most businesses must meet fixed financial charges (lease and principal payments) other than interest.
2. The TIE ratio ignores the fact that accounting income, whether measured by EBIT or net income, does not reflect the actual cash flow available to meet a business's fixed payments.

Cash flow coverage (CFC) ratio
A measure of the amount of cash flow generated by a business per dollar of fixed expense. Similar to the TIE ratio, but more inclusive.

These deficiencies are corrected in the **cash flow coverage (CFC) ratio**, which shows the amount by which cash flow covers fixed financial requirements. Here is Park Ridge's 2016 CFC ratio, assuming the business had $18,000 of lease payments, $13,000 of required debt principal repayments, and a tax rate of 35 percent:

$$\begin{aligned}\text{CFC ratio} &= (\text{EBIT} + \text{Lease payments} + \text{Depreciation expense}) \div (\text{Interest expense} + \\ &\quad \text{Lease payments} + (\text{Debt principal} \div (1 - T))) \\ &= (\$218 + \$18 + \$21) \div (\$16 + \$18 + (\$13 \div (1 - .35))) = \$257 \div \$54 \\ &= 4.8 \text{ times.}\end{aligned}$$

Sector average = 3.3.

Like its TIE ratio, Park Ridge's CFC ratio exceeds the sector standard, indicating that the business is better at covering total fixed payments with cash flow than is the average home health care business. This fact should be reassuring both to creditors and management, and it reinforces the view that Park Ridge has untapped debt capacity.

Asset Management (Activity) Ratios

The next group of ratios, the asset management ratios, is designed to measure how effectively a business's assets are being used. These ratios help to uncover whether the amount of each type of asset as reported on the balance sheet seems reasonable, too high, or too low in view of current (or projected) operating levels. Park Ridge, and all businesses, must borrow or raise equity capital to acquire assets. If they have too many assets, then their capital costs will be too high and their profits will be depressed. Conversely, if the level of assets is too low, then volume may be lost or vital services not offered.

Fixed-assets turnover (utilization) ratio
Total revenues divided by net fixed assets; measures the ability of a business's fixed assets to generate revenues.

The **fixed-assets turnover ratio**, also called the *fixed-assets utilization ratio*, measures the use of plant and equipment, and it is the ratio of total revenues to net fixed assets (net property and equipment):

$$\begin{aligned}\text{Fixed-assets turnover} &= \text{Total revenues} \div \text{Net fixed assets} = (\$3{,}996 + 89) \div \$81\\ &= \$4{,}085 \div \$81\\ &= 50.4 \text{ times.}\\ \text{Sector average} &= 63.1.\end{aligned}$$

Park Ridge's ratio of 50.4 indicates that each dollar of fixed assets generated $50.40 in revenue. This value compares unfavorably with the sector average of 63.1 times, indicating that Park Ridge is using its fixed assets less productively than the median home health care business. (The lower quartile value for the industry is 14.0; thus, Park Ridge is doing well enough to not fall in the bottom 25 percent of the sector.)

The value of the fixed-assets turnover ratio is highly dependent on the nature of the business. To illustrate, hospitals require a large investment in plant and equipment to treat patients, so they have relatively low ratios (about 2.5). Conversely, home health care businesses need minimal fixed assets to generate revenues because the services are provided in the patients' homes. Thus, they have much larger fixed-assets turnover ratios.

The **total assets turnover ratio** measures the turnover, or usage, of all of a business's assets. It is calculated by dividing total revenues by total assets:

Total assets turnover (utilization) ratio Total revenues divided by total assets; measures the amount of revenue generated by each dollar of total assets.

$$\begin{aligned}\text{Total assets turnover} &= \text{Total revenues} \div \text{Total assets} = (\$3{,}996 + \$89) \div \$1{,}220\\ &= \$4{,}085 \div \$1{,}220 = 3.3 \text{ times.}\\ \text{Sector average} &= 3.4.\end{aligned}$$

Each dollar of total assets generated $3.30 in total revenue. Thus, both Park Ridge's fixed-assets and total assets turnover ratios are below the sector averages, although the total assets turnover ratio is barely below. The bottom line is that the business may need to focus on generating more revenues for its asset base, particularly its fixed-assets base. However, it is also possible that Park Ridge's fixed-assets base is newer than the average home health care business. Newer assets have had less time to depreciate (e.g., their net value is higher); thus, the ratio can be affected by the age of a business's assets.

Note that another utilization ratio is the *current assets turnover ratio*, defined as total revenues divided by current assets. This ratio measures the amount of revenue generated by each dollar of current assets. When all three utilization ratios (fixed assets, total assets, and current assets) are examined, analysts can glean information about the financial productivity of all three major asset categories.

Days in patient accounts receivable The average length of time it takes a provider to collect its receivables. Also called *days' sales outstanding* or *average collection period.*

Days in patient accounts receivable is used to measure effectiveness in managing receivables. This measure of financial performance, which is sometimes classified as a liquidity ratio rather than an asset management ratio, has many names, including *average collection period* and *days' sales outstanding*. It is computed by dividing net accounts receivable by average daily revenue to find the number of days that it takes an organization, on average, to collect its receivables:

Days in patient accounts receivable = Net patient accounts receivable ÷ (Net patient service revenue ÷ 365)
= \$727 ÷ (\$3,996 ÷ 365) = \$727 ÷ 10.94 = 66.5 days.
Sector average = 37.1 days.

With a value of 66.5 days, Park Ridge is performing much worse than the sector average in collecting its receivables. Perhaps its payer mix is dominated by slow payers, or it is using manual rather than electronic billing. The lower-quartile value is 56 days, so Park Ridge actually falls in the bottom 25 percent of home health businesses. As discussed in chapter 7, businesses must collect their receivables as soon as possible. Clearly, Park Ridge should strive to increase its performance in this key area.

Other Ratios

Because of space constraints, and the fact that ratio analysis discussions can cause instant drowsiness, we have described only a few of the many financial ratios used in practice today (see "For Your Consideration: How Many Ratios Are Enough?" and "Critical Concept: Summary of Key Ratios"). Remember that to gain the most value from a financial ratio analysis, an operational ratio analysis should also be conducted, which will help explain the financial condition assessed. (Operational analysis is introduced in chapter 7.)

✓ FOR YOUR CONSIDERATION
How Many Ratios Are Enough?

In our discussion of financial statement ratio analysis, we highlighted 13 ratios commonly used to help interpret financial statement data. Although that may seem like a lot of ratios, our discussion just scratches the surface. For example, one of the most widely used sets of comparative data for hospitals (*Almanac of Hospital Financial and Operating Indicators*, published annually by Optum) provides data on more than 30 financial ratios.

Without putting in too much work, you could probably compile a list of 50 financial ratios. Yet studies have shown that about 90 percent of the information contained in financial statements can be uncovered using 10 or so carefully selected ratios, while 20 ratios would glean just about all of the important financial condition information contained in a business's financial statements.

How many ratios do you think are enough? Does it matter how the ratios are selected? Is there a cost to using more ratios than necessary? What is the disadvantage of generating too much data?

CRITICAL CONCEPT
Summary of Key Ratios

Ratio	Formula	Definition
Total (profit) margin	Net income divided by total revenues	Measures the ability to control expenses (dollars of income per dollar of revenue)
Operating margin	Net operating income divided by operating revenues	Measures the ability to control operating expenses (dollars of operating income per dollar of operating revenue)
Return on assets (ROA)	Net income divided by total assets	Measures the ability of a business's assets to generate profits (dollars of profitability per dollar of total assets)
Return on equity (ROE)	Net income divided by total equity	Measures the ability of a business's equity financing to generate profits (dollar of profitability per dollar of equity investment)
Current ratio	Current assets divided by current liabilities	Measures the dollars of current assets per dollar of current liabilities—a rough measure of liquidity
Days cash on hand	Cash and short-term investments divided by daily cash expenses	Measures the number of days that a business can continue to pay its bills without new revenue or financing
Debt ratio	Total liabilities divided by total assets	Measures the proportion of debt in a business's total financing
Capitalization ratio	Long-term debt divided by long-term capital (long-term debt and equity)	Measures the proportion of debt in a business's long-term financing
Times interest earned (TIE) ratio	Earnings before interest and taxes (EBIT) divided by interest expense	Measures the dollar of accounting income available to pay each dollar of interest expense
Cash flow coverage (CFC) ratio	Cash flow divided by fixed financial charges	Measures the dollars of cash flow available to pay each dollar of fixed financial charges
Fixed-assets turnover ratio	Total revenues divided by net fixed assets	Measures the dollars of revenue per dollar of fixed assets
Total assets turnover ratio	Total revenues divided by total assets	Measures the dollars of revenue per dollar of total assets
Average collection period (days in patient accounts receivable)	Net accounts receivable divided by daily patient revenue	Measures the average number of days it takes to collect a business's receivables

For a more comprehensive list of financial ratios, see the ratios appendix at ache.org/books/FinanceFundamentals3.

SELF-TEST QUESTIONS

1. What is the purpose of ratio analysis?
2. What are two ratios that measure profitability?
3. What are two ratios that measure liquidity?
4. What are two ratios that measure debt management?
5. What are two ratios that measure asset management?

13.5 COMPARATIVE AND TREND ANALYSIS

When conducting ratio analysis, the value of a particular ratio, in the absence of other information, reveals almost nothing about a business's financial condition. For example, if a nursing home management company has a current ratio of 2.5, saying whether this ratio is good or bad is virtually impossible. Additional data are needed to help interpret the ratio.

In our discussion of Park Ridge Homecare's ratios, the focus was on comparative analysis (benchmarking), in which the business's ratios were compared with sector average ratios (see "Healthcare in Practice: Some Hospital Ratios and How They Compare to Home Health Care"). Another useful ratio analysis tool is trend analysis, in which the trend of a single ratio is analyzed over time. Trend analysis gives clues about whether a business's financial condition is improving, holding constant, or deteriorating (see "Critical Concept: Comparative Analysis [Benchmarking] and Trend Analysis").

HEALTHCARE IN PRACTICE
Some Hospital Ratios and How They Compare to Home Health Care

To gain a better understanding of ratio analysis, we can examine some financial ratios for the hospital sector to see how they compare to the home health care sector.

First, we examine profitability:

	Home Health Care	Hospitals
Total margin	5.9%	3.8%
Return on assets	12.7	3.7
Return on equity	36.5	7.0

Here, we see that the home health care sector has a somewhat higher total margin than the hospital sector, so its ability to generate profits per dollar of revenue is slightly better. However, the difference is not substantial. Thus, although the types of services the two providers offer are different, their cost structures per revenue dollar are similar.

However, the home health care sector has a significantly higher return on its asset investment and an even higher differential return on its equity investment. This pattern means that the home health care sector (1) creates more revenues (but does not earn more on each dollar of revenue) per dollar of asset investment and (2) finances its assets with a higher proportion of debt. We can consider a few more ratios to confirm these assertions.

HEALTHCARE IN PRACTICE
Some Hospital Ratios and How They Compare to Home Health Care *(continued)*

Here is a look at asset productivity and capital structure:

	Home Health Care	Hospitals
Total asset turnover	3.4	1.0
Fixed-asset turnover	63.1	2.5
Equity multiplier (assets/equity)	2.8	1.8

These figures indicate that the assets of a typical home health care business are much more productive (in the financial sense) than hospital assets. For example, each dollar of home health care total assets (plant and equipment) generates $3.40 of revenues, while a dollar of hospital total assets generates only $1.00 in revenues. The underlying reason is that hospitals must have a large investment in land, buildings, and equipment to provide patient services, while home health care businesses can simply lease office space and start operations. This imbalance is confirmed by the stark difference in the fixed-asset turnover ratios.

Also, note that home health care businesses, on average, use more debt financing. Thus, each dollar of equity financing in a home health care business supports $2.80 of assets, while that same dollar of equity in a hospital supports only $1.80 of assets. The net result is that the total margin of a home health care business is leveraged up by asset productivity and debt financing to a greater extent than in the hospital sector, which creates a higher return on equity.

Finally, we examine liquidity:

	Home Health Care	Hospitals
Current ratio	1.9	2.2
DCOH	89.0	27.4

On average, hospitals have slightly more current assets relative to current liabilities as compared to home health care businesses; however, home health care businesses appear to hold more cash relative to operating expenses than hospitals. Of course, in general, hospitals are much larger in scale (assets and revenues) than are home health care businesses, and hence hospitals have higher levels of current assets and daily cash transactions. However, with the growth of large hospital systems, cash is often managed centrally and thus may not appear on the balance sheets of many individual hospitals.

(continued)

HEALTHCARE IN PRACTICE
Some Hospital Ratios and How They Compare to Home Health Care *(continued)*

The main point of this discussion is that basic differences exist in the financial and operational structures of different healthcare providers. Hospitals are inherently different from home health care businesses, which are inherently different from nursing homes, and so on. When performing financial condition analyses, the unique features of the sector must be recognized.

Note: This Healthcare in Practice is based on data in Risk Management Association (RMA), 2016, *Annual Statement Studies 2015–2016*, Philadelphia: RMA, and Optum 360°, 2017, *Almanac of Hospital Financial and Operating Indicators*, accessed December 14, 2017, www.optum360coding.com/Product/46985.

It is easy to combine comparative and trend analyses in a single graph, such as that shown in exhibit 13.4. Here, Park Ridge's ROE (the solid line) and sector average ROE (the dashed lines) data are plotted for the past five years. The graph shows that the business's ROE has increased substantially since it opened in 2012. After two years of being well below average, ROE was very close to the sector average for 2014, 2015, and 2016, but not so high as to be in the upper quartile. Although comparative and trend analyses are illustrated here with one ratio, other ratios can be analyzed similarly. For presentation purposes, charts often are used, with the comparative data color coded for ease of recognition and interpretation.

CRITICAL CONCEPT
Comparative Analysis (Benchmarking) and Trend Analysis

A single ratio—say, a debt ratio of 60 percent—does not tell much about a business's financial condition. To help interpret the ratios, analysts use comparative and trend analyses. Comparative analysis (benchmarking) compares a business's ratios with established values, such as industry averages; the ratios of leading companies in the industry; or those of primary competitors. For example, does the business use more or less debt financing than the industry average? Trend analysis focuses on changes in the business's ratios over time. For example, has the business's use of debt financing increased or decreased over the last five years? Calculating the ratios is not a big deal; a spreadsheet can easily do that. What matters is the interpretation of the ratios, and comparative and trend analyses are vital to this process.

EXHIBIT 13.4
Park Ridge Homecare: ROE Analysis, 2012–2016

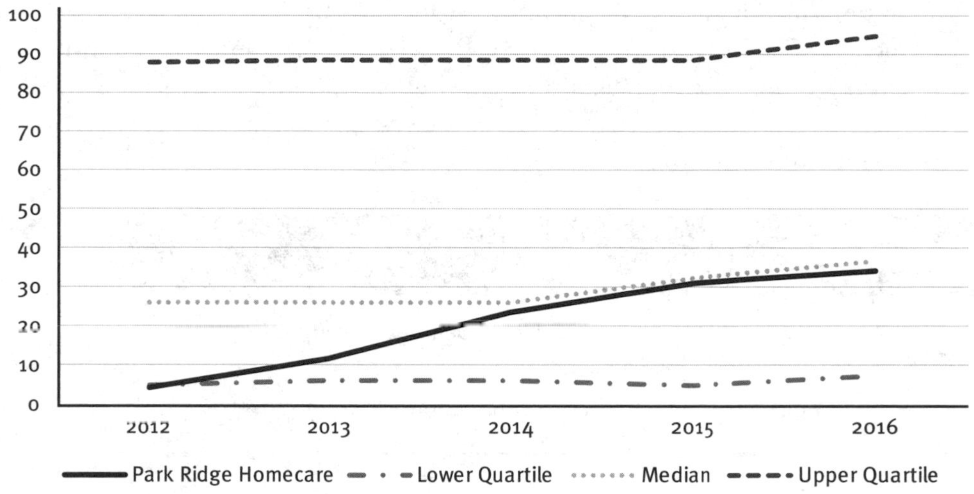

	Return on Equity (ROE)			
		Sector		
Year	Park Ridge Homecare	Lower Quartile	Median	Upper Quartile
2012	4.50	5.00	26.10	87.8
2013	12.10	6.2	26.3	88.5
2014	23.7	6.4	26.2	88.4
2015	31.4	5.1	32.2	88.2
2016	34.1	7.5	36.5	94.5

All comparative analyses require comparative data. Such data are available from a number of sources, including commercial suppliers, federal and state governmental agencies, and various industry trade groups. Each of these data suppliers uses a somewhat different set of ratios designed to meet its own needs. Thus, the comparative data source selected dictates the ratios used in the analysis.

In addition, there are minor, and sometimes major, differences in ratio definitions between data sources—for example, one source may use a 365-day year, while another may go by a 360-day year. Another source might use operating values as opposed to total values when constructing ratios.

Knowing the specific definitions used in the comparative data is imperative, because definitional differences between the ratios being calculated and the comparative ratios can lead to erroneous interpretations and conclusions. Thus, the first task in any ratio analysis is to identify the comparative data set and the ratios to be used. Then, make sure that the ratio definitions used in the analysis match those in the comparative data set.

Choosing the best available comparative data is a must. For example, industry averages should reflect businesses of roughly the same size and operating in the same geographic area as the one analyzed. In general, not-for-profit businesses should be compared to one another and not to for-profit businesses.

SELF-TEST QUESTIONS

1. How can comparative and trend analyses be used to help interpret a ratio?
2. Why is it important to be familiar with the comparative data set?

13.6 DUPONT ANALYSIS

Financial ratio analysis provides a great deal of information about a business's financial condition, but it does not provide an overview, nor does it tie any of the ratios together. DuPont analysis provides an overview of a business's financial condition and helps managers and investors understand the relationships among several ratios (see "Critical Concept: DuPont Analysis").

DuPont analysis, so named because managers at the DuPont Company developed it, combines basic financial ratios in a way that provides valuable insights into a business's profitability. The analysis decomposes return on equity, perhaps the most important measure of profitability (at least for for-profits), into the product of three other ratios, each of which has an important economic interpretation. The result is the DuPont equation:

$$\begin{aligned}\text{ROE} &= \text{Total margin} \times \text{Total asset turnover} \times \text{Equity multiplier}\\ &= \text{Net income} \div \text{Total revenue} \times \text{Total revenue} \div \text{Total assets} \times\\ &\quad\ \text{Total assets} \div \text{Total equity.}\end{aligned}$$

Again, we use Park Ridge Homecare's 2016 data to illustrate the DuPont equation. We have also included the sector average DuPont equation for later comparison. (Note that the ratios used in the analysis are rounded to the nearest tenth of a percent, so the multiplication results are not exact. Also, the sector averages in the following DuPont analysis differ slightly from the sector averages presented previously because the equation represents the average hospital's value on all four ratios, while the values presented above reflect the averages when the ratios are considered independently.)

$$\begin{aligned}\text{Park Ridge Homecare ROE} &= 34.1\% = 4.0\% \times 3.3 \times 2.6.\\ \text{Sector average ROE} &= 36.5\% = 5.9\% \times 2.2 \times 2.8.\end{aligned}$$

In the DuPont equation, the product of the first two terms on the right side is return on assets, so the equation can also be written as ROE = ROA × Equity multiplier. Park Ridge's 2016 total margin was 4.0 percent, so the business made a 4.0 cent profit on each dollar of total revenue. Furthermore, assets were turned over (or created revenues) 3.3 times during the year, so the business earned a return of 4.0% × 3.3 = 13.2% on its assets. This value for ROA is the same as was calculated previously in our ratio analysis discussion (13.4 percent) except for a rounding difference.

> **CRITICAL CONCEPT**
> DuPont Analysis
>
> DuPont analysis, which decomposes the profitability of a business into three components, uses this equation:
>
> ROE = Total margin × Total asset turnover × Equity multiplier.
>
> A business's profitability (as measured by ROE) is a function of these factors: (1) expense control, which is measured by total margin; (2) asset utilization, which is measured by total asset turnover; and (3) use of debt, which is measured by the equity multiplier. By analyzing the DuPont equation, managers can determine how each factor contributes to a business's profitability and hence can identify areas of strength and weakness.

If the business used only equity financing, its 13.4 percent ROA would equal its ROE. However, creditors and other suppliers of liability capital provided 60.8 percent of Park Ridge's financing, while the equityholders (the owners) supplied the rest. Because the 13.4 percent ROA belongs exclusively to the suppliers of equity capital, which makes up only 39.2 percent of total capital, Park Ridge's ROE is higher than its 13.4 percent ROA.

Specifically, ROA must be multiplied by the **equity multiplier**, which shows the amount of assets working for each dollar of equity capital, to obtain the ROE of 34.1 percent. Of course, ROE can be calculated directly: ROE = Net income ÷ Total equity = $163 ÷ $478 = 0.341 = 34.1%. However, the DuPont equation shows how total margin, which measures expense control; total asset turnover, which measures asset utilization; and financial leverage, which measures debt utilization, interact to determine ROE.

> ***Equity multiplier***
> The ratio of total assets to total equity, which indicates how many dollars of assets are supported by each dollar of equity financing.

Lori Gibbs (the CEO of Park Ridge) uses the DuPont equation to suggest how to improve its profitability (ROE) and hence financial condition. To influence the profit margin, Park Ridge must increase revenues and reduce costs. Thus, Lori can study the effects of raising charges to increase revenues, lowering charges to increase volume, moving into new services or markets with higher margins, entering into new contracts with managed care plans, and so on.

Furthermore, she can study the expense items and, working with clinical staff, seek ways to reduce costs. To boost total asset turnover, Lori can investigate ways of reducing investments in various types of assets. Finally, she can analyze alternative financing strategies to ensure that the optimal amount of debt financing is being used.

The DuPont equation also provides a useful comparison between a business's performance as measured by ROE and the performance of an average home health care business. The DuPont analysis shows that Park Ridge gets a lower return on its equity capital than does the average home health care business, a trend driven primarily by Park Ridge's lower profit margin. The business is getting slightly above-average utilization from its assets and uses only a slightly lower-than-average amount of debt financing. Thus, Park Ridge needs to do a better job of controlling expenses and increasing revenues. This shift will be important for the long-run financial performance of the organization, especially as it expands into a second location.

? SELF-TEST QUESTIONS

1. Explain how the DuPont equation combines several ratios to obtain an overview of a business's financial condition.
2. What role do asset and debt utilization play in a business's profitability as measured by return on equity?

13.7 OTHER ANALYTICAL TECHNIQUES

Common-size analysis
A financial statement analysis technique that uses percentages instead of dollars for income statement items and balance sheet accounts. Common-size analysis is especially useful when comparing one firm's financial statements to another (or to the industry).

Percentage change analysis
A financial statement analysis technique that expresses year-to-year changes in income statement items and balance accounts as percentages; shows which items and accounts are growing faster (or slower) than others.

Besides ratio and DuPont analyses, financial statement analysis frequently uses two additional techniques.

In **common-size analysis**, all income statement items are divided by total revenues and all balance sheet items are divided by total assets. Thus, a common-size income statement shows each item as a percentage of total revenues, and a common-size balance sheet shows each account as a percentage of total assets. The advantage of common-size statements is that they facilitate comparisons of income statements and balance sheets over time and across companies because they remove the influence of the scale (size) of the business. For an example of a common-size analysis, see the Healthcare in Practice box in chapter 12.

In **percentage change analysis**, the percentage changes in the balance sheet accounts, and income statement items from year to year, are calculated and compared. In this format, it is easy to see what accounts and items are growing faster or slower than others and thus to identify which are under control and which are out of control.

To illustrate, Park Ridge Homecare's operating revenues grew from \$2,666,000 to \$3,996,000 during 2016, or by \$1,330,000. This dollar increase in revenues translates to a \$1,330 ÷ \$2,666 = 0.499 = 49.9% increase. Over the same period, inventories increased by only (\$27 – \$22) ÷ \$22 = 0.227 = 22.7%. Thus, percentage change analysis reveals that revenues increased at more than twice the rate of inventories during 2016. Because inventories require both initial expenditures and carrying costs, the ability to grow revenues faster than inventories has a positive impact on profitability and hence financial condition.

The conclusions reached in common-size and percentage change analyses generally parallel those derived from ratio analysis. However, occasionally a serious deficiency is highlighted by only one of the three analytical techniques, while the other two techniques fail to bring the deficiency to light. Thus, a thorough financial statement analysis usually consists of a DuPont analysis to provide an overview and then includes several different techniques such as ratio, common-size, and percentage change analyses.

? Self-Test Questions

1. How are common-size statements created?
2. What advantage do common-size statements have over regular statements when being used to conduct a financial statement analysis?
3. What is percentage change analysis, and why is it useful?
4. Which analytical techniques should be used in a complete financial statement analysis?

13.8 LIMITATIONS OF FINANCIAL STATEMENT ANALYSIS

While financial statement analysis can provide a great deal of useful information regarding a business's financial condition, such analyses have limitations that necessitate care and judgment. This section highlights some of the problem areas.

First, many large health services businesses operate a number of divisions in different lines of business, which makes developing meaningful comparative data difficult. This problem tends to make financial statement analyses more useful for providers with single service lines than for large, multiservice companies.

Second, generalizing about whether a particular value is good or bad can be complicated. For example, a high current ratio may show a strong liquidity position (which is good) or an excessive amount of current assets (which is bad). Similarly, a high total asset turnover ratio may denote either a business that uses its assets efficiently or one that is undercapitalized and simply cannot afford to buy enough assets. In addition, firms often have some ratios that look good and others that look bad, which makes the firm's overall financial position, whether strong or weak, difficult to determine. For this reason, significant judgment and some knowledge of the organization's underlying operations are required when assessing financial condition.

Third, varying accounting practices can distort financial statement comparisons. For example, businesses can use different accounting (fiscal) years. If a business is highly seasonal, such as a walk-in clinic in a ski resort town, financial statement ratios in December can look dissimilar to those in July. In addition, firms can use different accounting conventions to value inventories, which can lead to ratio distortions. Other accounting practices, such as the classification of operating versus nonoperating revenues and expenses, can also create distortions.

Finally, inflation effects can distort a firm's financial statements. Recall that most asset values listed on the balance sheet reflect historical costs rather than current values. Inflation and depreciation have caused the values of many assets that were purchased in the past to be seriously understated. Therefore, if an old hospital that had acquired much of its plant and equipment years ago is compared to a new hospital with the same physical capacity, the old hospital, because of a lower book value of fixed assets, would report a higher turnover ratio. Furthermore, with lower depreciation expense, it is likely that the old hospital would report higher profitability. These differences in fixed-asset turnover and profitability are more reflective of the inability of financial statements to deal with inflation than of any inefficiency on the part of the new hospital's managers (see "For Your Consideration: Inflation Accounting").

Self-Test Question

1. Briefly describe some of the problems encountered when performing financial statement analyses.

For Your Consideration
Inflation Accounting

Inflation accounting (also called *replacement cost accounting* or *current cost accounting*) describes a range of accounting systems designed to correct problems arising from historical cost accounting under inflation. It was widely used in the nineteenth and early twentieth centuries but was mostly replaced by historical cost accounting in the 1930s after asset values were devastated by the Great Depression.

Historical cost accounting leads to two basic problems. First, many of the historical numbers appearing on financial statements are not economically relevant because prices have changed since they were incurred. Second, the numbers on financial statements represent dollars expended at different points in time. Thus, adding cash of $10,000 held on December 31, 2016, to a $10,000 cost of land acquired in 1969 makes little sense because inflation has caused the two amounts to represent significantly different levels of purchasing power. Under inflation accounting, the $10,000 cash would be added to the current market value of the land, say, $50,000, which equalizes the purchasing power of the two amounts.

During the past 50 years, accounting standards have encouraged companies to supplement historical cost-based financial statements with price-level (inflation) adjusted statements, but few companies have done so. In addition, during the 1970s, the Financial Accounting Standards Board reviewed a draft proposal that would mandate price-level adjusted statements. However, because of stringent opposition from companies, the proposal was never adopted.

What do you think? Would it be easy to estimate the current values of balance sheet assets? What are the advantages and disadvantages of inflation accounting? Should generally accepted accounting principles be revised to require inflation accounting?

THEME WRAP-UP: TECHNIQUES FOR EVALUATING FINANCIAL STATEMENTS

After a cursory ratio analysis, Lori knows that Park Ridge Homecare is basically on sound financial footing, although there are opportunities to strengthen performance. Park Ridge's return on equity is below the sector average, as are its total margin and operating margin. Thus, Park Ridge's expense control needs improvement. The business also needs to focus attention on its revenue cycle to speed up collections, as shown by its relatively high days in accounts receivable. Finally, Park Ridge could consider using a little more debt financing.

However, when all relevant factors are considered, Park Ridge's business model is financially sustainable. Given the right competitive environment, Lori should be able to start a second location without placing Park Ridge in financial jeopardy. She could probably take funds out of the short-term and long-term investment accounts and, with a moderate amount of new debt financing, acquire sufficient assets to start the new enterprise. If she applies the Park Ridge model to this second business, the new office is likely to become operationally self-supporting quickly. But Lori has to watch the expenses. Wish her lots of luck!

KEY CONCEPTS

This chapter presents the methods used by managers and investors to assess a business's financial condition as reflected by data in its financial statements. Here are the key concepts:

- *Financial statement analysis* uses data found in a business's financial statements to assess financial condition. *Operational analysis*, which uses data typically not found in financial statements, provides insights into why a firm is in a given financial condition.
- *Ratio analysis* is one technique designed to help interpret the data contained in financial statements, as well as other data. In essence, two data elements are combined to create a single value whose economic meaning can be easily interpreted.
- *Profitability ratios* show the combined effects of liquidity, asset management, and debt management on operating results. Profitability ratios are subdivided into margin measures and return measures.
- *Liquidity ratios* indicate the business's ability to meet its short-term cash obligations.
- *Asset management ratios* measure how effectively managers are using the business's assets.
- *Debt management ratios* reveal the extent to which the firm is financed with debt. These ratios are further categorized as capitalization ratios and coverage ratios.

- Ratios are analyzed using *comparative analysis*, also called *benchmarking* (in which a firm's ratios are compared with sector averages or other benchmarks), and *trend analysis* (in which a firm's ratios are examined over time).
- The *DuPont equation*, which provides a good overview of the factors that affect profitability, shows how the total margin, total asset turnover, and amount of debt financing (as measured by the equity multiplier) interact to influence a business's return on equity.
- In a *common-size analysis*, a business's income statement and balance sheet are expressed in percentages. This format facilitates comparisons between firms of different sizes and a single firm that grows over time.
- In *percentage change analysis*, the differences in income statement items and balance sheet accounts from one year to the next are expressed in percentages. In this way, it is easy to identify items and accounts that are growing appreciably faster or slower than average.
- Financial condition analysis is hampered by some serious problems, including development of comparative data, interpretation of results, and inflation effects.

Financial condition analysis has its limitations, but if used with care and judgment, it can provide managers with a good picture of a business's financial condition as well as identify those operational factors that contributed to that condition.

End-of-Chapter Questions

13.1 a. What is the primary difference between financial statement analysis and operational analysis?

b. Why are both types of analyses useful to healthcare managers and investors?

13.2 Should financial statement analyses be conducted only on historical data? Explain your answer.

13.3 One asset management ratio, the inventory turnover ratio, is defined as revenues divided by inventories. Would this ratio be more important for a medical device manufacturer or a hospital management company?

13.4 a. Assume that Old Gatorland and Badger Manor, two operators of nursing homes, have fiscal years that end at different times—one in June and one in December. Would this fact cause any problems when comparing ratios between the two businesses?

b. Assume that two companies that operate walk-in clinics both have the same December year end, but one is based in Aspen (a winter resort town), while the other operates on Nantucket Island (a summer destination). Would this difference in location lead to problems in a comparative analysis?

13.5 a. How does inflation distort ratio analysis comparisons, both for one company over time and when different companies are compared?

b. Are only balance sheet accounts or both balance sheet accounts and income statement items affected by inflation?

13.6 a. What is the difference between trend analysis and comparative analysis?

b. Which is more important?

13.7 Assume that a large group practice has a low return on equity. How could DuPont analysis be used to identify possible actions to help boost profitability?

13.8 Regardless of the specific line of business, should all healthcare businesses use the same set of ratios when conducting a financial statement analysis? Explain your answer.

End-of-Chapter Problems

13.1 a. General Hospital has a current ratio of 0.5. Which of the following actions would improve (increase) this ratio? (Hint: Create a simple balance sheet that has a current ratio of 0.5. Then, judge how the following transactions would affect the balance sheet.)

- Use cash to pay off current liabilities.
- Collect some of the current accounts receivable.
- Use cash to pay off some long-term debt.
- Purchase additional inventory on credit (i.e., accounts payable).
- Sell some of the existing inventory at cost (book value).

b. Now assume that General Hospital has a current ratio of 1.2. In this situation, which of the listed actions would improve this ratio?

13.2 Southwest Physicians, a medical group practice in Oklahoma City, is just being formed. It will need $2 million of total assets to generate $3 million in revenues. Furthermore, the group expects to have a total margin of 5 percent. The group is considering two financing alternatives. First, it can use all-equity financing by requiring each physician to contribute her pro rata share. Second, the practice can finance up to 50 percent of its assets with a bank loan. Assuming that the debt alternative has no impact on the expected total margin, what is the difference between the expected return on equity (ROE) if the group finances with 50 percent debt versus the expected ROE if it finances entirely with equity capital?

13.3 Park Ridge Homecare's financial statements are presented in exhibits 13.1, 13.2, and 13.3. In the chapter, we calculate selected ratios for 2016.

a. Calculate the business's financial ratios for 2015. Assume that Park Ridge had $18,000 in lease payments in 2015. (Use the ratio analysis discussion to identify the applicable ratios.)

b. Interpret the ratios. For the analysis, assume that the sector average data presented in the ratio analysis section are valid for 2015.

13.4 Consider the following financial statements for BestCare, a not-for-profit health insurer.

BestCare Health Insurer Statement of Operations, Year Ended June 30, 2016 (in Thousands)

Revenue	
Healthcare premiums	$26,682
Fees and other revenue	1,689
Net investment income	242
Total revenues	$28,613
Benefits and expenses	
Healthcare costs	$ 15,154
Operating expenses	
Selling expenses	3,963
General and administrative expenses	7,893
Interest expense	385
Total expenses	$27,395
Net income	$ 1,218

BestCare Health Insurer Balance Sheet, June 30, 2016 (in Thousands)

ASSETS	
Cash and cash equivalents	$2,737
Net premiums receivable	821
Other current assets	387
Total current assets	$3,945
Long-term investments	$4,424
Net property and equipment	$1,500
Total assets	$9,869
LIABILITIES AND EQUITY	
Healthcare costs payable	$2,145
Accrued expenses	929
Unearned premiums	382
Total current liabilities	$3,456
Long-term debt	$4,295
Total liabilities	$7,751
Equity	$2,118
Total liabilities and equity	$9,869

a. Perform a DuPont analysis on BestCare. Assume that the sector average ratios are as follows:

Total margin	3.8%
Total asset turnover	2.1
Equity multiplier	3.2
Return on equity	25.5%

b. Calculate and interpret the following ratios for BestCare.

	Sector Average
Return on assets	8.0%
Current ratio	1.3
DCOH (assume depreciation expense is $367)	41 days
Average collection period	7 days
Debt ratio	69%
Debt-to-equity ratio	2.2
Times interest earned ratio	2.8
Fixed-asset turnover ratio	18.5

13.5 Consider the following financial statements for Green Valley Nursing Home Inc., a for-profit, long-term care facility.

Green Valley Nursing Home Inc.
Statement of Income and Retained Earnings,
Year Ended December 31, 2016

Revenue	
Resident services revenue	$3,163,258
Provision for bad debts	110,000
Net resident services revenue	3,053,258
Other revenue	106,146
Total revenues	$3,159,404
Expenses	
Salaries and benefits	$1 ,515,438
Medical supplies and drugs	966,781
Insurance and other	296,357
Depreciation	85,000
Interest	206,780
Total expenses	$3,070,356
Operating income	$ 89,048
Income tax expense	31,167
Net income	$ 57,881
Retained earnings, beginning of year	$ 199,961
Retained earnings, end of year	$ 257,842

Green Valley Nursing Home Inc.
Balance Sheet, December 31, 2016

ASSETS	
Current assets	
Cash	$ 105,737
Short-term securities	200,000
Net accounts receivable	215,600
Supplies	87,655
Total current assets	$ 608,992
Property and equipment	2,250,000
Less: Accumulated depreciation	356,000
Net property and equipment	$1,894,000
Total assets	$2,502,992
LIABILITIES AND SHAREHOLDERS' EQUITY	
Current liabilities	
Accounts payable	$ 72,250
Accrued expenses	192,900
Notes payable	100,000
Current portion of long-term debt	80,000
Total current liabilities	$ 445,150
Long-term debt	$1,700,000
Shareholders' equity	
Common stock, $10 par value	$ 100,000
Retained earnings	257,842
Total shareholders' equity	$ 357,842
Total liabilities and shareholders' equity	$2,502,992

a. Perform a DuPont analysis on Green Valley. Assume that the sector average ratios are as follows:

Total margin	3.5%
Total asset turnover	1.5
Equity multiplier	2.5
Return on equity	13.1%

b. Calculate and interpret the following ratios:

	Sector Average
Return on assets	5.2%
Current ratio	2.0
DCOH	22 days
Average collection period	19 days
Debt ratio	71%
Debt-to-equity ratio	2.5
Times interest earned ratio	2.6
Fixed-asset turnover ratio	1.4

13.6 Examine the sector average ratios given in problems 13.4 and 13.5. Explain why the ratios are different between the health insurance and nursing home sectors.

GLOSSARY

Accountable care organization (ACO). An organization that integrates physicians and other healthcare providers with the goal of controlling costs and improving quality.

Accounting. The measurement and recording of events that reflect the operations, assets, and financing of an organization.

Accounting breakeven. Accounting breakeven occurs when all accounting costs are covered (zero profitability).

Accounts payable. Monies owed to vendors for purchased supplies. Payables arise when vendors offer trade credit (terms that allow the buyer to pay some time [say, 30 days] after the supplies have been purchased).

Accounts receivable. A current asset created when a service is performed but payment has not yet been received. The receivable is eliminated when the payment is collected.

Accrual accounting. A method of accounting that uses economic events, not cash transactions, as the basis for reporting.

Accrued expenses (accruals). Monies owed to various parties, such as to employees, for services rendered. Also includes interest owed to lenders and tax obligations.

Accumulated depreciation. The total amount of depreciation expensed over time against the fixed assets listed on the balance sheet.

Activity-based costing (ABC). An upstream approach to costing that relies on the premise that all costs in an organization stem from activities in or across departments.

Actuarial information. Data (including utilization data for the covered population) regarding the financial risks associated with insurance programs.

Agency problem. The problem that arises when the managers of a for-profit corporation are separate from the owners. In this situation, managers are motivated to act in their own interests as opposed to the interests of shareholders.

Aging schedule. A table that expresses a business's accounts receivable in increments according to how long it takes to collect each account.

Allocation rate. The numerical value used to allocate a cost pool to patient services departments (e.g., $40 per square foot of occupied space).

Ambulatory (outpatient) care. Care that is provided to patients who are not institutionalized. Typical settings include physicians' offices, outpatient surgery centers, and walk-in clinics.

Annual report. A report issued annually by a business that contains descriptive information about operations over the past year and several years of historical financial statements.

Average cost. Total costs divided by volume (e.g., if laboratory costs total $300,000 to conduct 15,000 tests, the average cost [per test] is $300,000 ÷ 15,000 = $20).

Average length of stay (ALOS). The average time an inpatient spends in the hospital (per stay).

Bad debt losses. Revenue that is expected, but never collected, from patients (or third-party payers) who have the capacity to pay.

Base case. In a capital investment analysis, the situation that is expected (most likely) to occur.

Base stock. The amount of inventory held to meet expected usage.

Basic accounting equation. The relationship between balance sheet accounts that requires the balance sheet to balance. That is, total assets must equal total liabilities plus equity.

Basis point. One-hundredth of a percentage point (e.g., 50 basis points equal 0.5 percent, or one-half a percentage point).

Benefit corporation (B corporation). A type of for-profit corporation that allows managers to consider social and environmental goals ahead of shareholder wealth maximization.

Bottom-up approach. A budgeting system whereby budgets originate at the department or program level and then are aggregated and approved by senior managers.

Budgeting. The creation and use of financial forecasts to plan for and control a business's operations.

Bundled reimbursement. The payment of a single amount for several procedures. When reimbursement is unbundled, separate amounts are paid for each procedure.

Business (practice) manager. The manager responsible for the finance function in a small healthcare organization, such as a medical practice with one or a few clinicians.

Business risk. The risk inherent in the operations of a business, assuming it uses no debt financing.

Call provision. A provision in a bond contract that gives the issuing company the right to redeem (call) the bonds prior to maturity.

Capital. For finance purposes, the funds used to acquire a business's assets, including land, buildings, equipment, and inventories. Note that in economics, capital generally refers to the assets owned by a business.

Capital budget. A plan (budget) that outlines a business's expected future expenditures on new capital assets, such as land, buildings, and equipment.

Capital gains. The profit that is generated when securities (or other investments) are sold for more than their purchase price.

Capital investment decision. The business decision involving which long-term assets (e.g., land, buildings, equipment) to buy. Such decisions often are referred to as capital budgeting decisions.

Capital rationing. The condition of having more acceptable projects than funds (capital) needed to undertake those projects.

Capital structure. The business's mix of debt and equity financing, often expressed as the percentage of debt financing.

Cash flow coverage (CFC) ratio. A measure of the amount of cash flow generated by a business per dollar of fixed expense. Similar to the TIE ratio, but more inclusive.

C corporation. A traditional for-profit corporation.

Centers for Medicare & Medicaid Services (CMS). The federal agency in the US Department of Health and Human Services that administers the Medicare and Medicaid programs.

Chargemaster. A provider's official list of charges (prices) for goods, supplies, and services rendered.

Charity (indigent) care. Care provided to patients who do not have the capacity to pay.

Chief financial officer (CFO). The senior manager (or top finance dog) in a large organization's finance department. Also called *vice president of finance*.

Claims denial. The refusal of a third-party payer to honor a submitted bill (claim).

Coinsurance. A sharing of costs between the patient and the insurer (e.g., the patient pays 20 percent of the costs of hospitalization).

Common-size analysis. A financial statement analysis technique that uses percentages instead of dollars for income statement items and balance sheet accounts. Common-size analysis is especially useful when comparing one firm's financial statements to another (or to the industry).

Community benefits. Services and initiatives taken by providers, such as financial assistance for uninsured patients of limited means and education programs, that enhance the health and well-being of the community.

Compounding. The process of finding the future value of a current (starting) amount or series of cash flows.

Comptroller (controller). The finance department manager who handles accounting, budgeting, and reporting activities.

Consigned inventory system. A system in which the supplier owns and manages the inventory until it is consumed (used).

Copayment. A fixed cost to the patient each time a service is rendered (e.g., $20 per outpatient visit).

Corporate taxes. Income taxes paid by for-profit (taxable) corporations to federal and state authorities.

Cost. A resource use associated with providing, or supporting, a specific service.

Cost allocation. The assignment (allocation) of overhead costs, such as financial services costs, from a support department to the patient services departments.

Cost center. A subunit in an organization that incurs costs but generates no revenues.

Cost-containment programs. State programs that require providers (primarily hospitals) to submit budgets each year for approval.

Cost of debt. The return (interest rate) required by lenders to furnish debt capital.

Cost of equity. The return required by owners to furnish equity capital.

Cost per discharge. The average cost of each inpatient stay.

Cost-to-charge ratio (CCR). A ratio used to estimate the overhead costs of individual services. Defined as the ratio of indirect (overhead) costs to charges (or alternatively, to service revenues).

CPT codes. Current Procedural Terminology (CPT) codes are used by clinicians to specify procedures performed on patients.

Credit enhancement (bond insurance). Insurance that guarantees the payment of interest and repayment of principal on a bond if the borrower (issuer) defaults. Insured bonds carry the rating of the insurer rather than the issuer.

Current assets. Cash and other assets that are expected to be converted into cash within one accounting period (often a year). Examples of noncash current assets include cash equivalents, short-term investments, receivables, and inventories.

Current liability. A payment obligation (liability) of a business that is due in the next accounting period, often one year.

Current ratio. Total current assets divided by total current liabilities; measures the number of dollars of current assets available to pay each dollar of current liabilities.

Dashboards. Gauges or visuals that present key information in a form that is easy to read and interpret.

Days cash on hand (DCOH). The number of days it would take to run out of cash if the business does not receive any additional revenues or financing.

Days in patient accounts receivable. The average length of time it takes a provider to collect its receivables. Also called *days' sales outstanding* or *average collection period.*

Debt capacity. The amount of debt in a business's optimal capital structure. A business with excess debt capacity is operating with less than the optimal amount of debt.

Debt ratio (or debt-to-assets ratio). A ratio that measures the proportion of debt (versus equity) financing in a business's total financing mix. Often defined as total debt (liabilities) divided by total assets.

Debt-to-capitalization ratio. Long-term debt divided by long-term capital (long-term debt plus equity); measures the proportion of long-term debt in a business's permanent (long-term) financing mix.

Deductible. The dollar amount that must be spent on healthcare services (e.g., $500 per year) before any benefits are paid by the insurer.

Default. Failure by a borrower to make a promised interest or principal repayment.

Direct method. A cost allocation method that allocates overhead costs directly to patient services departments. This method does not recognize services provided by one support department to another.

Discounted cash flow (DCF) analysis. The use of time value of money techniques to estimate the value of an investment.

Discounting. The process of finding the present value of an amount or series of cash flows expected to be received in the future.

Economic breakeven. Economic breakeven occurs when all accounting costs plus a profit target are covered.

Economies of scale. The business situation in which higher volume leads to lower per-unit cost.

Enrollee. A member of a managed care plan. Or, more generally, an individual who has (is enrolled in) a health insurance plan.

Equity multiplier. The ratio of total assets to total equity, which indicates how many dollars of assets are supported by each dollar of equity financing.

External audit. An examination of a business's financial statements by an outside party to ensure that the statements follow GAAP and are a fair representation of the economic status of the business.

Expense budget. A listing of the expected expenses of an organization, usually by department and service, and further broken down into components such as facilities, labor, and supplies.

Financial asset. A security such as a stock or bond that gives the holder a claim against the issuing business's cash flows.

Financial accounting. The field of accounting that focuses on the measurement and communication of the economic events and status of an entire organization.

Financial leverage. The use of debt financing, which typically increases (leverages up) the rate of return to owners.

Financial management. The use of theory, principles, and concepts developed to help managers make better financial decisions.

Financial plan. The portion of the operating plan that focuses on the finance function.

Financial risk. The additional risk placed on the business's owners (or the community) when debt financing is used.

Fixed-assets turnover (utilization) ratio. Total revenues divided by net fixed assets; measures the ability of a business's fixed assets to generate revenues.

Floating rate. A type of interest specified on a loan whereby the rate changes over time as interest rates in the economy rise and fall.

Form 990. A form filed by not-for-profit organizations with the IRS that reports on an organization's governance and charitable activities.

For-profit corporation. A legal business entity that is separate and distinct from its owners and managers.

Gatekeeper. A primary care physician who controls specialist and ancillary service referrals. Some managed care plans only pay for referral services approved by the gatekeeper.

General acute care hospital. A hospital that treats all conditions that require a relatively short hospitalization (e.g., fewer than 30 days).

Generally accepted accounting principles (GAAP). The set of guidelines, which have evolved over time, that prescribes the content and format of financial statements.

Government hospital. A hospital owned by a government entity. Federal hospitals are owned by the federal government, while public hospitals are owned (or funded) by state or local governments.

Gross fixed assets. The historical cost of a business's property and equipment.

Group policy. A single insurance policy that covers a common group of individuals, such as a company's employees or a professional group's members.

Healthcare Common Procedure Coding System (HCPCS). A medical coding system that expands the CPT codes to include nonphysician services and durable medical equipment.

Healthcare financing. The system that a society uses to pay for healthcare services.

Health services organizations. Organizations that provide patient care services. Examples include hospitals, medical practices, clinics, and nursing homes. Also called *providers*.

High-deductible health plan (HDHP). A type of health insurance that requires high deductibles but allows insured individuals to set up tax-advantaged savings accounts to pay those deductibles.

Horizontal system. A single business entity that owns a group of similar providers, such as hospitals.

Hybrid form. A legal business entity that has features associated with both partnerships and for-profit corporations.

ICD codes. International Classification of Diseases (ICD) codes are used by hospitals and other organizations to specify patient diagnoses.

Indemnification. The agreement to pay for losses incurred by another party.

Investment-grade debt. Debt with a BBB– or higher rating. Generally considered suitable (relatively low risk) investments for conservative individuals and institutions.

Investor-owned hospital. A hospital that is owned by investors who benefit financially from its operation. Also called a *for-profit hospital.*

Junk debt. Debt with a BB+ or lower rating. Generally considered to be more speculative than is investment-grade debt and hence inappropriate for conservative investors.

Just-in-time system. An inventory management approach in which items arrive just a short time before they are used, as opposed to sitting on the shelf for long periods.

Licensure. The process of granting "permission" for healthcare (and other) professionals to practice. Most professional licenses are granted by states with the goal of protecting the public from incompetent practitioners.

Limited liability company (LLC). A corporation that combines some features of a partnership with others of a corporation.

Limited liability partnership (LLP). A partnership that limits the professional (malpractice) liability of its members.

Limited partnership. A partnership in which the general partners have most of the control and unlimited liability while the limited partners have little control and liability that is limited to their initial contribution.

Liquid investment. An investment that can be sold quickly at a fair price.

Liquidity. The ability of a business to meet its cash obligations as they become due.

Long-term care. Care that is provided in either an institutional or outpatient setting that covers an extended period.

Long-term debt. Debt financing that has a maturity greater than one accounting period.

Marginal cost. The cost of one additional unit of output; in an outpatient setting, the cost (typically only for supplies) of one more patient visit on top of the existing volume.

Maturity. The amount of time until a loan matures (must be repaid). Short-term debt has a maturity of one year or less, while long-term debt has a maturity greater than one year.

Medical home (patient-centered medical home). A team-based model of care led by a personal physician who provides, or arranges with other qualified professionals to provide, continual and coordinated care throughout a patient's lifetime to maximize health outcomes.

Medicare Advantage plan. Managed care plan coverage offered to Medicare beneficiaries that replaces Parts A and B coverage.

Medicare payment percentage. Medicare discharges (or revenues) as a percentage of total discharges (or revenues).

Medigap insurance. Insurance taken out by Medicare beneficiaries that pays many of the costs not covered by Parts A and B. (Its purpose is to fill the gaps in coverage.)

Metric. A value used to assess one element of performance.

Mission statement. A statement that defines the overall purpose of the organization.

Net assets. The term used to designate the equity on a not-for-profit organization's balance sheet.

Net fixed assets. The current accounting (book) value of a business's property and equipment. Calculated as gross fixed assets minus accumulated depreciation.

Noncash expenses. Expenses that are listed on the income statement that do not represent actual cash outlays. The most prominent noncash expense is depreciation.

Nonoperating income. The income of a healthcare provider that is unrelated to the provision of patient services. The two most obvious examples are income from securities investments and income from charitable contributions (for not-for-profit businesses).

Notes payable. The balance sheet name typically used for a business's short-term debt, often bank loans.

Number of visits per physician. The patient volume of an outpatient facility on a per-physician basis.

Occupancy rate. The proportion (percentage) of hospital beds occupied.

Operating margin. Operating income divided by operating revenues. It measures the amount of profit per dollar of operating revenues and hence focuses on the profitability of a business's core activities.

Opportunity cost. The cost associated with alternative uses of the same asset. For example, if land is used for one project, it is no longer available for other uses, and hence an opportunity cost arises.

Organizational goals. Specified goals, including financial, that an organization strives to attain. Generally, organizational goals are qualitative in nature.

Organizational objectives. Quantitative targets that an organization sets to meet its organizational goals.

Other revenue. Revenue that is related to patient services but not directly tied to the provision of clinical services. One common example for hospitals is cafeteria revenue.

Outpatient revenue percentage. Outpatient revenues as a percentage of total revenues.

Out year. A future year beyond the next budget year.

Partnership. An unincorporated business that is created and owned by two or more people.

Patient capture. The concept that once a patient enters the system (e.g., a doctor's office), all services needed by that patient should be provided in the system.

Patient service revenue. The amount of revenue collected or expected to be collected as a direct result of providing patient services without considering potential bad debt losses.

Pay for performance. A reimbursement system that rewards providers for meeting specific goals (e.g., 90 percent patient satisfaction).

Percentage change analysis. A financial statement analysis technique that expresses year-to-year changes in income statement items and balance accounts; shows which items and accounts are growing faster (or slower) than others.

Personal (individual) taxes. Taxes paid by individuals to federal and state (in most states) authorities on wages, interest, dividends, capital gains, and proprietorship and partnership income.

Pooling. The spreading of losses over a large group of individuals (or organizations).

Postaudit. The feedback process in which the performance of projects previously accepted is reviewed and necessary changes are made.

Precertification. An insurer's authorization indicating its willingness to pay for a particular service when delivered.

Premium revenue. Revenue arising from capitated patients as opposed to fee-for-service patients.

Price per discharge. The average revenue on each inpatient stay.

Price setter. A provider that has the power (within reason) to set market prices for its services.

Price shifting. The act of charging more than full costs to one set of patients to compensate for charging less to another set. Also called *cross-subsidization.*

Price taker. A provider that has no power to influence the prices set by the marketplace.

Principal. The amount of money borrowed in a loan transaction.

Privately (closely) held company. A for-profit corporation whose stock is owned by a small number of individuals—usually the business's managers—and is not publicly traded.

Private not-for-profit hospital. A hospital that is not governmental but is operated for the exclusive benefit of the community.

Professional corporation (PC). A type of corporate business organization in which the owner or managers retain professional (medical) liability. Called a professional association in some states.

Professional liability. The responsibility of organizations and individuals who provide professional services, such as hospitals and physicians, for losses that result from malpractice.

Profit per discharge. The average profit made on each inpatient stay.

Profit (revenue) center. A subunit in an organization that both generates revenues and incurs costs, hence creating profits.

Project liquidity. The ability of a project to pay for itself from the cash flows that it generates. Project liquidity is measured by payback; the shorter the payback, the more liquid the project.

Proprietorship. A simple form of business owned by one person. Also called *sole proprietorship.*

Prospective payment. A reimbursement system meant to cover expected costs as opposed to historical (retrospective) costs.

Provider panel. The group of providers—say, doctors and hospitals—designated as preferred by a managed care plan. Services delivered by providers outside of the panel may be only partially covered, or not covered at all, by the plan.

Publicly held company. A for-profit corporation whose shares are held by the general public (a large number of shareholders) and traded on an exchange, such as the New York Stock Exchange, or in the over-the-counter market.

Qualitative risk assessment. A process for assessing project risk that focuses on qualitative factors as opposed to a statistical analysis of profit variability.

Random loss. An unpredictable loss, such as one that results from a fire or hurricane.

Ratio analysis. The process of creating and analyzing ratios from the data contained in a business's financial statements and elsewhere to help assess financial condition.

Real asset. Property and equipment, such as land, buildings, and machines, used to create a business's cash flows.

Receivables quality. A subjective measure of the speed and likelihood that a business's receivables will be collected.

Reciprocal method. A cost allocation method that fully recognizes all services provided from each support department to other support departments.

Relative value unit (RVU). A measure of the amount of resources consumed to provide a particular service.

Relative value unit (RVU) method. A method for estimating the overhead costs of individual services based on the intensity of the service provided as measured by RVUs.

Relevant range. The range of output (volume) for which the organization's cost structure holds.

Residual earnings. The earnings (profits) of a business after all expenses (including interest on debt financing) have been paid.

Restricted account. An account with funds restricted to specific uses by donors.

Restrictive covenant. A provision in a loan agreement that protects the interests of the lender by restricting the actions of the borrower.

Return on equity (ROE). Net income divided by the book value of equity (net assets), which measures the dollars of earnings per dollar of equity investment. ROE measures the rate of return to the owners of the business.

Return on investment (ROI). The profitability of an investment, measured in either dollars or percentage (rate of) return.

Return on total assets (ROA). Net income divided by the book value of total assets; measures the amount of profit per dollar of investment in total assets. ROA indicates the financial productivity of a business's total assets.

Revenue budget. A listing of the expected revenues (including both operating and nonoperating) of an organization, usually on a monthly, quarterly, and annual basis and broken out by department, service, and payer.

Risk-adjusted discount rate (RADR). A risk adjustment method that changes the discount (opportunity cost) rate to reflect the unique riskiness of the project being analyzed.

Risk-free investment. An investment that has a guaranteed (sure) return. In other words, the probability of earning the return expected is 100 percent.

Risk transfer. The passing of risk from one individual or business to another (usually an insurer).

Safety stock. The amount of inventory, above the base stock, held to meet unexpected usage increases or delays in receipt of reorders.

Salvage value. The estimated value of an asset at the end of its useful life.

Schedule H. An attachment to IRS Form 990 filed by not-for-profit hospitals that provides additional information on the hospital's community benefit activities.

S corporation. A for-profit corporation with a limited number of shareholders that, after filing an application with the Internal Revenue Service, is taxed as a proprietorship or partnership.

Securities and Exchange Commission (SEC). The government agency that regulates the sale of securities and the content and format of financial statements.

Semifixed costs. Costs that are fixed, but not at a single amount throughout the entire relevant range.

Short-term investments. Securities that are held in lieu of cash. Typically very safe, short-term securities with maturities greater than 90 days but less than one year, such as Treasury bills.

Simple budget. The original budget, unadjusted for actual volume.

Specialty hospital. A hospital that treats patients with a common characteristic or condition, such as a children's or a cancer hospital.

Stakeholder. A party that has an interest—typically financial—in an organization. For example, owners (in for-profit businesses), managers, patients, and suppliers are some stakeholders of healthcare businesses.

Standard. In variance analysis, the budgeted (expected) value established at the beginning of the budget period.

Step-down method. A cost allocation method that partially recognizes services provided from support departments to other support departments.

Stockholders (shareholders). The owners of a for-profit corporation by virtue of holding one or more shares of the company's stock.

Stockless inventory system. A system in which suppliers deliver small quantities of inventory directly to the using departments; a refinement of the just-in-time system.

Stockout. The situation in which a needed inventory item is not available at the provider.

Straight-line method. A method for calculating the depreciation expense of a long-lived asset that assumes the loss of value is constant over time (follows a straight line).

Strategic value. The value inherent in a capital investment that is not captured in its cash flow estimates. For example, a project may provide a foot in the door in a new service area that could lead to other profitable investments.

Sunk cost. A cost that has already occurred or is irrevocably committed. Sunk costs are nonincremental to capital investment analyses and hence should not be included.

Target capital structure. The capital structure that a company strives to achieve and maintain over time. Generally the same as the optimal capital structure.

Terminal value. The cash flow assigned to the last year on the time line of a long-life project to account for the value lost because the cash flows were truncated.

The Joint Commission. An accreditation body for hospitals and other health services organizations.

Time line. A representation of time and cash flows. It may be an actual horizontal line or cells on a spreadsheet.

Times interest earned (TIE) ratio. Earnings before interest and taxes divided by interest charges; measures the number of times that a business's interest expense is covered by the earnings available to pay that expense. This ratio provides insight into how much earnings could fall before the business has trouble meeting its interest payments.

Top-down approach. A budgeting system whereby the finance staff prepares the budget for senior management approval, after which it is sent to department and program heads for implementation.

Total assets turnover (utilization) ratio. Total revenues divided by total assets; measures the amount of revenue generated by each dollar of total assets.

Total costs. The sum of fixed costs and total variable costs.

Total (full) costs. The sum of direct and indirect (overhead) costs. Thus, full costs include both direct and overhead costs.

Total (profit) margin. Net income divided by all (both operating and nonoperating) revenues. It measures the amount of total profit per dollar of total revenues.

Total variable costs. The variable cost rate multiplied by volume (e.g., if a walk-in clinic has a variable cost rate of $15 per visit and experiences 10,000 visits annually, total variable costs for the year equal $15 × 10,000 = $150,000).

Trade-off theory. A theory proposing that a business's optimal capital structure balances the costs and benefits associated with debt financing.

Traditional costing. The top-down approach to costing that first identifies costs at the department level and then (potentially) assigns these costs to individual services.

Transparency. The ability of outsiders to know what is happening in a business.

Treasurer. The finance department manager who handles capital acquisition, investment management, and risk management activities.

Trustee. An individual or institution, often a bank, that represents the interests of bondholders.

Underlying cost structure. The relationship between volume and an organization's total costs. Often called *cost structure*.

Underwriting. The selection and classification of candidates for insurance.

Values statement. A statement of the core beliefs that underlie the culture of the organization.

Variable cost rate. The added cost for each additional unit of service (e.g., the variable cost rate at a neighborhood walk-in clinic is $15 per patient visit).

Variance. In accounting, the difference between what actually happened and what was expected to happen.

Vertical system. A single business entity that owns a group of related, but not identical, providers such as hospitals, medical practices, and nursing homes.

Vision statement. A statement that describes the desired position of the business at a future point in time.

Volume. The amount of services provided (e.g., number of visits, number of inpatient days). Also called *utilization*.

INDEX

Note: Italicized page locators refer to figures or tables in exhibits.

ABOUT THE AUTHORS

Kristin L. Reiter, PhD, is a professor and associate chair in the Department of Health Policy and Management of the Gillings School of Global Public Health at the University of North Carolina at Chapel Hill, where she specializes in healthcare finance. She is also a research fellow in the Cecil G. Sheps Center for Health Services Research and an investigator with the North Carolina Rural Health Research Program, both at the University of North Carolina at Chapel Hill.

She received a bachelor of science degree in accounting from Northern Illinois University, and a master of applied economics and a doctorate in health services organization and policy (with a concentration in corporate finance) from the University of Michigan. Prior to joining academia, she worked in public accounting, serving not-for-profits and clients in the insurance industry.

Dr. Reiter teaches undergraduate- and graduate-level courses in healthcare accounting and financial management and is involved in research projects examining hospital financial performance and the business case for quality. In the past 10 years, she has served on the audit, finance, and advisory committees of several healthcare professional associations. She is a coauthor of more than 50 peer-reviewed articles, and she has presented to academic and professional audiences in the United States, France, and Canada.

Paula H. Song, PhD, is an associate professor and the director of the residential masters program in the Department of Health Policy and Management of the Gillings School of Global Public Health at the University of North Carolina at Chapel Hill, and she is a research fellow at the Cecil G. Sheps Center for Health Services Research at the university.

Dr. Song's research and teaching interests cover areas such as healthcare financial management, investment strategies in not-for-profit hospitals, and business case evaluation for health initiatives. Dr. Song received her doctorate in health services organization and policy, as well as master's degrees in health services administration and applied economics, from the University of Michigan.